Warriors and Heroes of a Different Kind: Battling Kidney Failure

Priscilla Stanbury

Interior design and typesetting by Facile Web&Graphic
Cover design by Jazmin Welch

ISBN 978-1717396747
Printed in Canada
FIRST EDITION

Profits from the sale of this book will be donated to St. Paul's Hospital Foundation for renal research and to the Scleroderma Association of BC for research.

For Roland,
My fellow renal patients
And the heroes in our midst

The woods are lovely, dark and deep,
But I have promises to keep,
And miles to go before I sleep,
And miles to go before I sleep.

—Robert Frost, *Stopping by Woods on a Snowy Evening*

Contents

Foreword   7

Prologue   9

Chapter 1. Kidney Failure!   13

Chapter 2. Living with My Transplant   41

Chapter 3. A Pothole in the Road   65

Chapter 4. Second Kidney Failure   95

Chapter 5. Friends along the Way   128

Chapter 6. Kidney Failure Explained   157

Chapter 7. Among the Nocturnal Elite   195

Chapter 8. Receiving a Transplant   215

Chapter 9. Some Solutions to Transplant Challenges   248

Chapter 10. Some Research Projects   254

Epilogue   271

Appendix 1: Transplantation: From Root to Route, a Layper-   282
son's Overview

Appendix 2: Some Milestones in Kidney Transplants: From   308
Yesterday to Today to Tomorrow

Notes   312

Glossary   329

Sample of Emergency Diet Meal Plan   333

Resources   334

Acknowledgements   339

About the Author   343

Foreword

Over twenty years ago, scleroderma was the primary cause of Priscilla Stanbury's kidney failure, more accurately described in her case as "a scleroderma renal crisis." Scleroderma or systemic sclerosis is a very rare auto-immune connective tissue disease that has an estimated prevalence of 276 cases per million. There is no known cause or cure. It can be deadly.

Priscilla received a kidney transplant lasting many years that failed three years ago. Her book is not just about the chilling effects of a subset of a rare disease affecting relatively few. Instead, it will be of interest to all renal failure victims, and others. That failure has many potential causes, including diabetes, hypertension, polycystic kidney disease, congenital abnormalities and even failed transplants.

In addition, millions are affected by one or more of the many autoimmune diseases and other collagen vascular diseases such as rheumatoid arthritis and systemic lupus erythematosus. Her book will also be of interest to readers inspired by the warriors and intrepid fighters described so vividly in the book. Their struggle to strive for and attain fulfillment in their lives in spite of the deleterious effects of their disease is uplifting. Their most common feature? Endurance. In Priscilla's case, she chooses to endure in "happiness rather than misery." In her words, she lives in the present while accepting and dealing with her bodily condition.

That condition now consists in part of relentless neuropathic pain, serious Raynaud's disease challenges, deteriorating mobility and dialysis in the hospital three nights a week for eight hours each time. Life depends on functioning kidneys. Dialysis is a renal (kidney) replacement therapy. It is an invasive treatment. Basically, it removes excess fluids from the body, replacing a key function of the previously healthy kidneys.

Priscilla finds that the benefits of nocturnal dialysis for her outweigh the downsides of attending day sessions. In her words, she has better toxin removal and improved blood results. Factor in thirty-two hours of hemodialysis a week, with travel to and from the hospital and recuperation after each treatment, as well as the other conditions cited above, and then ask the question, "How has she found the time and energy to write a book about scleroderma and renal failure?" Perseverance beyond description helped. In addition, doing so was to some degree cathartic. Too, she wants, as we do, to encourage readers to donate a kidney and save a life. Her book may help others volunteer.

Priscilla was born in England to Canadian parents and emigrated to Canada at an early age. She is well-educated. She has been a special needs lecturer in England, and has taught in several departments in British Columbia university and college settings for seventeen years, working primarily with students with learning disabilities. She received a peer-nominated *Exceptional Service Award* for her work in Vancouver. She was awarded the Scleroderma Association of BC's (SABC) prestigious *Gurmej Kaur Dhanda Memorial Scleroderma Community Service Award* in 2016 with the citation that she is " . . . an exemplar, survivor, SABC Director and author." She retired as a director when her disease made it impossible to continue. Not only has Priscilla been active in SABC, she has become our friend.

Priscilla is not a professional writer nor does she have formal training as a researcher in the medical field. We find her writing engaging, insightful and varied. Medical references have been vetted by professionals in Canada and Europe. Doctors and professionals have praised her for undertaking to write this book. One, a nephrologist, told her it was a noteworthy undertaking. A Belgian consultant stated that it would be ". . . of benefit to thousands of patients everywhere."

A particularly engaging feature of her book is the inclusion of a chapter introducing us to her "friends along the way." In many ways, this is a book of stories about them as well as other dialysis and transplant recipients, a diverse, courageous and supportive group that adds greatly to our overall understanding of the impact of renal failure, in particular. In addition to all those cited above, medical specialists, general practitioners and nurses will surely benefit from reading about this group and, in particular, about Priscilla Stanbury, who has directed that proceeds from her book be divided between scleroderma and renal research.

Joan Kelly, Co-founder, Scleroderma Association of BC and Bob Buza, Past-President, Scleroderma Association of BC and Scleroderma Canada.

Prologue

This is my quest

—Mitch Leigh and Joe Darien, *The Impossible Dream (The Quest)*

"One in ten Canadians will develop some form of kidney disease during their lifetime."

These words swirled around in my head as I lay in the hospital bed during a dialysis session. I was willing the session to end so I could return to the comfort of my home. No trivial slogan for me. The message was real and redolent with meaning. I was one of the statistics, as were my ten hemodialysis companions in the room. We few were but a fraction of the total number when considering the community dialysis centres and other hospital provisions, not only in my province, but also in the rest of Canada. Kidney disease has often been referred to as the "silent killer" because it is not always easy to detect without the full-blown symptoms of actual kidney failure. How many of my friends were aware of, or cared about, these statistics? On my days off I wondered how I could interest other people in thinking about the ramifications of these statistics.

Since experiencing my second kidney failure and being in company with other dialysis patients, I had become more aware of the battle my companions faced. I had heard moving stories of their hardships and challenges. Two patients in particular stood out for me. One was a woman whose partner was facing many health issues, exacerbated by a meagre income caused by his inability to work. They lived a grim life. Their home consisted of one room with one small hot plate, and a toilet and sink. Food was limited. Any food they had needed to be kidney dialysis-friendly, a challenge in any circumstances.

The other patient was a fairly young man who had been on and off dialysis since 1985. He had a transplant that lasted five years, further dialysis, then another transplant that lasted eleven years before failing again. Each kidney failure created additional complications for him, so that he was now no longer eligible to receive another transplant. He would have to spend the rest of his life on dialysis.

The swirling words of the headline persisting in my thoughts, refusing to abate, now intermingled with the plight of these two patients, created a question for me. What to do? How could I not only spread this message but also help my fellow patients? For obvious reasons, I couldn't donate a kidney. My finances, while not tight, were insufficient to make any dent in the much-needed resources to alleviate some of the challenges of diagnosing kidney disease or providing medical assistance for patients and treatment.

Stuck in this quandary, I was approached a few days later by a research assistant asking if I wished to participate in a special survey being carried out by my own hospital. I would be one of five hundred patients to be interviewed. Was I interested? "Yes," was my immediate reply. The survey's theme revolved around how much we patients understood about kidney transplants. Easy questions were gradually replaced with more difficult, ethical ones that required some deep thinking on my part. Having completed my interview, an idea suddenly captured my attention. I would write a book about kidney failure to raise awareness of kidney disease and hopefully encourage more people to become donors. No sooner had this thought occurred than I immediately perceived the book in its entirety, chapter by chapter.

The problem: I am not a writer. If asked, I would describe myself as the least articulate person I know and certainly not a writer, and I wasn't sure I had the discipline needed to take on a book, but I had a mission. The fact that I have completed my manuscript surprises no one more than me. Whether or not I have achieved my mission remains to be determined.

Once I had decided upon my course of action, I worked on the assumption that the more people I told, the greater responsibility I had to achieve my goal of finishing the book. The most interesting results from announcing my intentions to everyone I encountered were the responses I received. Fellow patients were eager to participate, something that only served to add a greater dimension to my manuscript. Without their stories, my book would have been very much less than what it is. As well, the more I talked about it, the more I learned about kidney disease and kidney failure.

As word spread that I was writing a book, patients I had never met began to approach me and ask questions about it. One person I happened to meet while waiting for my ride home from dialysis sought me out. "Have you included these facts in your book?" he asked, reeling off a series of questions. Fortunately, I was able to assure him I had.

Seemingly satisfied, he replied, "I see you have everything covered. Thank you for doing this for us." When I asked him if he would like to have his story included, he declined.

A number of patients likewise wished not to contribute because, as they explained, "I live with this situation every day of my life. I do not wish to be reminded of it." I respected their decisions.

This book is a compilation of my experience and of my fellow patients' experiences, combined with technical information. Although the emphasis is on the personal aspect, I could not avoid including medical information since it all works hand in hand with our condition and treatment. All personal stories have been adapted to serve the purpose of explaining aspects of kidney failure. Names and identities have been altered to protect individuals' confidentiality. I have opted not to name doctors or the location of my treatment in order to universalize my material. Some readers may find this an impersonal method, but to me, it felt important. On the other hand, for my friends, family and others with whom I am associated, I used their real names.

The book includes two appendices devoted to specific kidney-related material. One describes the history of kidney transplantation from its inception to today's practices, and the other identifies milestones in kidney transplants since the first successful kidney transplant. I hope readers may be interested. Spread throughout the chapters are boxes containing pertinent medical facts elicited from history or from current information. It also felt important to include a chapter on some contemporary research to explain how kidney failure may be tackled in the future.

I wish my readers a thought provoking read, and an informative one. Above all, I wish for readers to consider those whose lives have been affected by kidney disease, and how we could work cooperatively to improve their lives, as well as encourage others to live as healthily as possible so that they may avoid becoming another statistic.

Priscilla Stanbury, September 2017

Chapter 1 | Kidney Failure!

Let's start at the very beginning
A very good place to start
—Richard Rodgers and Oscar Hammerstein, *Do Re Me*

A shock

The ambulance, its familiar British "hee haw" siren piercing the quiet suburban neighbourhood, had arrived. I remember being in a terribly dishevelled state as the paramedics carried me down the stairs from my bedroom and loaded me first onto a gurney, then into the waiting ambulance. My husband, Christopher, stood on my right side talking to Sue, a neighbour from across the road, who, jolted by the sound of the siren, had rushed to see what was happening. Once I was safely secured and the doors clanged shut, with its engine revving, the ambulance, siren blaring once more, gathered speed and hurtled off to meet the early morning traffic on its way to the emergency department of my local hospital.

Upon arrival I was rushed down a corridor to a spot near a curtained area. Barely aware of something having been deposited on my chest, I lay in a haze waiting for medical attention, feeling absolutely wretched, fighting back uncontrollable pangs of nausea, fearing that I would spontaneously spew out whatever remnants I had left in my body following several days of continual vomiting. My head throbbed with such intensity I could hardly bear its pressure. How long my wait was I do not know: seconds, minutes, hours perhaps? Time becomes fluid when ill.

Then movement occurred. A figure in white emerged from behind a curtain. Coming towards me was the most magnificently golden-haired, beautifully sculptured young male doctor I had ever seen. A real Adonis! My potential saviour! Almost too rich a sight for me to behold. Even with my diminished sense of reality, I had the presence of mind to appreciate the irony of my situation. Here I was in anything but a glorious state being seen to by such a dazzling physician. How I yearned for a tender response from him, longing for him to lay his healing hand on my mine, stroke my brow and say some soothing words that would instantly rescue me from my plight and heal whatever was ailing me. Instead, he unceremoniously picked up whatever had been placed on my chest and read aloud: "Kidney failure."

Well! This was the first time, it seemed to me, I had heard mention of such a grave condition, especially ascribed to me. Furthest thing from my thoughts. My family was healthy: parents aging but without any particular medical concerns, two siblings in excellent health. I came from strong stock. I had survived most childhood ailments, including recovering from two bouts of bronchial pneumonia and, in my late teens, glandular fever. Kidney failure? Never. True, I had recently been diagnosed with an autoimmune disease that had so far not really affected my day-to-day life. I had gradually accepted that diagnosis more as an inconvenience than as a life-affecting illness. Above all, I remained a healthy person.

Surely this marvellous-looking doctor was mistaken in his assessment. I was suffering from nothing more than a particularly nasty bout of flu. His words were an insult to my well-being. I bolted upright, most indignantly replying, "No one has ever said anything like that to me, ever!" before promptly collapsing back on the gurney.

The response: "I am sending you to a ward." Obviously I wouldn't be going anywhere that day. How I had arrived in such a condition was beyond my befuddled and addled brain. It requires a little explaining.

Some personal background

I am a Canadian, from Vancouver, but having been born in England it had always been my desire to return to my birthplace. I was able to do this in the early 1970s following university and after having paid off my student loan of $10,000 within a year of graduating. I bought a one-way ticket to a new venture. The new venture had by now become an old venture. Along the way, much to my surprise, having avowed to mix with as few Canadians as possible, I unexpectedly met one at a particularly Canadian event in January 1980: the annual Maple Leaf Ball sponsored by Canada House, the diplomatic centre for Canada in London.

I was shown to my table where I found myself seated next to a tall fellow wearing glasses and attired in a formal Nova Scotia dress tartan kilt. An uncommon mode of evening wear for Canadians but not so unusual for those hailing from Nova Scotia, nor for this individual, as I was soon to discover. My dinner companion was a most convivial fellow, full of good spirits, and immediately introduced himself as Christopher. Indeed, as I thought, he had come from Nova

Scotia. I was at the ball because of my status as a Canadian student in London, having decided to return to university for post-graduate studies. Christopher was there in his capacity as primary designer for a Canada House PR publication *Canada Today*. Apparently both of us had been residing in London for a few years.

We spent an entirely enjoyable evening together, getting on well. When the band had struck its last chord, I thought that was that, but Christopher hesitated, stalling me in the process. He was most intent upon securing my telephone number before I left. I casually gave it to him, not thinking then that this would mark the beginning of a significant relationship. We were married a year later and our son, Roland, was born towards the end of our first year of marriage.

The lead up

Now, nearly a decade later, we were living in a south London suburb. Christopher was still working as a graphic designer with Canada House, and I, in my early forties, was lecturing in a local college, teaching students with learning disabilities. Our seven-year-old son, Roland, was enjoying his primary school life, which included extracurricular activities such as swimming, learning to play a flute and being a member of the local Beaver Cubs group. We were healthy. Nothing unusual had been happening; life was life with its customary ebbs and flows.

As autumn 1989 turned to winter, I began to notice my hands and arms had become swollen and less flexible. I was moving a little more sluggishly and feeling much more tired. I paid scant attention to these symptoms, although by the following January, I thought I had swollen glands. I made an appointment to see a GP at my local clinic. I explained my symptoms.

"Have you noticed anything else different?" the doctor asked. I explained, "My hands are frequently swollen, I walk rather sluggishly and I'm always tired, but I haven't noticed any other symptoms." He examined my throat and glands and then said, "I believe you have an autoimmune disease called lupus. But we need to do a blood test. Because it is an expensive test, we have to wait until there are other similar tests. This will take about a month. We will get back to you."

I lost no time in consulting with our friend and neighbour, Sabi, who lived a couple of houses from us. While tiny in stature, Sabi was, by contrast, hugely vibrant and vivacious in nature. She was an anaesthetist and, having passed the medical requirements needed to practice in the United States, was due to depart soon for a new life. She helpfully explained my condition. "It is a condition that occurs when our immune system, our defender against disease, decides our own cells are foreign and begins to attack them."

Sabi also supplied me with pages and pages of information about lupus. Lupus, I learned, was a particular, chronic autoimmune disease manifesting symptoms such as painful inflammation, swelling and damage to the joints. It caused skin to redden and blotch, damaging kidneys, blood, heart and lungs, and in some cases attacking the brain. It seemed a most unkind and severe condition. Having digested this new information, I began waiting for my results.

My reaction to all this was muted. I was living in a kind of limbo. Nothing had been confirmed. It was difficult to perceive what changes might occur. I could either have been absorbed by sheer panic or have thrived on a pure belief in my well-being. I chose the latter, so sure was I of my continued good health. Three weeks later I received a call from the GP's office, requesting me to come in. I went, not quite knowing what to expect. As I entered the office, my doctor immediately asked me how I was feeling.

"Hah," I thought, "something is up." Doctors rarely ask a patient how they are feeling. Usually they ask, "What can I do for you?"

Before I could respond to his question, he said, "I am right: you have an autoimmune disease. But I am wrong: it is scleroderma." The doctor gave me a little more information about this autoimmune disease and said I was being referred to a specialist. Upon hearing the latest diagnosis, Sabi announced it was a more positive diagnosis than lupus. In retrospect, though, I doubt anyone with lupus would agree with her.

Scleroderma is called both a rheumatic disease and a connective tissue disease. The term "rheumatic disease" refers to a group of conditions characterized by inflammation and/or pain in the muscles, joints or fibrous tissue. A connective tissue disease is one that affects tissues such as skin, tendons and cartilage. In some forms of scleroderma, the manifestation is hard, tight skin, but in other forms, the problem goes deeper and can affect blood vessels and internal organs.[1]

Sometime in June I met with the specialist, a rheumatologist at my local hospital. He wore the ubiquitous white coat, was middle-aged and possessed a matter-of-fact manner. During our consultation, he had a tribe of doctors-in-training examine me. Moving my hair aside, he said to them, "Look at her forehead. Do you see it bears no lines? This is an example of how scleroderma tightens the skin."

That struck me as a funny thing to say since I was still relatively young. Inwardly I thought, "Perhaps it just means I am still young." He also said, "In some cases scleroderma can contribute to kidney failure." He took both blood tests and urine samples, neither of which showed anything out of the ordinary. He thought I would be fine, but did ask me if I wished to have any medications. I declined. I made a follow-up appointment for six months later.

Hearing the scleroderma diagnosis, and needing to come to terms with its physical effects and possible consequences on my professional and family lives, was enough to absorb. The idea that I might be susceptible to kidney failure was even more daunting. As with many of us, I was woefully ignorant about kidney failure. I had heard of it and understood that it had serious ramifications, but it seemed light years removed from my current place in time, so well was I doing with my new condition. So often, my nose almost needs to be pressed up against a window for me to relate to something. I needed to be either personally involved or else know someone who is involved, for it to be meaningful. This information was simply words that were "full of sound and fury, signifying nothing."[2]

During a family dinnertime in September, in the midst of chatting, I suddenly exclaimed, "I am seriously ill and may be laid low in January." No response: the words fell some place in mid-air, never captured. We carried on talking. The thought was but a momentary stop in the flow of conversation, hotly fogging its surroundings briefly like steam emitted from a boiling pot only to evaporate moments later.

Christopher and Roland probably thought me a little odd, though. I have no idea what possessed me to say what I did. I was doing relatively well with scleroderma, work and family life running hand-in-hand. I can only surmise that intuition plays a larger part in our subconscious than we are aware, and somehow we instinctively know when we are really ill. However,

I brushed the thought aside, dwelling no more on my outburst. My life carried on pretty much as usual.

I did have some issues, however, with swallowing and found myself more fatigued than usual. Walking seemed a little more laborious. I had my follow-up appointment with the consultant in November, complete with blood and urinary tests and once more nothing unusual showed up. Further proof, I was sure, of my relatively good health.

In February 1991, almost a year to the day after my scleroderma diagnosis, I experienced some peculiar symptoms. For about a month, I had been feeling less well than I had previously. I kept thinking I was about to come down with flu one day, only to feel better the next. It was a time of year when many were suffering the effects of a flu virus so mine was not particularly unusual. I also remember experiencing extremely itchy skin. During a meeting, I was suddenly aware that one of my colleagues had been staring intently at me as I was in the act of scratching one of my shins. I had been completely oblivious to my actions, having been totally absorbed in the process of trying to remedy my incessant itchiness. My ear lobes were often terribly itchy as well. Sometimes I noted that I needed to use the washroom less frequently than usual. I thought it simply meant that I had developed a greater capacity to hold fluid than I had in the past or maybe I had been drinking less than I normally did.

I had been to the doctor the week before our mid-term break because I thought I might have a recurrence of something like glandular fever. My doctor ordered a blood test. This was on a Friday. On the Sunday night, the eve of my blood test, I decided to celebrate my not having to work the next day. I invested a great deal more effort into our evening meal, especially since my culinary skills were haphazard at best, and embarked on cooking a special treat: a roast dinner, complete with dessert.

As I was excitedly preparing what was going to be this fabulous meal, I began feeling dreadful and could not settle. It was a most odd sensation. I couldn't decide whether I wanted to lie down, sit down or walk around the living room. Something just didn't feel right, really didn't feel right. Surprisingly, one of my colleagues called me and asked how I was. She said she had been moved to call because she hadn't thought I had looked well that week. I explained that I thought I had a virus and was due to have a blood test the following day. We talked a while longer, then said our goodbyes. In due course, our dinner was prepared and eaten. However, I don't remember if it had been the spectacular meal I had wanted it to be. Later, bedtime was just like any other night. I slept well.

The next day, Monday, I dragged myself to the local hospital for my blood test, and dragged myself back home, buying some grapes on the way. They were all I felt like eating, and I did so while sitting at the dining room table. Both Christopher and Roland were out and not expected home until early evening. Midway through the afternoon, I began to feel really unwell and simply had to lie down. I got into bed, where I remained for the next three days, growing increasingly ill: first, a blinding headache, followed by extreme nausea, then violent vomiting. My nausea was completely unpredictable, spontaneous and literally projectile. I recalled scenes from *The Exorcist*.

Fortunately, this all happened when GPs still made house calls. On the third day, Wednesday, Christopher called our local doctor's office to explain my condition. The doctor's first reaction was that Christopher should take me to his office at once. Christopher said that would be very difficult because I could hardly get out of bed and was continually being sick. The doctor assured Christopher that he knew I wasn't overreacting because I had been to see him infrequently. He knew that I was ill. He told Christopher he would come at the end of his morning session. He arrived as planned.

When he first saw me, he said, "I think you have a very bad flu virus. I am giving you anti-nausea pills to stop you being sick. Stay home for the week. Give the medication time to work." He also asked Christopher to call him by 9:00 am the next day, whatever my condition. He would again come after his morning session, at noon.

I did not improve; the pills were of no effect. Christopher, at 9:05 am, was about to call when there was a knock on our front door. It was the doctor. His immediate reaction upon seeing me was to rush me to the hospital. Would I like to go by our car or by ambulance? I opted for an ambulance because of my persistent nausea. I was alert enough to remember his telling me he was going to reassure eight-year-old Roland that all was going to be okay as he watched me suddenly being carted off in an ambulance to hospital. I recall him saying something like, "Mummies aren't expected to be ill, and it can be upsetting and confusing for children to see them when they are. Their world no longer appears stable." The mother in me welcomed his thoughtful concern for Roland.

Later I learned that Sue, our neighbour, had commented to Christopher, as I was being loaded into the ambulance, "I have never seen anyone looking so grey."

Christopher replied, "Yes, I think 'Cilla (as he called me) is quite ill." Kindly, Sue agreed to look after Roland while Christopher followed behind the ambulance in our car. Sue became a stalwart support to Roland during my stay in hospital. This conversation had taken place on the day the ambulance had rushed me to hospital, my present residence.

Hospital life

Once on the ward where I had been sent, I experienced a sudden urgent need to use the washroom. There, I voided blood clots both orally and posteriorly. This shocked me. I expressed my surprise to the nurse who nonchalantly said, "It is simply an indication you are ill." Too stunned to reply, I returned to my bed. The nurse wrapped a blood pressure cuff on one arm and inserted an intravenous needle into the other and an oxygen filter in my nose. With tubes straggling around me, I was obviously staying put.

When Christopher returned with Roland a little later to see me, Roland said nothing to me about his feelings. However, on the way home, he tearfully asked Christopher, "Is mummy going to be all right?" The last time he had seen me, while obviously unwell, I looked the same old mum. This was the first sign for Roland that my condition had greater ramifications for him than he had ever considered, and for Christopher, too, in his role as prime parent and caregiver.

I don't remember much of ensuing events but as the day wore on, I became acclimatized to my situation, and my thoughts turned to work. It was by now Thursday; classes would resume on Monday. I needed to prepare something for my colleagues. I couldn't leave things hanging in the air. I asked the nurse for some paper, a pen and something on which I could write. She was surprised by this request. Her first response was, "You should simply rest."

"Can't," I said. "This is extremely important for me." As requested, she returned with paper, pen and something to write on. I immediately began to scribble notes about the work I had been doing. I had not only been teaching several classes but also managing a number of projects in various venues in the community. All required attention.

I don't know how I managed to muster the strength or energy to write intricate details of lesson plans and information required to monitor the project work. All I can say is that I probably did what anyone would have done given the same circumstance and the obligation to keep work operating smoothly. It took me many hours. I wrote late into the night. Suddenly looking up, I noticed one of the night nurses, while doing her rounds, merely shaking her head at seeing me sitting up beavering away in the dim bedside light. When finally finished, I had completed fourteen full pages of notes for my colleagues. The next day Christopher rushed my precious document to the college's vice-principal so everything could be in place for the following Monday. I had a reputation for notoriously bad handwriting, yet I gather whatever I had written had not only been legible but also made sense. Both follow-up project work and classes continued without a hitch.

My memory of the next two days is a blur. I understand that the hospital wanted to confirm I had kidney failure before transferring me to another hospital. That determined, on Monday I was sent by hospital transport to a hospital specializing in kidney disease. Although I felt very unwell, I was still puzzled as to why the doctors seemed so concerned. I said, "I don't need to be here. I am fine."

One of the doctors told Christopher, but not me, "Indeed if anyone needs to be here, it is Priscilla." I must have been in shock. I could not register what was happening to me. My mind was disconnected from my body. My sudden change in condition had been difficult to absorb.

At the second hospital, I had a kidney biopsy to determine the cause of my kidney failure. This entailed me having to lie face down on the bed while a doctor inserted a needle into one of my kidneys to remove a small sample. Afterwards I was required to remain in this position for about eight hours to prevent any damage to my organs. I lay alone in a cell-like, windowless room, my head towards the rear of the room, my feet door side. I have no recollection of my thoughts; I must have simply followed orders.

Halfway through this ordeal, I became aware of the sound of clattering footsteps echoing in the empty room. I turned my face sideways so I could see whose feet they were. A face bent down close to my mine. It was not the face of a medical attendant but that of a man in clerical garb, his collar indicating he was a Roman Catholic priest. He was looking for a particular patient and merely happened to enter my cell—oops—room by chance, to find out if I were the person he had come to see.

I am not Roman Catholic, neither particularly religious nor a regular church attender. I would not have actively sought clerical advice, but for some reason my subconscious being welcomed his presence. Much to my surprise, I began silently quoting a line from *The Rime of the Ancient Mariner*: "O shrieve me, shrieve me, holy man!" In reality, I merely asked him to say a prayer for me, which he did. It seemed to be of some comfort. Christopher, being a Roman Catholic, was delighted to hear I had been willing to do this.

The biopsy results attributed my kidney failure to my underlying condition of scleroderma. I had what is medically termed a "scleroderma renal crisis." It literally happened overnight, as kidney failure can do, and left me completely bedridden for almost six months. All of the symptoms I had experienced during the preceding month turned out to be classic signs of kidney failure.

Days came and went. I was once again in a room by myself. I was still mobile, although I spent most of my time bedridden. One night I woke up in the early hours of the morning and was completely taken aback, for there were snakes contentedly curled up by my feet. I immediately jumped up and raced to the nurses' station to let them know about this appalling state of affairs. The nurse on duty calmly told me, "Go back to bed." Like a child I obeyed, and I must have gone back to sleep with the snakes still *in situ* on my bed. Later I learned that hallucinating is part and parcel of being very ill.

I underwent numerous tests to determine the extent of damage caused by my scleroderma. I cannot remember what tests I had, other than there seemed to be quite a number of them. My blood pressure had been dangerously high, something in the range of 250 over an equally high number. The nurses were not keen to let me bathe or wash my hair.

One day I was sent via hospital transfer to a larger hospital for some tests. Following my tests, the porter pushed my wheelchair to a small partition by the hospital's front door where I waited for my return ride. I must have looked absolutely unkempt: glasses perched precariously on my nose, dressing gown in disarray, unwashed hair hanging limply around my ashen face. My body slumped in the wheel chair. I was a mere shadow of my former self. Now I was reduced to rubble.

I felt simply awful, fighting back the horrible effects of nausea, terrified I was going to be sick in broad view of everyone striding in and out of the main door. I realized that a few days before, I would have been one of those same people, walking in a similar manner, healthy and robust. My fragility struck me. My fate could happen to anyone. I pledged to myself that I would never again let anyone I met pass by without giving them great respect. I have not always kept my pledge, but it is never far from my thoughts and has certainly influenced many of my views.

On subsequent visits to the same hospital for further tests, nurses accompanied me. On one occasion, during our return to my base hospital, I felt tired and had a strong urge to close my eyes. I did. From some distant place, I heard a faint trace of a voice saying, "Stay with me, stay with me." I didn't want to open my eyes. It took real effort for me to extricate myself from my dreamlike state. When at last I did, I found the nurse bending low, scrutinizing my face.

"I just felt sleepy," I said.

"No, you were definitely failing." She had noticed an obvious change in my appearance. I was kept under constant surveillance during the remainder of our journey. I must have been in a much more perilous state than I realized and was moved to a version of an intensive care ward, very close to the nurses' station, where my condition was constantly monitored.

On another occasion, when I was more sentient, this time in my home hospital, following an endoscopy test for which I had been sedated, a porter had been called to wheel me back to my ward. I must have received a heavy dose because I was still feeling the effects, akin to being drunk. The drug unleashed my inhibitions and loosened my tongue. For some reason I was mesmerized by the porter's hands and focused all my attention on them. I told him, "You have beautiful hands. I just want to kiss them," not once, but repeatedly. I was relentless in my pursuit, even trying to kiss them when returned to my room.

A few hours later, having recovered both my decorum and dignity, red faced, I shamefully admitted my anti-social behaviour to the nurse, who, upon hearing my tale, burst out laughing. I received my retribution on my back in the form of hives that kept me awake for hours from their itchiness. It turned out I was allergic to the drug used to sedate me.

Initially, I lived in a stupor. The nurses were both my protectors and warders. Protectors, because they were there to keep me safe and aid my recovery; warders, because I was like putty in their hands. I was totally compliant. I remember thinking that how I was behaving must have been very similar to ways in which many prisoners of war had behaved during their internment. Any physical or mental resistance I had had was now vanished, leaving me like an empty shell. Had the nurses put a collar around my neck and led me like a dog, I would have obeyed. Had they told me to lie on the floor or stand in the corner, I would have done so. It was a really bizarre situation in which to be. I was cognitive on one hand, but not on another. I was a stranger to myself.

As my condition improved, I was moved to a ward with other patients. Hospital wards are busy, sometimes chaotic, places. Nurses perform their duties, doctors do their rounds, visitors come and go. Normally, I would have engaged in conversation with my fellow patients or taken an interest in my whereabouts; however, in my current state I was totally oblivious to my surroundings and my ward mates. I have no idea how many others shared the ward or the nature of their illnesses. I continued to live in a nether world, an isthmus between reality and vagueness. I had sufficient capacity to realize that I was behaving out of character but lacked the ability to rectify it.

I do, though, recall the day I was finally allowed to have a bath. Two nurses wheeled me into a bathroom containing the largest bath I had ever seen. "It's brand new," they explained. "It can tilt and turn and be temperature controlled, and it has a door in its middle to permit easy access for immobile patients." This was a wonderful treat.

I was helped into the bath, the door closed and sealed, and the water turned on. As the nurses washed me, and especially my hair, I wallowed in the sensuality of the warm soapy water gently caressing my whole being. It was pure joy, my craving for the luxury of feeling clean again now satisfied. Throughout the remainder of my stay in hospital, as my well-being improved, and with it my cognition, bed baths became routine care for me. I was never again bathed in this tub.

One Sunday, I woke up suddenly, labouring for breath. The duty doctor's response was ominous. "You may have a blood clot in your lungs from having been bedridden for so long. I will order an x-ray for you tomorrow." Somehow I wasn't convinced he was right in his diagnosis but didn't challenge him. When Christopher and Roland visited me later in the day, I didn't mention the suspected blood clot. Our conversation was preoccupied with domestic matters: catching up on what Roland was doing and the day-to-day business in which they were involved.

The following morning I was taken for an x-ray. The results showed I had a massive amount of fluid in my lungs but no blood clot. When kidneys fail, they are no longer capable of removing excess fluid. It accumulates in different areas of our body such as in our feet, legs, hands, stomach and lungs. As soon as the doctors had seen the x-ray results, someone rushed me, bed and all, to the corridor by the nurses' station. With little fanfare, the doctor immediately inserted a tube into my upper right chest area and proceeded to drain several litres of fluid. The actual amount escapes my memory, but it was considerable.

While this was going on, Roland, who was at school, uncharacteristically broke down in tears. When his teacher asked him what was wrong, he replied, "Something is not right with my mum." Christopher was called. He collected Roland, rushed home and called the hospital only to learn Roland's intuition had been spot on: I had been in crisis. When I heard what had happened, it increased my belief in thought transference and that inexplicable things do occur, especially between those in close bonds.

Although my condition had created chaos in our family's life, Roland, until that point, had remained calm and collected, taking my situation in his stride. He later told me that he had felt secure and safe because of the warm support he had received from Sue, who had two sons close to Roland in age, as well as from his friends, teachers and even head-teacher, who, on occasion, had hugged him and said comforting things.

Even though I remained in hospital for almost two months, I have only superficial memories of the medical staff who looked after me. The nurses were distinguishable by their different uniforms denoting the hospitals where they had received their training. Some had frilly caps and cuffed sleeves, while others wore coloured belts or blue dresses with white pinafores, and still others dressed simply in plain white uniforms. All wore dark blue capes when off-duty. I must have engaged in some conversation with them, but in my memory, they are a sea of faces, coming and going, providing my care.

A stream of doctors attended to me, too. Most were also just faces, but three stood out. First was the resident nephrologist, a young New Zealander with a distinguishing accent, who was completing his training. He removed the fluid from my lungs. I cannot remember his name. He was shorter than most of the other doctors, had a warm, caring, personable manner and was friendly, chatty and exceptionally approachable. I liked him immensely.

Months later, following my discharge, Christopher and I were back, walking down a hospital corridor to one of my many medical check-ups, when we encountered this doctor. As he was about to walk past us, I said, "Hello" or some other greeting. He stopped in his tracks, stared at me and then said, "Goodness, I would never have recognized you. You look so much better than when I last saw you." We exchanged pleasantries, and then carried on, my transformation a testament to the effects of dialysis.

The second doctor, a consultant as most doctors are called in British hospitals, must have been a rheumatologist mostly interested in my scleroderma. I often saw him later at one of the clinics I attended. I felt him to be really in my corner, and certainly someone who supported me when I wished to be discharged from hospital. He was portly, most likely in his mid-forties. When he visited me, he would grab a chair, sit really close to me, almost holding my hand kindly, and caringly speak to me in hushed tones. I felt special in his company, truly cared for.

The third consultant, probably one of the head nephrologists, was tall and wore glasses. In his early forties and very personable, he also possessed a kind, caring bedside manner. He tended to me later when I received my transplant.

During my two-month stay in hospital, my physical strength ebbed more and more, though my mental state improved a little. However, I remained in a fog, most of my thoughts vacuous. My weight dropped considerably, and I continued to feel overwhelming spontaneous outbursts of nausea and a constant sour taste in my mouth. The nausea resulted from the high level of toxins in my body: when our kidneys fail and can no longer filter waste, our creatinine and uremic levels rise, causing a build-up of toxins. The effects: both nausea and a ureic-like taste in the mouth.

It is hard to pinpoint what keeps us going and our spirits up, but I do know support of others plays a huge part. Often I was too ill to appreciate the different visitors who came. I recall one colleague who happened to be in the hospital's vicinity decided on the spur of the moment to visit me. I could see she obviously felt unnerved by my physical appearance and weakened state, not having seen me since my kidney failure, and she didn't know how to react. She said something like, "I had no idea how sick you were. I'll come back another time." Then she abruptly left, never to be seen again.

One of my very dear friends, my soul sister Sarah, frequently visited me. I had been immediately drawn to her. We first met many years previously while I was teaching in a social services centre, and she was providing support to my students. Sarah is tall and graceful, her lovely features topped off with a mass of dark brown hair. I thoroughly enjoyed spending time with her. During her visits she often spent her time massaging my feet, and she even shaved my legs. We shared many common interests, most importantly a similar sense of humour that would find us curled up, hugging our stomachs in pain after laughing intensely over some little joke. So comfortable was I with her, that I felt confident enough to give baby Roland his first bath in her company.

Sarah recently shared the thoughts and feelings she had experienced during the time I was in hospital. She told me that each time she drove to the hospital, she never knew whether I would be alive or dead. Though she felt gloomy, she remained eager to see me. To help calm her worries she would play a George Michael album, *Without Prejudice*, as loudly as she could. Those songs still carry profound memories for her. Each track expressed a particular emotion that had a special relevance for her. Singing along with the song voiced these emotions, so by the time she reached the hospital, she had released her feelings, leaving her able to function calmly. Interestingly, Sarah's memories of seeing me in hospital have not remained prominent. She remembers her helpless feeling as she observed the severity of my illness. She also remembers her tremendous concern for Roland, so young, so vulnerable, should something worse happen to me. During her journey home, Sarah would replay the music again, this time more quietly and calmly, feeling less driven. She would arrive home exhausted yet comforted that I was still alive, and still hopeful all would be well.

How can we ever repay our friends' generosity and kindness during times of crisis? I owe a life-long debt of gratitude.

I received a tremendous number of well-wishes and cards from friends, family and colleagues, in the end something in the order of over two hundred cards. These, Christopher and my friends posted on the walls around my bed. It was amazing that so many people were concerned for my well-being. I owed it to them to get back on my feet and back to work!

My treatment

At some point, the medical staff decided the best treatment was for me to do continuous ambulatory peritoneal dialysis, or, as it is called, CAPD. I had a tube inserted into my peritoneal cavity. Part of the tube was inside my abdomen while the remaining few feet dangled outside with a plug attached so that fluid could flow into my peritoneal cavity and then be drained out. I have little recollection of the procedure or how it affected me. I was taught how to perform the dialysis myself.

The principle of peritoneal dialysis is to cleanse the kidneys using a chemical solution that sits in the peritoneal cavity. Its purpose is to capture water and waste from the blood and filter out toxins. To do this, clean solution is inserted through the abdominal tube and remains in place for several hours, collecting toxins. At the end of a specified time, referred to as dwell time, the dirty solution is drained out of the tube into an empty bag and replaced once more with clean solution. Peritoneal dialysis is a gentler form of dialyzing since it is a continuous process. The bags containing the solution resemble clear, giant hot water bottles, each with a long tube that could be attached to my own peritoneal tube.

CAPD would enable me to dialyze both at home and at work. To be able to work was of paramount importance to me since I was a major wage earner. I wanted to return to work in September. It was now late March and I was still considerably ill. The doctors were dubious that I would ever return to work, let alone in September. Once all my other tests had been completed, and I had been set up with CAPD, I begged to go home.

When my consultant visited me on one of his rounds, again sitting close to me and speaking in his customary hushed voice, I told him, "I am in mourning and need to be in the comfort of my own home in order to recover more effectively."

"I am astounded and impressed you are able to recognize your feelings in this way. Of course, you must go home. I shall get your discharge organized immediately," he responded.

True to the consultant's word, I was immediately discharged and entered an unknown future. Initially though, I frequently needed to return to the hospital, as my CAPD regimen needed tweaking. What took longer to assuage was my state of mind regarding my sudden and unexpected altered condition. I was in mourning. The mourning process played an important part in my adaptation from my former ways to the new reality confronting me. It took me some months to overcome the loss of my old life.

Shortly before I was discharged, the same consultant in company of his residents supported me again when he said to them, "This patient is a prime example of someone who needs a transplant. A transplant would dramatically improve both her and her family's prospects. Five years ago we would never have considered a transplant because we would have believed scleroderma would reject a kidney. Fortunately times have changed and our thinking with it."

Home and recuperation

Once home, I was far too weak to do anything for myself. I could barely lift my head from my pillow. I remember lying in my bed, looking out of the bedroom window, observing a chestnut tree as it gradually transformed from barren branches to buds to leaves. A special care assistant provided by the British National Health Service came for about four hours every day to bathe and dress me and prepare my breakfast and lunch. This was an absolute godsend. My wonderfully chatty, kind aide, named Betty, had come from Nigeria. She was a tremendous support, not only to me but also to Roland and Christopher. She was a truly lovely person who became more of a friend than simply a caregiver, remaining with me for well over four months.

At some point, a sofa bed was made up for me in the living room so I could be more involved in everyone's comings and goings. I was either semi-carried or well-supported as I weakly made my way down the stairs. Having made it downstairs, I was better placed for visits. Nola, one of our immediate neighbours in our row of townhouses, was an eminently affable woman. We had become great friends, and when gardening would share those convivial, over-the-fence, gossipy conversations known for their friendliness, comforting banality and pleasant sociability. Nola would, in the same spirit of camaraderie, stop by either on her way home from work in the evening or on weekends.

Nola's visits were extremely important to me. Not only did they represent my connection with the outside world, but they also represented the reality of day-to-day life. Our conversations ranged from trivial neighbourhood gossip, a reminder of our former banter, to meatier subjects. The substance was irrelevant; what was more meaningful, and something that had never occurred to me before, was the importance of that frequent outside contact. At one point I told Nola, "I am like a desert, dry and arid, and your visits represent an oasis of hope for me. I somehow crave to know all the minor details in your life. There is another world out there, something vibrant and pulsing, of which I long to be a part." Nola's visits were like a halfway house for me in my convalescence.

Gradually I was able to get up on my own and began to bathe and dress myself. Life was slowly taking on more shape. My dear friend Sarah, she of the bubbly humour, came over every Sunday and prepared our evening meal, which we would plan in advance each week. We had many wonderful laughter-filled evenings together, not to forget good meals, too. One of the meals, a stew, stands out, because we lived on this for an entire week! Christopher had bought the ingredients, of which there were a lot. Sarah then prepared our copious quantity of stew.

Food, which plays such a significant role in our lives, had been a forgotten substance during my sojourn in hospital. I have few memories of being served meals and even fewer of eating them. They must have been quite bland. Once home, though, my desires changed. We watched a TV program involving a number of amateur cooks competing against each other to make the best meals, our mouths salivating as we anticipated the taste of the finished products. Sarah would try to emulate some of the meals while she prepared ours, the results often causing uproarious laughter. Sarah's visits were joyful for Roland, too, as they created a veneer of routine. On the surface, we were a happier crew. Those evenings shielded us from the worrying circumstances confronting our family.

During my initial recovery, food restrictions were slightly less stringent than they would be later since the aim was for me to try to gain weight. I was shockingly thin. Dietary restrictions are a salient part of kidney failure. Once kidneys fail to cleanse waste material, the body is no longer able to process some food nutrients. Food containing high levels of potassium, such as bananas, potatoes, avocados, mangoes, tomatoes and numerous others, are not filtered effectively. This can lead to an overload of potassium, damaging the heart. Likewise, food containing high levels of phosphorus, such as peanut butter, beans, chocolate and dairy products, can accumulate in the body, stripping calcium from bones, causing them to weaken. I was only permitted to eat potatoes once a week after having soaked them for several hours.

As my kidney failure continued, my diet became more restricted. Mealtimes were difficult, as was entertaining, because of the limited number of things I could eat. Dining out was challenging since menu choices were far from being kidney-friendly. I was allowed to drink half a cup of liquid a day. This was the early 1990s. Since then some changes in dietary practices have taken place. Then, I was required to drink a liquid phosphate binder before each meal, the purpose of which was to gather unabsorbed phosphorus. All food contains traces of phosphorus. I had a choice of two flavours, either peppermint or liquorice. No matter which one I chose, the taste was the same: ghastly. I had a perpetually bad taste in my mouth. Today, the liquid binder has been replaced with taste-free tablets.

Another best friend, Jane, someone I had known since we were two when our parents, also closely connected, had introduced us, now resided in California but had moved to Scotland for two years with her three teenage girls when her husband, Bill, had been sent there by his optical company. Jane and I had been born at the same time, merely days apart, she in Vancouver and I, in England. Although separated by distance, our friendship had remained solid. Now we were both in the UK, we were able to see more of each other.

After dropping off her three daughters at the American School in Surrey,

Jane stayed with us twice for several days before returning to Scotland. As with Sarah, her primary thoughts were for Roland's welfare. Jane made it her mission to ensure he was receiving the attention he deserved. Jane is one of my most elegant, urbane friends. Her entire demeanour—from posture and physical features to hairstyle and dress—oozes natural glamour. Some evenings, while lying in bed fighting back my endless nausea, I wistfully admired her graceful poise as she sat beside me working on a needlepoint.

Around Easter, wanting to do something special with Roland, Jane decided they would make Easter cookies. They must have baked dozens and dozens of bunny-faced cookies, since everyone feasted on them for what seemed ages, except, sadly, me because of my restricted diet. Too soon, Jane's visits ended. She and her family returned to the United States shortly after I had recovered sufficiently to return to work but before we could visit them in Scotland.

When I became more independent and able to do things for myself, I revived a neglected skill: crocheting. I started out with a three-coloured blanket. By the end of my convalescence, I had completed three enormous blankets. When I had recuperated sufficiently to return to my working life, I never crocheted again. It had served its purpose of providing some rehab activity for me.

One day, while crocheting during an afternoon dialysis session, I had a vivid déjà vu moment. I recalled something that had been said to me about being very ill. I wracked my brain, trying to remember the situation. Eventually, from some long-forgotten corner, the source flashed before me.

Almost eighteen years previously, when I had been living in central London, I had shared a flat with a diminutive, friendly, self-contained seminary student who was training to become a Roman Catholic priest. In his spare time my flatmate performed psychic readings over the phone. Returning home from a particularly rigorous interview for graduate studies, I passed his room while he was giving a reading. I wasn't eavesdropping, merely walking down the hallway. What he was actually saying, I didn't hear.

Later that evening, as we encountered each other in the kitchen, we exchanged pleasantries. I told him about my difficult interview. He began to describe, in precise details, both the location and building where it had taken place.

I was amazed, "Yes, you have identified it perfectly."

Silence for a moment, then he said, "Pfft, you're in." Meaning I had been accepted. We chatted awhile longer. Then he began to tell me things about myself, nothing of much importance, just things he could see. One was to do with someone wearing glasses (who, years and years later, turned out to be Christopher).

Then he said something more portentous, "When you are in your forties, you are going to have a serious illness."

I said, "No, I have had pneumonia twice as a child, and will be fine."

"No, this is very much more serious, really serious."

We talked a bit more and that was that. True to his words, I received my college acceptance. I moved closer to the college and soon forgot everything he had said. I never considered it further until that moment when I was performing my dialysis. Incredible, I thought, and once more mused over the powers of the paranormal.

Ever present in my mind was my return to work in September. Medical staff remained skeptical, but I was determined. In my desire to follow through with my intentions, I discovered I was extremely goal-oriented and fiercely competitive with myself. Once I focused on something, I was determined to see it through.

At first, my return to public life required that I be in a wheelchair. Christopher would drive us to our destination, unload the chair and help me wobble into it. Roland would then take over. He loved pushing me. He was in charge! And it was important for him to feel he was part of the family core. My illness weighed heavily on him. His world had been shaken, the bond between mother and child tested, as my GP had predicted.

Roland remembers now that, while he felt a certain degree of security because of the great support he received, he knew underneath his composure he could not explain how he felt. It was a mixed reaction between anger that this had happened, and grave concern that all would be right. Pushing me in my wheelchair was his way of being in control of an uncontrollable situation. It represented his own way of mourning the passing of a life and the growing acceptance of a newly imposed one.

My chair was heavy for a young child to push but Roland, happily smiling, would weave me awkwardly in and out of the other pedestrians as they busily conducted their affairs. He thoroughly enjoyed being able to steer me according to his fancy. Even then, Roland had a tremendous sense of fun and could appreciate the humorous side of things. He had a wonderful way of expressing it. Our journeys usually involved raucous laughter as he encountered unforeseen obstacles and struggled to move on. Just hearing Roland chortling his delightful laugh brought pleasure to my ears.

When Roland was in good spirits, I felt much happier, too. It is hard being a mother unable to provide the nurturing a child requires. In the early stages of my kidney failure and subsequent severe illness, I lived in a daze, not absorbing much of what was happening around me. I was preoccupied with simply surviving. As my health improved, so did my ability to interact with Roland more actively and be supportive at that important time.

I became more supportive of Christopher, too. He not only needed to provide the solace for Roland and look after his daily activities, but also to care for me, whether it was visiting me in hospital, driving me to endless appointments once home, preparing evening meals or performing all the household tasks. He bore much of the brunt of my illness.

Caregivers are often forgotten as concern is focused on the invalid. They become secondary in peoples' eyes but in reality are the glue that holds a family together. Any improvement in my health was a bonus for Christopher and relieved his concerns. I noticed he, too, became less anxious and more of his usual placid self as our lives were slowly restored to their former domesticity. One of his strengths was his loyalty and faithfulness during times of stress and unexpected challenges. I will always carry with me the memory of his unstinting kindness and devoted helpfulness as he needed to assist me in ways not usually expected of husbands.

While recovering at home, I would dream of being able to lead a more ordinary life. Our outings provided me with just that. I could actively participate in the daily trappings of life. With Roland's help guiding me I could enter shops. I would like to think that, during this time, I acquired a greater appreciation for the challenges wheelchair users face on a daily basis. It was sometimes entirely degrading and rather appalling, but also humorous, to find myself in a store, nose to counter and eyes slightly above the rim, arms waving wildly while I tried to catch the sales assistant's notice so I could pay for a purchase. Eventually my flaying arms would capture the sales clerk's attention and I could complete my transactions.

Return to work

My nausea held sway over my destiny well into July and then suddenly stopped. The built-up toxins must have finally cleared. Things were looking up. About two weeks before my desired return to work, I tried my hand at driving again, short journeys at first to feel comfortable. I made an appointment to see my GP about a week before work began to get medical clearance for my return full-time. The doctor was most concerned that I not only wanted to return to work but especially to full-time. Before he agreed he insisted that I make a follow-up appointment in a month's time, which I did. At this appointment, he asked me if I had had any idea how ill I had been. I must have mumbled something coherent because he seemed satisfied.

I believe this doctor saved my life. To him I owed my future well-being. After we had left England and were back in Canada, I felt it behooved me to send a thank you letter to him. I also thought a First Nations artifact would be an appropriate gift to enclose and something different to display on the clinic's walls. I received a thank you in return and, indeed, my gift had been hung on a wall.

I did return to work in early September. One of the challenges for me was the need to perform dialysis at work. My employers were most accommodating and even organized a changing room for me in the head branch of the college. As it turned out, I never used this facility. I would simply perform my dialysis wherever I was. In the 1990s the common practice was to perform dialysis every six hours but for me this was not possible. I had to exchange my solution every four hours irrespective of my surroundings. The times were 8 am, 12 pm, 4 pm, 8 pm, 12 am, and then dry overnight, the common name for this state.

The hospital supplied me with a travelling bag for the dialysis solution. The bag had an attached plug so that I could warm my solution, which was important because using a cold solution could be a shock to my body. During the dialysis, I needed to exchange the fluid inside me with the clean, warmed solution. First I removed the fluid within me by placing the draining bag on the ground or low enough so the fluid could easily drain out.

Then I placed the new bag of solution above shoulder height so it could flow in easily. I tried using several devices, from hooks to clothes hangers.

My procedure took almost a full hour to complete and required scrupulous attention to hygiene and careful manipulation in attaching the bag's tube to my body tube. It could not be hurried lest I accidentally got a kink in the tube running from the bag of dialysis solution. No matter how well I tried to complete the process effectively, I often ended up with wind in my peritoneal cavity. It was excruciatingly painful and usually manifested itself in referred pain in my right shoulder. It would take me about three dialysis sessions for my condition to return to normal.

When I had my monthly follow-up appointment, my GP admitted he was surprised I was coping so well. He had never expected me to work full-time. He told me, "Research has shown when organizations treat returning workers benevolently, the worker fares very much better and becomes productive in a shorter period of time than would otherwise be the case."

My day always started with checking my weight, taking my temperature and recording the results in a journal. This was to keep track of any possible fluid retention and to check for potential infections. A possibility of site infections was always prevalent because of the tube in my abdomen. I next needed to meticulously cleanse my site with a special solution and then cover the site opening with a large adhesive bandage, medically termed a Mepore bandage, ensuring the tube's covering was well-cleansed, too. Baths were out, but careful showering was permitted.

Although I was able to do dialysis at home, I required both solution and medical supplies in order to do so. The solution was packed in sturdy cardboard boxes. Each box contained a day's supply—about five bags a day. The delivery company, an international firm called Baxter, delivered not just one week's supply at a time but a month's. In other words, boxes and boxes! Fortunately, we had a garage in which to store the boxes. They were lined up, floor to ceiling, covering several walls. We were hard-pressed to find space for our car. Christopher, thank heavens, brought me my daily boxes and disassembled them for the garbage. When asked of his memory of this time, he just shook his head and muttered something about "*Those boxes.*" I can only imagine how difficult it must have been for those whose premises were small and had limited space.

Being on dialysis meant that activities had to be carefully planned in advance. Spontaneity does not exist for those with renal failure. During my recovery period in the summer school holidays, Christopher and I were fortunate to be able to send Roland to his cousins in the States. Before he arrived at the airport on his return, we needed to stay overnight in a hotel so that I could do my dialysis.

On a different occasion when we wished to visit the Museum of London that had just opened, I knew that I would have to exchange my fluids sometime during our visit. I had to call ahead to organize a room in which to do this. The museum kindly made their first aid room available for me. When it was time to perform dialysis, I was directed to the room; Christopher and Roland continued with their sightseeing. Since I was also due to attend a two-day conference later in the year, again I needed to organize a suitable place in which to do my dialysis. As well, I needed to contact Baxter to ensure I would have supplies waiting for me at the conference.

Travel was possible, but likewise necessitated quite a bit of organizing beforehand in order to have supplies at hand. While I never travelled during this time, I heard tales of people sitting on the beach in warm places such as Spain and simply draining in cold solution to keep themselves cool.

During my dialysis treatment, my body's physical appearance changed. First I developed a moonface. My face became round and rather pudgy. I looked entirely different than I had prior to kidney failure. I presume it was a result of the kind of chemicals used and the strength of the dialysis solution, since today, happily, I see fewer people with moonfaces. Another change was apparent in my abdomen; because of the fluid retained, it had increased in size so that I needed to wear loose clothes. Gone was sleek, close-fitting apparel. I also felt quite bloated most of the time because of the fluid I bore. Overall, I felt my sense of femininity had been plundered. What was once secure was no longer assured. We lose a vital part of our very being, of who we are or were, when an illness requires us to make unwanted changes in habits, dress and lifestyle. We exist as best we can.

Additionally, I was experiencing greater levels of fatigue from my kidney failure and dialysis. I was already tired from the effects of scleroderma so this was a double whammy. For me, the combination of working full-time and managing a family was about all I could do. I had little free time to enjoy life's pleasures. Apart from our venture to the museum, grocery shopping and my daily work, I hardly left our home.

While I had been placed on the wait list for a kidney transplant, and knew I would eventually receive one, I had little sense of how long a wait it would be. Years could pass before a suitable match could be found; I was prepared for the long wait. I was also unaware of what might be transpiring behind the scenes. I had had blood tests to find my blood type, and a stress test and chest x-rays, but nothing more. I attended a dialysis clinic every three months for check-ups. Miraculously, though, fortune smiled brightly!

Receiving my new kidney

Only nine months after my kidney failure and my subsequent need to do dialysis, I was offered a new kidney. I distinctly remember the phone call. It came on November 19, 1991, a Thursday night, at 11:00 pm. The hospital had a kidney. Would I come immediately? No time for second thoughts. Drop everything, grab an overnight bag and run.

It is slightly over 60 years since the first successful kidney transplant was performed.

Fortuitously, our niece, Alexandra, who had accompanied Roland on his return from his summer holiday, was staying with us. A bright 17-year-old who had just graduated from high school and was in limbo while she decided on her next course of action, Alexandra had been sent to help us. Roland would be cared for while I spent time in hospital. I only had time to make one phone call to my vice-principal. It was late, but thankfully she was still up. As soon as she recognized my voice, she knew my reason for calling.

We arrived at the hospital after midnight. All was quiet, somewhat different. Being admitted as a walk-in patient late at night was unusual. I was immediately given a liquid immunosuppressant called cyclosporine to drink. It would begin the anti-rejection process. Surgery was scheduled early that morning. I must have slept well. I remember nothing more until I was called for my operation and wheeled to the OR.

There, a number of doctors settled by my side. How wonderful they all seemed, so reassuring. Fear, anxiety, nervousness and excitement all play a part in the build up to surgery. Most people react in one of two ways to these feelings preceding surgery: either being deadly silent or talking incessantly. Mine is the latter. I would have to be in a comatose state to be mum. Simply lead me towards an OR, or mention surgery, and I am the most animated, garrulous person you could possibly meet. I shudder to think of things I have probably said before being anaesthetized.

Early on in my pre-surgery state—pre-gloves, pre-oblivion—the anaesthetist must have touched my arm. As he did so, I noticed how soft and gentle his hands were. Of course, I couldn't resist mentioning this. His colleague said, "That's because he never washes dishes," most likely joking. Whatever the purpose of his reply, it did make me think about the important role hands and touch play in the medical field.

I was anaesthetized and surgery was duly performed. But success was not to be had. The surgeons had worked for five hours trying to attach the new kidney, but something had happened to the vessels when it was retrieved from my deceased donor. My new kidney would not function.

No tears, just great disappointment for me. All I wanted to do was heal and return home. To my surprise, I was continuously given an immunosuppressant throughout the weekend, but no dialysis. On Sunday, a nurse came by and said, "The consultant needs to take another blood test."

Probably routine, I thought. Sunday evening a "Nil by mouth" sign was placed above my bed. Something was up. For some reason, I felt optimistic. Sure enough, early Monday morning my tall, personable consultant approached my bed with a number of minions in tail, as was customary in England. He said, "I have good news and I have bad news. The bad news is the transplanted kidney doesn't work and you could remain here for a couple of weeks while you heal. Alternatively, the good news is you can have another transplant and be out of here by Saturday. What is your preference?"

I would have been a fool to turn down the offer but all I could remember was the severe pain from the first surgery. I weakly asked, "What do you suggest?"

"Transplant," immediately responded the consultant. Once again, off I went to the OR.

Almost immediately upon my recovery, pain aside, I felt entirely well. The kidney was working! It was the most amazing feeling. I felt completely reinvigorated. I had had no idea how unwell I had been. It is hard to gauge the effects of illness because it becomes a way of life, a norm. Rarely do we compare our state of health with others. We can tell when we feel rotten but not necessarily appreciate real wellness unless a major change occurs. This was that moment.

I was bedridden, in some discomfort and suddenly desperate to use the washroom. I had been given a large volume of water to drink. I hadn't voided anything nor had I needed to do so until then; failed kidneys often mean no urine output. I don't remember not having to use the washroom during my kidney failure, but suddenly needing to do so was like an immediate surge of electricity through my system. The rapid sensation of having a full bladder impelled me to run as quickly as I could before I had an accident. All this occurred because my kidney was functioning and my creatinine had dropped from around 500 to 20 micromoles per litre (μmol/L). No wonder I felt better.

The consultant had been right. I was discharged on Saturday. Once more I could reclaim my own sense of place in society, first as a wife and mother in the home, and secondly, unhindered by the trappings of ill health, as a professional member of the work force.

A renascence had happened. Exciting and unknown prospects lay before me.

Chapter 2 | Living with My Transplant

Come on baby let the good times roll
—Earl King, *Let the Good Times Roll*

Early days

I arrived home mid-afternoon on Saturday, slightly weak but feeling wonderful, and bearing a precious gift: a new kidney. I had been given a rebirth. While I had been in hospital, I had felt safe; home, however, was a different matter. Would my kidney fail? I was to return to the hospital early Monday morning for a check-up. The next forty-eight hours were a worry for me. I kept a watchful eye on my need to use the washroom. Was I drinking enough? Voiding enough? Was my kidney still working? When I had my check-up, the result was, yes, all had been fine. It took me months to feel relaxed about my transplant. Every evening prior to a blood test and for the next few days afterwards, I was edgy, waiting for a recall from the hospital in case something was wrong. Actually, this feeling continued for the duration of my transplant's life—well over twenty years. One can never be complacent with a transplant.

Transplant patients require an armload of medications. These may include blood pressure pills and other meds for particular conditions. In my case, it meant taking pills to control the effects of scleroderma in addition to a number of immunosuppressant pills, because a transplant is a foreign body and will forever remain so. The body's natural inclination is to rid itself of any foreign object, so immunosuppressant medication must be taken every twelve hours in a strict regimen.

The medical procedure with new transplants includes twice-weekly checkups at a transplant clinic for at least the first month, followed by weekly check-ups, gradually tapering to monthly, and so on. A well-functioning kidney requires four-monthly check-ups.

While on peritoneal dialysis, I had only needed to visit the hospital periodically. Now, with a transplant, I would require more frequent visits to a clinic, something I found hard to accept. I am embarrassed to say, indeed, I felt some frustration that I would be forever connected to doctors and clinics. This was a lifetime commitment. Welcome to the world of double chronic conditions!

I also confess that for many years I never fully endorsed or accepted that I had, and would always have, kidney disease. The reasons are threefold. First, events happened so quickly for me. One minute I was okay, the next very ill and then so much better because of a transplant, almost as though nothing had happened. I had had little time to reflect on my condition. Second, getting back to work and maintaining an ordinary life was forefront in my thoughts. Third, I seemed to manage well with scleroderma and had always felt so able to deal with any challenges. Nothing could stop me in my tracks. Events would show how wrong I was.

Every month I needed a full blood test in addition to testing for kidney function. Because each medication is essentially lethal, it is important to monitor them; with any physiological change, the medications could be detrimental to my health. The doctors need to check potassium, phosphate, creatinine, calcium, hemoglobin and glomerular filter rate (GFR) levels. Each is vital to kidney function.

With weekly check-ups in place, and recovery going smoothly, my Christmas that year was not only a celebration and feast but also a fun-filled, entertaining time. For the first time in nine months, I was able to host a party; we had eight for Christmas dinner. Our gathering consisted of the three of us, my niece and two of Christopher's friends, and my good friend Sarah and her mother. We ate and drank to our hearts' desire, table laden and champagne corks flying. It was the beginning of many dinner parties to come over the years.

I wanted to get back to work as soon as I could, because I had tasks waiting for me to complete. Since my early days working with the college, I had been appointed to the position of the special educational needs coordinator. It was my role to work with faculty, helping them integrate students into their classes. Part of my role included providing workshops as well as initiating new projects and working with community organizations.

Fortunately, I was able to return to work in January 1992 after a six-week absence that had really been less because of the Christmas term break. My return coincided with the beginning of the new term so it felt as though I had hardly been away. I managed to complete my weekly check-ups without too much interruption to my working schedule. As winter morphed into spring, the frequency of check-ups reduced. The need for me to attend the clinic was now monthly, enabling us to travel.

Christopher and Roland had gone to Halifax, Nova Scotia, to visit his family and were to join me in Vancouver, my hometown, for three weeks later in August. Before travelling abroad, and to test my newly acquired freedom, Sarah and I decided to try a short trip to Suffolk, the area known as Constable Country after the painter of *The Hay Wain*,[1] and to Norfolk. Several days before Sarah and I were due to depart, I had my usual monthly blood tests and shortly afterwards I received a call from the hospital asking me to repeat the tests. This was new. Something was amiss. Was my kidney not functioning well? I immediately lapsed into despair. My next-door neighbour, Nola, knowing I was on my own and anxious, invited me to stay between tests and results. This was comforting and helped alleviate my stress. Her gesture is best described as "The best portion of a good man's life: his little nameless unremembered acts of kindness and love."[2] My results were fine, it turned out, and we could embark on our venture unfettered. The weather was superb and our little adventure was great fun. My desire to travel had been whetted. On to Vancouver.

Travelling had proved successful, and everything was progressing smoothly, so smoothly we decided to spend the first autumn midterm break in Portsmouth. All went well until our last night when we had a blip in the plans, causing an unwelcome hiatus from my work. Mercifully, my work was primarily administrative, so I did not need to organize class coverage, but still it put a spanner in the works.

We were sitting in the foyer of our hotel, waiting to go into dinner. I went to look at the menu and must have tripped over my husband's foot. He was 6′2″ and wore a size 14 shoe, so tripping over it was not such an oddity. As I fell, I heard a crack and landed with a thump on the ground. I was immobilized. An ambulance was called, and once more, off I went to hospital. I had broken my hip. Because Christopher accompanied me to hospital, the hotel staff sprang into action and looked after Roland. We owed them an enormous amount of gratitude.

I had been taken to a naval hospital in Portsmouth. I do not remember much pain, probably because I was kept in traction that night, and then operated on the next day. When travelling with a transplant, it is important to carry medical documents in case something happens. Over the years my package gained in size. I also recall the doctors in England telling me that if I needed medical help anywhere in England to make sure, wherever I was, that they were called. I asked the doctors to contact my hospital in London prior to their performing surgery. This they did.

Because the scleroderma had affected my lung function, the doctors did not want to anaesthetize me. Instead they gave me a local injection. What looked like a plastic sheet was draped over my lower body to protect the area from germs. I couldn't see what the surgeon was doing and was numb, but I could hear a noise that sounded like a Black and Decker drill working on my nether regions. Indeed, it was a drill. My body had become like a piece of furniture. I had a large plate, somewhat resembling a door hinge, inserted into my hip.

Hip fractures usually occur later in life; consequently, I was placed on the geriatric ward. I was the youngest patient. As a result of my kidney transplant and the need to avoid getting an infection, I was prescribed a really strong, four-day dose of antibiotics. I felt godawful, almost as though I were having kidney failure all over again. I was both physically sick and unwell. I was hardly able to lift my head off the pillow. The nurses needed to carry me to a bath and wash me themselves. Happily, after the four days I was perfectly fine. I remained in hospital for fourteen days. My hip, a pivotal joint, required lengthy immobilization.

I have a couple of memories from my stay in that hospital. One relates to a nurse telling me that the previous night a young naval officer had been brought to the emergency department suffering from firework burns to his face, the night before having been Guy Fawkes Night.

In 1605, a member of a group of provincial Roman Catholics protesting the Protestant faith tried to blow up the Houses of Parliament. The plot failed. Guy Fawkes was hanged, and the day, November 5, remembered ever afterwards with fireworks and the burning of a Guy Fawkes effigy.

The second was the food. Hospital food has never been known for its taste or appearance, but for some reason, the meals were absolutely delicious, so good, in fact, that I wrote a note commenting on the wonderful fare I had had. Christopher told me that indeed it was said guests staying at a Holiday

Inn beside the hospital clamoured to use the cafeteria. Maybe this being a naval hospital, sailors merited a better quality of food.

We were fortunate in having friends in Portsmouth where Christopher could stay between his visits to me and his need to commute to London. They were extremely hospitable, too. When I was discharged from hospital, still fairly immobile and weak, we were able to stay the night with them before embarking on the journey home.

Once home, I obviously required follow-up treatment that included physiotherapy and check-ups to ensure my hip surgery had been successful. I also had my transplant clinic to attend. My transplant consultant referred me to a bone specialist to ascertain the cause of my hip fracture. Test results pointed to weakened bones and the onset of osteoporosis. I was still in my mid-forties. Medical opinion was that the massive amount of prednisone, an immunosuppressant medication, I had been given early on in my initial transplant treatment had stripped me of calcium, thus weakening my bones. I was given hormone replacement therapy via an under-skin patch, a therapy that I continued for many years until studies showed that it could lead to cancer.

Work was high on my agenda. I was desperate to get back. Because I needed time to convalesce, I couldn't attend in person. My employers were supportive and permitted me to work from home while I recovered. I could monitor projects and even hold meetings. Our living room became my office by day. My hip healed and my mobility improved, but I had to use a cane for several years after that to help me walk.

When I was able to return to work in January 1993, it was to the gloom of gathering storm clouds. Mutterings of potential educational cuts were making their rounds. One Saturday in early March I returned home from visiting one of the projects I had organized to find an ominous-looking envelope on our doorstep. Sure enough, my position was going to be cut from a full-time to a part-time job. In effect I would lose over half my pay and would need to reapply if I wished to continue. Part of my role as special educational needs coordinator was to oversee the integration of our students into mainstream college courses. It had taken years to finally have our students recognized as being the capable students they were and given opportunities to extend their educational horizons. The work I had been doing would be affected drastically, reducing the quality and service. Our students' needs would be relegated to the back burner, not a positive step if we were to continue moving forward with providing them opportunities to be integrated in classes with others and accepted as real members of society, something so longed denied to them.

Therefore, my receipt of the ominous envelope informing me that my position was being amended meant that my work and our family life would need reassessing. Christopher and I spent that weekend in one long discussion weighing what I should do. I loved my work and my students and was caught between wanting to hang on to compete with a colleague for the part-time position or taking a plunge to explore new ventures. We finally reached a decision. It was time to return to Canada. Although Christopher hailed from Nova Scotia and I from Vancouver, for my work, Vancouver seemed the obvious choice. All this could happen because I had a functioning kidney.

The day before the deadline, I duly handed in my resignation along with other colleagues who needed to reapply for their positions. That Friday, the phone rang around noon. Christopher answered. The call was for me. I took it. It was my principal. "Are you really sure you want to do this? Won't you please, please reconsider?" I thanked him for his call but said I had made up my mind and would abide by my decision. He wished me all the best and we hung up.

This had come from one of the very people who had cut my position. I was now being asked not to leave. I said to Christopher how complimented I felt. If I never, ever experienced anything like this again, it would be sufficient to keep me going forward for a long, long time. Emboldened by my kidney transplant, I was empowered to take risks. Nothing could stop me.

My leaving party was a spectacular affair and totally unexpected. Everyone in the college attended. I was overwhelmed by my colleagues' kind words. I left work feeling good about myself. A new life awaited. We put our house on the market, sold it, packed up our belongings to be shipped to Vancouver and, after Roland's school finished for the summer, travelled around England seeing as much of it as we could. Roland's teachers and classmates were sorry to see him leave, too. It was an emotional time for all of us.

When I told my nephrologist about our move to Canada, she asked, "Are you really sure you should do this? You are going to need follow-up and support. It is imperative that the medical system look after you." I reassured her the medical treatment would be absolutely fine in Canada and, in particular, in Vancouver. I was given my medical notes and a nine-month supply of medication to tide me over until I had found a doctor in Vancouver. Christopher asked for some documentation to present at Customs, as we would be bringing a massive amount of drugs into Canada. My doctor's reaction was that a letter was unnecessary. "No one would touch these drugs with a barge pole, unless they had to," she said. And sure enough, this was the case when we landed in Vancouver.

Settling in

In early September, on our way to the airport, we sold our car to the dealer from whom we had purchased it, and continued our journey via taxi. With one-way tickets, we boarded the plane and bid adieu to what had been my home for twenty-two years. We had learned closer to our departure date that my father's health had begun to deteriorate but that it was not crucial we arrive earlier than planned. It was a surprise, therefore, to be greeted at the airport in Vancouver by my sister and stepmother bearing sad news. My father had died during our flight. It had not been the joyous landing we had anticipated, and it was particularly hard for Roland who had been worried about what the future might be like for him in his new setting.

The next month was a blur because we needed to spend time with my stepmother, enroll my son in a school, find a nephrologist for me and find a place for us to live. We were living a nomadic existence, staying with my stepmother, friends and Christopher's brother, Bruce. We eventually found an apartment to rent very near Roland's school. I made an appointment with my father's doctor so I could be referred to a nephrologist. Although I had grown up in Vancouver, I did not know how the transplant medical system worked. My father's doctor said, "I am going to refer you to one of the local hospitals. The doctors there really know what they are doing. They are a good bunch."

I made an appointment to see the nephrologist, who said, "I feel optimistically cautious your kidney will function well." I was to return to the clinic in three months. That settled, having found accommodation and Roland established in school, I needed to focus on finding work. The Transplant Clinic provided access to a social worker, who said, "I have just the place for you. It is an employment agency specializing in working with people with particular challenges. You'll fit in because of your autoimmune disease and kidney transplant." It was helpful advice. At the agency I learned how to create a resume and compose a cover letter, practice interview techniques, grasp the concept of networking and gather a collection of organizations I could use for networking purposes.

One family event, in particular, stands out for me during our first autumn in Vancouver. It was Hallowe'en. Roland knew nothing about the North American tradition of dressing up and knocking on doors, soliciting candy. With most of our belongings in storage and still wearing the clothes in which we had arrived in Vancouver, we hunted around for a costume. We managed to cobble together an odd mixture of clothing and created a cross between a pirate and a vagabond. We helped Roland dress, supplied him with a bag for his treats and went off in search of loot for him.

Our first port of call was his granny's house. We instructed him to go to the door, knock on it and call, "Trick or Treat!" This was met with great enthusiasm and much fuss by his granny. Because she was family, though, and he was accustomed to being received enthusiastically, I don't think much registered with Roland. We had him repeat the same process with her next-door neighbour, a good friend of the family. Roland shyly approached the door, rang the doorbell and said the magic words. When he was given candies, even before the door was closed, he turned to us, his face lighting up in amazement.

"Mum, Mum, Dad, Dad. She gave me sweets," he exclaimed, bounding back to our car. A light bulb flashed in his head. He had been initiated. There was no stopping now. By the end of the evening, he returned home with a bag heavy with treats. This was the perfect antidote to Roland's sad introduction to his Canadian life. Vancouver had its rewards after all.

With proceeds from the sale of our house in England, and some help from the Bank of Mum and Dad—Christopher's parents—we bought a townhouse and took possession of it on New Year's Eve. Much to our surprise, the house was devoid of light bulbs, so we lived in the winter grey and dark for a day or so. We had to deal with a larger problem, as well. One of the downsides of kidney failure, and in spite of receiving a transplant, is that for insurance policies we are deemed to have a "life-threatening illness" and are therefore ineligible to apply for life insurance. However, most mortgages require applicants to take out life insurance. Fortunately, I was able to apply for life insurance through my work when I was employed, but this continued only so long as I was employed.

Seeking employment and a new future

My quest for work began in earnest after we had moved into our new home. My experience in England enabled me to apply for a variety of jobs from teaching to community work. One of the people whom I met in my search, a person who worked with students with disabilities, shocked me by suggesting I had better ditch my cane—even though I still needed to use it—if I were to secure employment. I wondered whether attitudes were that different here in Canada. To bolster my spirits during the soul-destroying job search, I made a list of things I would get when I finally secured employment, including items Roland would like. They became goals that kept me going through the rough times. I have forgotten most of them, but I do remember that getting a cat was one. Never having had an animal before, I was sure that with work we could afford to look after one.

In February 1994 I accepted a month's substituting in the basic education department of a local college. I continued to apply for other work only to hear the same unwelcome message: "No Vancouver experience." My cane, although prophesized to be a deterrent, turned out not to be. My so-called lack of "Vancouver experience" was. Eventually, I was offered a short-term contract with a college in Langley where I gained further local experience since I worked there on a part-time basis for almost two years. Next, I was hired by an adult education institute to teach Grade 10 English to summer school students. I had never taught this subject before but had the good fortune to meet with the person who customarily taught it. Five days a week, for three hours every evening, I was responsible for twenty-five students, primarily second-language speakers.

We were able to enroll Roland in a summer arts school program so this gave me time to prepare classes during the day. In spite of the overwhelming preparation work I needed to do, I looked forward to my class each day. The students themselves were enthusiastic, too, and worked hard to achieve good results. Finally, the six weeks came to an end. I said, "We have now come to the last class. I have enjoyed working with you all. You have been wonderful students. I thank you very much."

There was much clapping, after which one of the students stood up, leapt onto a chair, looked around at the other students and said, "I am speaking for all the class." The rest of the students nodded in agreement. "I just want to say you are the best teacher we *never* had," followed again with considerable clapping. Even though my student had confused *never* with *ever,* I must have passed muster, since I was invited to return the next summer. I had opportunities of summer work at this institute for several years, but did not need to follow them after I had secured more permanent work.

Close to the end of August that first year back in Canada, we were down to our last one-thousand dollars. Both Christopher and I had been living on short-term contractual work. I noticed that a local college was advertising for a part-time instructor in their then-called Adult Special Education Department. This was my field, and the job was my heart's desire. I applied, was interviewed and sure enough a couple of days later I received a phone call from the coordinator. Yes, I was hired. Thus began my teaching career at this college where I remained until my retirement.

A year after I began teaching at the college, with my kidney now four years old and still doing well, I was able to take on further classes. Sometime in the spring of that year, Christopher and I decided to separate. We had been growing in different directions. It was an amicable breakup, but a split is never simple or straightforward. It was a challenging time, and impacted not only our lives but Roland's as well. His world had been shaken for the third time. However, as the pattern of separation gradually formed our lives, Roland confessed to me that he thought the separation had actually improved our lives, and he began to embrace his new life, spending his time between the two of us. He felt he received more quality time with Christopher and me than he had when we had been together. Once the divorce had been finalized and the dust of separation settled, the three of us began to enjoy a more compatible existence than we had previously. Christopher and I remained on very good terms.

While I was waiting for our divorce to be completed, I needed time to reflect. We had been together for over thirteen years, and now I was experiencing a change in my lifestyle. I immersed myself in self-awareness reading material and also revived a long-held interest: learning how to do reflexology. I enrolled in a course and learned the theory behind reflexology, the practice of how to locate body parts on a foot and hand, and then how to address whatever part needed attention. Sometimes our instructor would demonstrate techniques on us. On one occasion, while working on my right foot, she came to an abrupt stop, looked at me quizzically and said, "Your kidney is not where it should be. It is lower down on your foot."

"Yes," I said. "I have had a kidney transplant. My new kidney is in my groin." I explained that when kidney transplants are carried out, the new kidney is surgically attached on either the right or left side of the abdomen.

> In 1951, a group of French doctors known as the French School, also referred to as the French Transplantation Club, developed a method whereby the transplanted kidney was inserted into the right iliac fossa, the space in the pelvis or ilium, and connected to the iliac vessels. This was a most innovative technique and is the method widely used today.

Mine was transplanted on my right side. I can sometimes feel a slight bump under my skin. Whenever friends, relatives or colleagues learn I have had a kidney transplant, they ask questions such as, "Do you still have your kidneys?" "How many kidneys do you have?" "Where is your kidney?" "Can you eat anything?" Many assume that kidney failure means a loss of one kidney as opposed to both and that a transplant involves more than one kidney, along with removal of the native kidneys. However, it is not common to remove native kidneys. They are only removed if there is a health risk as in cancer or cysts. Although in kidney failure both kidneys stop working, we only need one kidney to function adequately; one transplanted kidney is sufficient to enable us to live full lives. As well, following a transplant, we can eat most things, always bearing in mind a constant need to maintain good potassium and phosphorus levels.

Other conditions

Kidney patients rarely have only one condition. They often have co-morbid conditions, that is, other health problems in addition to their kidney failure or as a result of their kidney failure. For me, my underlying condition of scleroderma always lay in the background. I joined the Scleroderma Association of BC (SABC) shortly after our return to Vancouver. I had learned about this association in a visit to my GP, who, rather scathingly, suggested that joining might not be positive for me. At that time, medical opinion did not favour such gatherings. The medical community believed such gatherings consisted of groups of individuals who would moan about their condition rather than work towards eradicating negative impressions of their diseases.

Being obstinate when told "No," I listened not to the voice of a professional but to my own curious one. What a surprise it was for me to discover that the group, having been founded by a few women in the early 1980s, consisted of people who were anything but a lot of moaners. Instead, I found energetic, vocal and committed people devoting their efforts not only to educating those suffering the effects of scleroderma, but also to working towards improving the quality of care provided by medical personnel, while at the same time pushing the boundaries of research. Today, as a result of the efforts of the founders, scleroderma has a strong national organization dedicated to educating the public about this disease, advocating for improved treatments and raising vast sums of money to aid research into its causes, develop new treatment methods and acquire the most up-to-date medical equipment for diagnosis and treatment.

> Since the early 1980s, the Scleroderma Association of BC (SABC) knows of at least 400 people in British Columbia who have succumbed to this disease. The median nation-wide survival is eleven years. It is one of several connective tissue disorders characterized by spontaneous over-activity of the immune system resulting in the production of extra antibodies into circulation. In scleroderma, the activation of immune cells produces scar tissue in the skin, internal organs and small blood vessels.[3]

As a consequence of my scleroderma, I have needed to see a number of other specialists, often on a monthly basis, to confirm that my condition is stable. My symptoms include considerable joint pain and compromised lung function, as well as digestive and intestinal complications. I require medication for my gastroesophageal reflux disease (GERD). Most people who have scleroderma also experience cold hands, feet and nose. In fact, any exposed extremity can be affected. This is caused by collapsed blood vessels and results in poor circulation. The tips of my toes and fingers become cold and numb, making it difficult to use them. Even on a hot summer day, if I sit in a shady area, my fingers will be affected. This is called Raynaud's disease.

As far as my own condition is concerned, I feel I have had a relatively easy time in comparison to many others who not only show visible signs of the disease, but also experience greater lung compromise, considerable digestive disorders, skin discolouration and challenges with fingers and toes. One form of the disease can contribute to the formation of calcium deposits under the skin that leak a chalky, white liquid from the fingers, in particular, and form open, oozing sores. Many scleroderma patients require finger amputation to offset the effects of this extremely painful condition known as calcinosis.

The people I know bear the indignities of their condition with grace and resilience. Rosanne, whom I met through my involvement with the SABC, is its president, and a positive illustration of the dynamism so often displayed by those affected with scleroderma. She first noticed in 1992 that her thumb had "gone cold" while downhill skiing, one of her favourite sports. Worried that she might develop something more serious such as frostbite, she made an appointment to see her GP. Her GP diagnosed Raynaud's disease and informed her that it could become more severe, leading to her developing oozing sores, ultimately causing her to lose her fingers. Her response, was, "Oh, great!"

A few years later, after observing further concerning symptoms, she once more visited her doctor who confirmed she had scleroderma in addition to Raynaud's. So far, her Raynaud's disease has not progressed beyond making her hands, feet and body core perpetually cold. She describes this as continually experiencing "a painful coldness to the core." To counteract these effects, Rosanne wears gloves and socks both indoors and out, a heated vest and heat pads on her feet. She has been treated with Viagra. "Yes, Viagra," she says, to shorten episodes and maintain blood flow to her extremities.

She has observed her body change as her skin tightens, hands swell and fingers curl uncontrollably. She also has painful calcium deposits on her fingers. Roseanne says, "My face is so tight it restricts me from opening my mouth, requiring me to cut my food into very small pieces. Reduced esophagus elasticity is making it more difficult to swallow and results in my having severe acid reflux. I'm fortunate, I have very little scar tissue forming in my lungs to compromise my breathing capacity. The overall tightness in my skin feels as though I am a medium-sized body living in a constricted-size skin."

Determined to make the most of her life, she and her husband have cycled tandem around various countries to see as much of the world while she can. They are credited with having raised over $100,000 for the SABC during the past few years through their annual Scleroderma Ride for Research. Rosanne is a vibrant, fun-loving person who is fighting to retain a fully functioning life in spite of her debilitating condition.

A goal realized and a tale with it

One of the goals that kept me going when I was seeking employment unexpectedly did come to fruition. One night I received a phone call from an acquaintance asking, "Would you like a cat, a two-year-old neutered ginger tom named Garfield?" His owners were moving into a pet-free complex. We said yes and inherited our second-hand cat. Garfield was a delightful, sweet-natured cat. He liked people and always joined our parties, making himself at home with any guest. But he was territorial, and after Roland and I moved into a garden condo with a front gate, he would sit at the gate and snarl at any dog passing by, irrespective of its size.

Garfield lived on easy street for many years. He was the only cat on the block until one day another feline appeared in the apartment building beside us. The cat, named Luke, was a sleek, black tom whose fur appeared translucent in the sunlight. He quickly found Garfield. Luke was fearless. "Pugilist" was his middle name. He had venom coursing through his veins, shining fiercely in his eyes and spewing from his mouth, too. Once he had discovered Garfield, his sole purpose in life was to seek and destroy our cat. Garfield, though, was not always the poor victim. He could land a sizeable claw as well.

One summer evening a group of us were having dinner on our patio. It was still fairly light out. Garfield happened to be inside, sitting on a table watching us through a window that was a good distance from the ground. All was peaceful when, from the bushes on the other side of the garden, a black feline appeared. It was Luke. As soon as he spotted Garfield across the patio, he was riveted. His eyes locked onto Garfield. Crouching low and quivering in attack mode, he proceeded to launch himself, like a rocket flying into the air, flinging himself spread-eagled at the window, hissing loudly as he did so. He clung there for a moment but his mission was a failure. Garfield, no doubt, sped off to the safety of some dark corner inside as Luke dropped to the ground. Without looking up or around, head low, ears pinned to it, eyes down, belly to the ground, tail flat, Luke slunk off back to the bushes from whence he had come. We couldn't help laughing at the spectacle.

Whenever I saw Luke and Garfield in close proximity, I would, as surreptitiously as possible, remove Garfield and take him inside. Around five o'clock on a Thursday evening in early May, the patio doors were open when I heard a slight noise outside. I found Luke and Garfield sitting immediately in front of the door, nose to nose, staring at each other, muttering growls. A fight was brewing, claws would soon be extended, teeth lashing out and fur flying. At once I grabbed Garfield. No sooner had I done this than Luke jumped into the air and sank one of his incisors into the bottom of my right thumb. The pain was instant, searing and intense. I yelped and dropped Garfield who proceeded to strike out at Luke. There must have been a very quick exchange between the two because Luke was soon gone.

I picked my defender up again, giving him a quick once-over. There was a slight scratch on him. I then cleaned my wound with antiseptic lotion. It was hardly visible. I didn't think much more of it. As the evening wore on, however, my hand started hurting and began to swell. The swelling continued throughout the night. In the early morning, Roland came home from film school where he studied animation, thanks to a scholarship. I showed him my thumb. "Yikes," he said, "you need to get that looked at."

He would have happily taken me to hospital then, but I said I would go in the morning. I am not sure how much sleep I had that night, but when I woke in the morning, Roland had already left for school. I phoned a colleague who lived very close to me to ask her if she wouldn't mind taking me to a local hospital whose emergency department treated minor injuries. I thought I might have fractured my hand somehow when I dropped Garfield.

Debby kindly drove me to the hospital. I assured her I would be fine, so off home she went. It wasn't long before a nurse came, took my information and then left. Very shortly afterwards, a doctor came, examined me and, without saying much, left. Although I still thought I had sustained a fracture, another doctor came and informed me I could have an infection from the cat bite. Well, that made sense. A little later a third doctor attended me and asked me various quite personal questions. This doctor, an infectious disease specialist, wanted to establish the source of infection. Soon I was told I would be admitted to hospital, given intravenous antibiotics and remaining in hospital for several days.

Normally with this kind of infection, I would have been prescribed a course of antibiotics and sent home. I was different, however. I had a transplant and would require more careful attention. Kidney recipients can live ordinary lives, but there are complications. We have a weakened immune system as a consequence of taking anti-rejection medication and are easily susceptible to infections. We cannot be given just any medication. For example, we cannot take anti-inflammatory drugs such as ibuprofen or usual antibiotics. These do not mix well with the immunosuppressant medications. All our medications need to be carefully researched and prescribed in particular doses.

I was, therefore, admitted to the hospital and immediately started on a course of intravenous antibiotics. In those days before cell phones, I tried to have Roland contacted at school. Eventually, he was found and came to the phone. I told him what had happened, and that I was going to be kept in for several days. He asked me, "Do you need anything? Can I do anything?"

"No, just keep an eye on Garfield," I said. I did not want Roland to lose time from his studies. Although I had arrived at the hospital unprepared to stay, I adapted to my new environment, preparing to receive my intravenous antibiotics twice a day, six hours apart. I have no idea why, but I was sent to a geriatric unit where I was visited by a number of doctors, including, to my amazement, a plastic surgeon who had been specifically called from another hospital. The surgeon wanted to ascertain whether or not I might need surgery, but following his examination, he felt it would not be necessary. I wasn't ill so it felt peculiar to be in a clinical setting. Also, I had been wearing the same clothes since my arrival. By Sunday, I was beginning to feel that a change of underwear might be a welcome addition to my hygiene. My friends who would have gladly brought me fresh apparel all seemed to be away or not close by. I wondered if the hospital might let me go home to change.

I was sitting in the patients' lounge, having finished my first treatment, when the infectious disease doctor came to see me. I asked if I could go home. He responded, "I don't think you are taking this seriously enough. I had a patient who was a musician. He and his friends were clearing out a house. Everything had been removed. The musician happened to open a cupboard door and found a cat there. It had been locked in, and was obviously distressed. It lashed out at the musician, biting him on the thumb. This bite resulted in him losing his thumb." I felt duly chastised and sheepishly said all I really wished to do was get a change of clothing.

The hospital agreed to my request on condition that I sign a waiver releasing them from any responsibility for subsequent reactions that I might have and that I promise to return for my six o'clock treatment. It felt rather strange returning home by bus, my intravenous needle still in my wrist. Once home, I checked Garfield for signs of infection from his injury, but seeing none, embarked on my clothing renewal. I had a shower and put on clean clothes. It was bliss. I do not know how people manage to live in the same clothes for days at a time. For me, three days had been enough. I packed a bag, and was just about to make my return trip when Roland arrived home. He drove me back to the hospital where I remained for several more days, enjoying my clean attire. Upon my discharge late on Tuesday afternoon, the doctor who had been primarily responsible for my care told me to call him if I noticed anything unusual. I said I would, but didn't anticipate a need arising.

When I returned to work, I regaled my colleagues with my adventure. Thursday of that week, I noticed some unusual blotches on my arm above the bite mark. I thought they would disappear. On Friday morning, however, they were worse. As directed, I called the hospital ward to speak to the doctor who had discharged me. He came to the phone. I explained the peculiar blotches on my arm. He said, "Excuse me," and put the phone down. Several minutes later he returned and told me to report to the emergency ward. I was expected and would be given further instructions.

I drove to the hospital, went to the emergency department, introduced myself and, as told, had been expected. I was directed to the second floor, where I was also expected. "Cardiac Unit," I read on the sign above the ward. "*Heart,*" I thought. Having been in a number of different wards in different hospitals, I wasn't surprised to find myself there. I went to the nurses' station where several nurses glanced up at me briefly and then continued with their work. I stood there for a few minutes, still getting no reaction. This was peculiar. I excused myself, said my name and mentioned the doctor who was to meet me. One of the nurses immediately apologized and said, "I am so sorry. No patient ever walks into this unit."

She at once found the doctor, who ushered me down a long corridor to an examining room. He looked at my arm, left me and upon his return said I would be re-admitted for observation. I explained that I had driven there and again had to ask if I could go home to collect an overnight bag. The doctor reluctantly agreed. At home, I left a note for my Roland, letting him know where I was and asking him to feed Garfield. After I had returned to the hospital once more, the doctors worked on resolving the cause: I had developed a delayed allergy to the antibiotics and was given another round of intravenous treatment. The doctors treated me even more cautiously because of my compromised immune system. I was discharged on the Sunday.

Strangely enough, I hardly ever saw Luke again. I did meet his owner later and let him know what had happened. He said, "Luke is an interesting cat." Garfield, though, lived with us for over fifteen years—or should I say, we lived with him. He gave us much pleasure over the years, as well as some blood-curdling moments. One evening, Garfield had an encounter with another cat that fled down the busy road we lived on. Garfield was determined to follow. As he ran across the street, I envisioned him being flattened by a car. Miraculously, he made it safely across the road. I called Roland to help me rescue him. We waited for a break in traffic and arrived breathless to find Garfield hiding under a car. As we were about to catch him, he ran back across the road. Our hearts were in our mouths.

When we arrived home, there was Garfield, sitting quite happily by the patio doors as though nothing unusual had taken place, looking at us as though to say, "Where have you been?" Often, his rash behaviour required a visit to the vet, invariably on a Friday just after the clinic had closed. Off we would go to the animal ER, paying a hundred dollars just to walk in the door. My colleagues soon tired of my cat tales, and whenever I mentioned another vet visit, they would groan and roll their eyes saying, "Not again."

We were notorious!

Garfield and I had something in common: we both had an autoimmune disease. His was a skin disorder called pemphigus foliaceus. His skin would blister, then scab, and his hair would break off in strands. When the disease was diagnosed after a series of blood tests followed by a biopsy, the vet prescribed the same steroid medication for him that I was taking. Mine was for anti-rejection, his for his autoimmune disease. We both took prednisone every other day. I took two 5 mg pills, while Garfield took one. I administered his dose the same day I took mine. The routine worked beautifully until his death. For some reason I lost track of days, not from mourning but rather from a change in habit. It took me many years to get back on track. Today I keep a note on my calendar lest I lose track of the days.

While it was easy for me to swallow pills, Garfield was a different matter. I would usually give him his pill around his dinnertime when he was hungry and most receptive to being picked up and cuddled. I would pick Garfield up, holding him closely to me, sit on a chair, use my thumb and forefinger to pry open his mouth at the back of his jaw, pop in the pill and hold his mouth closed for a moment to ensure he had swallowed it. I had countless hours of practice, and you would think practice would improve my quality of administration. I followed the vet's instructions to the letter, priding myself on my speed and accuracy. Invariably, when I released Garfield and stood up, I would find the wretched pill sitting on the chair. Back to the drawing board.

Garfield eventually succumbed to kidney failure, as do many cats. His symptoms mirrored those of humans: loss of weight, nausea, vomiting, loss of appetite, frequent urination and extreme fatigue. Cats normally sleep about eighteen hours a day. Garfield's sleep pattern exceeded this. To determine if he had kidney failure, the vet followed similar tests, drawing a panel of blood to check his creatinine levels, among other things. On the Friday prior to his demise, I had taken him to the vet to have his levels checked. The blood results were quickly returned. His creatinine was good, still in the normal range, but over the weekend things changed dramatically, akin to my first kidney failure. His symptoms were much more evident on Monday. Roland and I returned to the vet. This time, the vet told us another blood test would likely show a huge spike in creatinine level. He also told us Garfield was probably feeling wretched, but hard to assess because cats are incredibly stoic. This was the end. Roland and I reluctantly had Garfield euthanized at home the next day. We mourned the loss of a precious family member for some time.

Follow-up care and side effects

I continued to do well with my kidney. I attended clinics every three months for a check-up. I followed a standard procedure. First I had my blood test taken a week prior to my appointment. Then at the appointment, I signed in, weighed myself to check for any considerable weight gain and waited to see my assigned nurse. The nurse checked my blood pressure and temperature, noted them on a paper and asked me if I had anything to discuss with the doctor. This was also noted. While waiting to see the doctor, I often met with a dietician who monitored my blood results for potassium, phosphate, iron and calcium levels. Although I could eat anything, I still needed to be cautious lest my potassium and phosphate levels rose. The doctor, who had received a copy of my blood results, would review them with me. If something was not doing well, I would immediately be told. The doctor also ordered further testing should it be necessary. All things being well, I could leave, booking my next appointment usually for three months' time. The clinic also had a pharmacist with whom I could discuss my medication.

There are some side effects to my medications. I am more susceptible to skin cancer as a result of my immunosuppressant drugs and need to be careful of sun exposure. It is true that anyone can have skin cancer; my medication simply exacerbates my risks. I had my first bout of skin cancer towards the end of my twentieth year of having a transplant. I noticed something that looked like a pimple on one of my shins. I simply thought it might be a bite or some mark that would clear up on its own. It remained the same for some time then turned into a scab. I assumed I might have scratched it when getting dressed or shaving my legs. A little while later the scab turned into a rash. I thought it odd so when I next had an appointment with my GP, I showed him. He thought it looked suspicious and took a biopsy. I was called back to see him. He told me it was skin cancer and needed to be removed. He referred me to the local skin clinic.

Because Roland and I were going to Mexico for a week's holiday, my GP suggested I cover the scab with a bandage until I had been seen at the skin clinic. I did not wait long for my appointment. When the doctor examined me and performed his own biopsy prior to removing the cancer, he informed me that it was the "spreading kind" and definitely needed to be removed. The skin clinic is an interesting place where a clear procedure is followed. First, the doctor removes as much of the cancer as possible and then does a biopsy of the tissue to make sure all the cancer has been taken. Patients remain in the waiting room during this part of the process. I met a number of people who were having cancers removed. One woman told me this had been her seventh time.

After the doctor had examined my specimen, I was recalled to the surgery and informed that the cancer had been successfully removed. I was given some cream to put on the site every day until it healed, and was given the doctor's home number in case something wasn't right with my wound. Following my surgery, I went to work. This was a Friday. The next day I thought my wound looked a little peculiar. It seemed to be oozing pus rather than being red and inflamed. I hesitated to call the doctor. The following day my wound looked even more peculiar, oozing further pus, and had begun to be painful. This time I did call the doctor at home, and he told me to go to the clinic the next day. There, the doctor looked at my leg, left the room and returned with a colleague. They concurred that my wound was infected and prescribed antibiotics. I was to continue applying the cream for as long as the wound remained open. Healing took well over a month.

As a consequence of the risk of transplant patients getting cancer, the clinic has the support of a dermatologist who examines long-term transplant recipients every six to eight months. This leads to early cancer detection. I have had a number of biopsies that have indicated potential cancer spots since my first experience.

Another side effect of kidney disease, in particular, is weakening bone structure. Kidney failure itself can cause renal bone loss. The result can be early onset of osteopenia and osteoporosis, which I have, and as a result have broken a number of bones: foot and ankle, as well as my earlier hip injury. Taken over a long time, prednisone can shorten life so some patients are reluctant to take it. Initially one of my rheumatologists prescribed calcium tablets for me, but the doctors felt it would not be advantageous for me to use them to bolster my calcium levels. Instead I used them as a phosphate binder. The binder's role is to soak up excess phosphorus that may not be absorbed and is most commonly used by patients on dialysis. Some patients take Tums or other forms of phosphate binders. I also need to ensure that I have yearly flu shots because of my compromised immune systems.

A working life

As the years passed and colleagues retired, I secured more work, eventually becoming a tenured instructor, gaining greater job security. Was I a good teacher? I cannot say, but I loved my work and enjoyed all my students. I did, though, have some definite failings. I can attest to at least three of them. The first: an inability to recognize my students. On the first day of our program, we would have our students introduce themselves and write a name card that they would then place on the table in front of them. Our classes were small because of the nature of the students' learning needs. Having been with the students throughout the day, I would feel I had gotten to know everyone and their names pretty well. I was forever confident that I would remember who everyone was at my next teaching session. Oh, how vanity teases the truth. Without fail, I would be thrown off-course because not only were the students wearing different outfits but also they were sitting in different places. Out came the cards again! The programs we offered were finite in length. It was rare to have new students attend after about the second week. Fortunately this coincided with my ability to recognize everyone. Once the students accustomed themselves to the class, they invariably sat in the same seats and often arrived before we did.

On one occasion, the program was well into its second week. As I entered the classroom, I greeted the students but noticed a new male student sitting in the back of the room in the same seat in which another male student usually sat. The familiar student always wore a cap. I was puzzled. I hadn't been told to expect a new student. I kept my bewilderment contained while I thought how to handle this new situation. Then, my brain kicked in. I realized it was the same student but without his proverbial cap. He looked entirely different. Privately, I enjoyed my blunder.

My second frailty lay in my recalling students' names. I had a propensity for calling students by the wrong name. I would explain my weakness at the beginning of each program and apologize in advance. I would say, "I know your name; please forgive me if I call you by the wrong name," and with the student's correct name on the tip of my tongue, out came the wrong name. Some of my students were very understanding, others not so.

I remember confessing my problem to another one of my colleagues who told me, "This is my worst nightmare too. If a student's name is Mat and I get it into my head his name is Matthew, I am plagued for the rest of the year. I can never get his name right." It seemed we were more likely to confuse our male students' names than our female students' names. I have no answer to this. But I did feel a little less shamed with my colleague's similar disclosure.

My third weakness related to spelling. I have never been a consummate speller, and as with my name challenges, I would explain to my students that I sometimes had difficulty spelling words correctly. I asked them to excuse me if they saw me writing a word on the board as this enabled me to check if I had spelled it accurately. As I believe that the best method of teaching is to empower the students rather than the teacher being the expert, I would often solicit their help too. Our students varied greatly in their writing skills. Some struggled even to form words, while others were extremely literate and wrote really well. There was always someone in the class who could help me.

We, the faculty, were evaluated every five years to ensure our teaching skills were up to scratch. The evaluation process was carefully monitored and followed a precise formula. Both faculty and students were part of the process and invited to write their comments, in addition to giving us scores from one to five, with one being "excellent." I was fortunate. I usually received favourable responses from all parties. During one of my evaluations, I was given the students' submissions to read over. They were positive; however, one student in particular, who had given me an excellent evaluation, wrote this comment: "*Lern* to spell!"

My transplanted kidney enabled me to do things that would have previously been impossible for me to do had I remained on dialysis. At the college, which gained university status while I worked there, I taught in both the business and continuing education departments as well as in my own department. I served on a number of sub-committees, represented my department as Union Rep and chaired the university's Professional Development Committee for many years. I was a member of a provincial networking organization and chaired its annual conference committee for several years. I also applied for special funding, organized and managed a number of special projects, and co-coordinated my department in the last two years before my retirement.

Interestingly, of approximately five hundred faculty, there were four of us who had had transplants: two of us had had kidney transplants, one a heart transplant, and the fourth a liver transplant. The university health benefit department sponsored two Organ Donor Days each year for many years, coinciding with the province's Organ Donor Week. Those of us who had received transplants assisted with the donor booth. We were always pleased to see the number of students, faculty and staff who stopped by to sign up as donors. We appreciated the supportive environment of the university.

Additionally I was a member-at-large on the board of the SABC for many years until health issues dented my involvement, and I volunteered with a number of other organizations.

Being able to work meant that I could help Roland participate in ex-tra-curricular activities during his adolescent years, provide him with his own holidays to various parts of the world and contribute towards his post-secondary fees. The benefits of my kidney transplant were not only en-joyed by me but also transferred to Roland as well. An entire family gained from the benefit of my kidney transplant, not just me the recipient.

I could travel freely. Roland and I enjoyed many excursions together both within and outside Canada. I could do anything at the drop of a hat and eat pretty much anything I wanted to. Never far from my thoughts was the restricted diet that I had had to follow before my kidney transplant. No morsel of food ever passed my lips without this memory in the back of my mind. I also never forgot that this blessing, the kindness of my donor, might not last forever. I cherished every moment of my kidney's life.

Chapter 3 | A Pothole in the Road

If you're going through hell, keep going.
—Attributed to various sources

First signs of a fissure

"Your kidney is failing," said the nephrologist during one of my appointments in mid-December 2007.

"No. It cannot be. Absolutely not," I fervently replied.

"Not so." The doctor showed me a chart tracking my creatinine levels. Before my eyes I could see a *red* line—at least to me it seemed red—slowly wending its way upwards. I was stupefied. To me it represented nothing more than a blot on the landscape. I was informed that I most likely wouldn't notice any difference or experience any symptoms at this stage.

"How long will it be before it fails?" I asked.

"Hard to say," was the response. We discussed the likelihood of another transplant. The probability seemed unlikely. I pictured the year 2015. Why, I have no idea, but it seemed years ahead.

The doctor's words entered one ear, hovered a moment in the middle and hastily exited the other ear. I carried on as before, with only a vestige of some doubt in the back of my mind. Roland and I had planned to spend that Christmas in Las Vegas, our first of several visits. Off we went to enjoy ourselves amidst the slot machines and extravaganza.

My kidney was nearing its sixteenth year that September. I had been leading an active life, my professional career in full swing. I'll admit that I slowly had become aware that things weren't exactly right. It was difficult to pinpoint exactly what. Maybe I wasn't voiding the same quantity that I had been accustomed to, or perhaps I had to use the washroom less frequently. I wondered if these symptoms were an omen of a failing kidney but quickly brushed the thoughts aside. The risk of kidney failure was ever present; I had adapted to the uncertainty.

The other differences related indirectly to my kidney health. I had been taking immunosuppressant medication for so many years that I had developed an increasing susceptibility to infections. I had had two urinary tract infections (UTIs) in the past two years. Such infections are not uncommon in women, anyway, but more prevalent for those whose immune systems are suppressed and whose ureter was shorter following a kidney transplant. I had needed two antibiotic prescriptions to treat the infections. Because the effects of antibiotics are usually cleared via the kidney, regular use of them stressed the kidney, especially a transplanted one. Each prescription would cause my creatinine level to rise, and then it would drop once I had completed the course of antibiotics.

Sometime later, after December 2007, most likely around the time of my monthly blood test or while awaiting the results, which is when I usually felt my most vulnerable, I must have told friends and colleagues about my failing kidney. Their reactions seemed casual. I didn't really feel I had a problem. Why should they? I had been managing my scleroderma well, was energetic and seemingly healthy, so I assumed I could manage my kidney transplant, too.

The fissure begins to widen

What captured my attention in the next few years was unrelated to my kidney function but may well have had some impact upon it. First, in 2008, the "retirement" word began to tickle my brain. Second, Roland was in the final stages of his animation studies at university and would soon be ready to test his wings in the wider world. As well, conditions around our garden condo had changed. Traffic noise had increased; we could hardly open a window without an assault from the din emanating from the road. The trees, very small when we moved in, having grown, now shut out a good portion of light. The garden upkeep had become less enjoyable. A change in address, therefore, appealed to me.

Bad idea, as it turned out. I am normally prudent, but with my kidney still functioning well, or so I thought, I threw caution to the wind. I bought another condo before selling mine. The new condo, the perfect property for me, was more expensive than my current one, but the sale of my present condo would pay for most of it. However, no sooner had I completed the transaction than the market crashed, and with it the value of my own condo that sat unsold for five months while I watched my money disappear in the abyss. My garden needed constant attention and I had to keep the old condo in good order until it sold in a buyer's market. We had two weeks to dispose of potted plants, pack our belongings and clean. No sooner had we moved into our new condo than I realized it was absolutely unsuitable for our needs. We were stuck. I couldn't sell it in a flattened market. We had to stay put. Thus began our winter of discontent, accented by major snowstorms, so unusual for Vancouver.

Some normality returned when classes resumed in January 2009 after the holidays. Then, adding to further aggrievement at end of the month, one Saturday as I was crossing a main street, my right foot simply buckled underneath me. I fell, my left hand reaching for anything to grab. Lying curbside, I realized I was clutching desperately onto the bottom of a pair of jeans, a man's. Embarrassed, in pain and unable to move, I uttered some apologetic words. The stranger, thankfully, showed understanding. An off-duty paramedic appeared, calmed my frayed nerves and called an ambulance. I was transported to hospital with a broken right ankle.

Following x-rays and examinations by a number of orthopedic surgeons, I was admitted with "an unstable fracture." To reinforce the fracture, a pin would be inserted into my ankle on the Monday. I called Roland, who was by now working, to apprise him of my accident. He is accustomed to receiving alarming phone calls from me. He accepts them kindly and considerately, but no wonder the thought of exploring the world would appeal to him! Likewise, I needed to disturb a colleague's weekend respite in order to organize a substitute during my absence from work.

After the surgery, one of the surgeons said to me, "I have never worked on such soft bones as yours." That gave me pause. I was off work for four months. I had to use a wheelchair rather than crutches until my fracture was stable and sufficiently healed for me to start walking. I could dress, wash and use the washroom on my own, but cooking and other household chores were beyond me. A number of friends came by with some wonderful meals, but Roland did most of the cooking. He would make my breakfast, prepare a lunch for me before heading to work and then cook the evening meal upon his return. Together we collected our groceries, he once again being my handler, steering me through the store while I reached things from the shelves. Because he had to care for me, Roland missed many social interactions. I am indebted to him for his unconditional dedication and love. He is one member of the quiet army of family members sacrificing personal and leisure pursuits to care for a needy parent. An illness plays heavily upon a family's resources, emotionally, physically and financially. Most of us have little experience of such a life. Those who provide the solace and care deserve applauding.

My convalescence completed, I had just returned to work in mid-May when I experienced my second mishap. This one would prove to be even more serious. Again it was a Saturday. I had just completed my errands and noticed the car's gas tank was low. Feeling fatigued from my first week's work, I debated whether or not I should have Roland fill the tank when he got home. I won my own argument. I would do the deed. At the station, I paid for my gas in the shop and was walking gingerly back to my car when I was momentarily distracted. My left foot clipped the side of a wire basket containing cans of oil. The inevitability of my fall flashed before my eyes, there being nothing for me to grab onto. With a huge whack, I landed flat on my face, my arms folded in front of my chest. Stunned, I cried out, "I have broken every bone in my body."

A good Samaritan rushed to my aid and helped me up. It seemed I had not broken anything, but I had fractured one of my front teeth and pierced my front lip. My arms and hands were numb but I could stand and walk. An ambulance was called. Yet again, off to the hospital. I was examined in the ER and my lip repaired. I had x-rays of my left arm to see if I had broken anything, but no x-rays regarding possible damage to my neck. Apart from my left arm being very sore, it had not been broken. The doctor thought I might have chipped a bone and gave me a sling to wear for a few days. Both my hands were incredibly numb.

Roland came to my rescue and drove me home in his car. Meanwhile, my car, with a full tank of gas, had been moved to the side. And the large tub of ice cream I had purchased? By the time Roland had seen to me and returned home with my car, the ice cream had melted, reduced to a runny mass of liquid in the trunk. Poor, long-suffering Roland: he had not only me to care for, but also had the task of completely cleaning the trunk.

On the Monday, my dentist gave me a temporary front tooth. Other than my face being badly bruised and my hands and arms still somewhat numb, I was all right. It so happened that on Wednesday of that week I was being honoured by the university for my fifteen years of service. There was a large turnout at the service luncheon that year, with awards being presented to a number of staff and faculty who had served at least fifteen years and up to forty years. When my turn came to receive my recognition, pen and pin, I knew my recent injuries were obvious, but there was nothing I could do about them. Swallowing a giant breath, I went up to collect the university's pen and appreciation pin gift. Following the presentations came the photographs of our different years' groups. I hoped if I stood in the background my face might be a little less exposed. I confess I have never looked at a copy of the picture taken on that occasion.

As that summer passed, I seemed to take a long time to recover. My hands still prickled, a couple of fingers were numb and my elbow remained sore. Also, we felt we were passing the time mourning losses. We bade a sad farewell to our beloved cat, Garfield. On top of that, Roland lost one of his young American cousins, Rollo, to a tragic accident a few weeks later. Rollo had completed his MBA and had just accepted a job in Massachusetts. After attending Rollo's funeral, Roland spent a week in Florida with his other cousins and their family.

We decided to commemorate our life with Garfield. We arranged a memorial tea party in August, exactly a month to the day after his demise. We invited a number of friends who had known Garfield, along with a United Church minister to provide the spiritual side for our gathering. We had created a little shrine for him with pictures and other memorabilia. We began our tribute with a glass of bubbly, followed by the minister's talk that included quotes from St. Assisi, patron saint to animals, and lots of stories of Garfield and other cat tales. We then had tea and fancy sandwiches filled with ingredients Garfield liked. Thank heavens, Garfield had an eclectic taste and enjoyed food like salmon, eggs, cucumbers and tuna. We followed the sandwiches with goodies that Garfield would have savoured, too. We sent everyone home with a goody bag filled with Garfield's favourite candies—small, coloured peppermint drops. While Garfield enjoyed human food, he only received such delicacies on a rare occasion, mostly dining on his crunchies—so-called by his vet—and the usual cat mush.

Meanwhile, also in August, I had developed another UTI and was given a series of antibiotics. This UTI continued without a break for three years. Any woman who has ever had a UTI can attest to the discomfort and sense of illness it causes. I had tests to determine the origin. None was found. I seemed to acquire allergies to any antibiotic I took and was finally referred to both a gynecologist and an infectious disease doctor who eventually found an antibiotic I could take, and who continued to check on my condition every six months for the next several years. The UTIs varied in their effects. Sometimes I could no longer quell my urine flow. It would, unabatedly and forcefully, stream down my legs, often for several hours at a time. To say the least, this was most embarrassing. My recurrent prescriptions caused my creatinine levels to skyrocket and then plummet upon completion of the prescription. It was as though I were suspended on a yo-yo string. Eventually, my creatinine levels continued skywards, marking a significant deterioration in my kidney function.

I also started having intestinal problems and paid many visits to my gastroenterologist, who prescribed various treatments, none of which relieved my symptoms. The orthopedic surgeon, meanwhile, concerned about my osteoporosis and recurring fractures, referred me to an endocrinologist. In November, the endocrinologist started me on a fairly new medication called Forteo, the purpose of which was to increase the levels of calcium in my bones, thus minimizing the effects of osteoporosis. I was required to self-inject the medication in my stomach daily for eighteen months. It was an expensive medication, thankfully covered by my work medical plan. Shortly after I began the treatment, my walking, already affected by my broken hip years ago, began to cause me more challenges. While I had had a slight limp after my hip fracture, I was now finding my legs, the right one in particular, less flexible, achy and more difficult to bend, especially as I got into a car. I thought it might be related to the new medication. The endocrinologist ruled out this possibility but discontinued the medication since he felt it could be jeopardizing my kidney function. I ended up using Forteo for only nine months.

Worried about my decreasing mobility, I had also seen my GP, who, unable to find a cause, referred me to my rheumatologist, who likewise could provide me with no answer. Visits to other doctors over the next few years never seemed to resolve my situation. In hindsight, I wished I had told my infectious disease doctor—whom I firmly believe may have been able to help me—about my mobility issues. I had implicit trust in this doctor's general ability to diagnose conditions.

From 2009 until 2012 it seemed as though I were to live perennially with these issues: UTIs, limited mobility and intestinal problems. I spent most of the time feeling unwell. It was as though I were plagued. I had fallen down a rabbit hole of unwellness and couldn't get out. They were difficult years for me, too, because I had had increased work responsibilities since the fall term in 2010 and needed to be on top of them. I was really distressed. Somehow I managed to appear competent. Thankfully none of my colleagues was aware of my internal struggles. Having lived with scleroderma for years, I had learned that while we might share some personal, temporary feelings or trials and tribulations with our colleagues, talking about recurring health problems was of little purpose. No one wants to hear a prolonged dialogue about continual ailments, not because of lack of care, rather more because of an inability to know how to help. One of my colleagues used to say when in a classroom, "We are in a zone." This was equally true of the workplace. We were there to accomplish tasks, not to commiserate.

Work, fortunately, was a distraction. Though I was in pain and struggling to stay on top, it was a great mood elevator; when at work I needed to be focused and fully engaged in university life. Interacting with my colleagues was pleasurable and interesting. We are all energized in different ways; for some it is accomplishing a task, for others sharing ideas and for others still, engaging in a new activity. Being with other people energizes me. No matter how ill, worried or niggled I am by something, as soon as I am in company with another person, I am uplifted. Entering work in the morning was my salvation.

Having saved sufficient funds, in May 2010, Roland ventured forth for destinations afar. His aim was to attend the World Cup in Africa after visiting England, France and the Middle East en route. I accompanied him to the airport. We had had a number of separations over the years but this time was different. He had no return date. With uncontained motherly tears slowly creeping down my cheeks and Roland's eyes equally brimming, we bid our fond farewells at the departure gate. When I regained my composure, I watched as Roland, his face full of excitement and smiles, passed through security and left the nest. I was saddened, but I thought, "It is as it should be," and returned home to my routine and health challenges.

Adding insult to my current torment, in November 2011, I noticed the pin that had been holding my broken ankle in place was starting to protrude. I met with the orthopedic surgeon the following March. He said it could easily be removed, but probably not until sometime in June. Meanwhile, the real estate market had improved so I could sell the dreaded condo that I had carelessly chosen. Fortunately, Roland, having completed his grand tour, returned home briefly in late April before preparing to depart once more, this time to Belgium to be with a young Belgian, Veerle, whom he had met on safari in Africa. Romance was in the air.

He helped me with my condo search. I did not want to make another costly mistake! The completion date for the sale of the condo was set for the middle of May. Roland assisted with the packing, but when moving day arrived, we had yet to find another home. Roland camped in an apartment owned by Christopher. I had been invited to stay with an old school friend and former colleague, Penny. One of the calmest, most patient and wisest of people I have ever met, she has an ability to ease a burden and proved to be a most solicitous host. She so enjoys looking after others that I was not even expected to cook any meals. My only contribution: to shop for the ingredients Penny requested.

I did soon find a condo, with Roland's approval, and was able to take possession in early July. Coincidentally, Veerle, Roland's girlfriend, visiting California, decided to come to Vancouver for four days while on her journey home to Belgium. She arrived on the day I moved into the new condo. With most things still in packing boxes, we three spent her time in Vancouver living like campers. It was a great way for me to meet her because formality simply didn't exist. Veerle has an infectious sense of fun, she's sociable and she adapted easily to our camp-style arrangement.

In the meantime, my ankle surgery that had been booked for June was deferred to July and then to August. That meant I needed to miss three weeks of work. Roland was due to leave for Belgium in the middle of August and would not be returning for months. My Seattle cousin, Deborah, another patient person, came and stayed with me for a few days following my surgery.

The fissure becomes a pothole

Around this time, my hands, already prickling occasionally, presumably from my earlier fall, began to cause me additional trouble. My fingers started tingling, and the tingling in my hands was beginning to become more bothersome and painful. I realized the cause of this was neck-related but to what extent I couldn't say. Some years previously, I had been diagnosed as having a "little arthritis" in my neck, but at the time I was told it was nothing serious. I thought it might relate to this. Also, I felt continually tired from the relentless UTIs. As well, I was making little progress with my walking. The only time I actually felt well was while I was off work, recovering from my minor surgery. Then, my walking seemed a little easier, and my tingling hands, less obvious.

As soon as I returned to work in early September, the symptoms returned with an even greater vengeance. Later in the month I was due for one of my three-monthly transplant check-ups. I was in a bad way. When I told my nephrologist about my hands and my arm problems, he suggested I have some physiotherapy to help relieve the symptoms. It was also during this visit that I told my nephrologist I was really struggling but wanted to keep going until the end of the year. His reply: "We'll help you get through." He also explained that part of his role was not only to treat patients but also to heal them. I was encouraged by his words and his telling me to always ensure I saw him when I had my appointments. Tall words, since I never saw him again until July of the following year.

My appointment had been in the morning. I returned home and collapsed on my living room sofa, absolutely exhausted, but I needed to go to the university later that evening for our annual parents/caregivers' and students' evening. This evening was arranged after classes had been in session for several weeks to provide information about the course work and work experience component, as well as give opportunities for students and parents to meet each other. That night, it was my turn to welcome everyone and introduce my colleagues. I didn't know how I would lift myself off the sofa, let alone drive back to work and perform my tasks. But I did. All went well. I continued to think my symptoms were fatigue-related and would eventually disappear once I had retired.

As suggested by my nephrologist, I started having physiotherapy. Dee, the physiotherapist, worked tirelessly to relieve my neck, hand and arm symptoms, which were becoming more persistent and painful. I never seemed to make any progress. In January, Dee finally said, "I think there is something else going on. Go to your GP, ask to have an x-ray and bring me a copy of it so I can see what's happening." By the time I had had a neck x-ray, I had spent well over a thousand dollars on physiotherapy, some, but not all of which was covered by my medical plan. The x-ray, taken in April 2012, revealed collapsed cervical discs from stenosis. My GP confirmed nothing could be done. Because I had continued to complain about my walking, he referred me once again to my rheumatologist; an appointment was set for June. As asked by my physiotherapist, I obtained a copy of the results from him.

In March, I had finally decided to retire, my decision driven largely by my continuing health issues. The pain in my arms had become excruciating. Something was seriously wrong, but what, I had no idea. It was a struggle to keep going. When I informed my colleagues I was going to retire, they initially thought I was joking. I had always appeared so robust, enthusiastic and eager to work that this was anathema to them, so well-hidden had been my concerns, but they finally accepted my decision.

The last major task I performed before retiring was to introduce the concept of a university-wide peer mentorship program for students with autism. The purpose would be to provide continual support to these students while attending university, by pairing them with other students who would act as their guides and mentors. I did my research and planning and then met with my dean, my co-coordinator colleague and faculty from two interested departments. The meeting was a success, my idea fully embraced. My proposal had been accepted. With my pending retirement, my role had been accomplished. I was able to pass on the daunting task of organizing the peer mentorship program.

My actual retirement date was July 31, but I finished work after the term had ended in May and I had completed my Professional Development requirements in June. Between the end of May and my appointment with my rheumatologist in June, my walking deteriorated to a shocking degree. In a space of three weeks, I regressed from increased limping, to dragging my right foot, to once more using a cane and, finally, to needing a walker. At my retirement tea party, I remember hugging the walls as I shuffled to the party room, filled with colleagues, staff, administrators and friends who had come to bid their adieus. Three of us retiring together had asked only to receive a few words from our dean who would, in turn, give each of us our university gifts. I was to be last. While my other colleagues were being feted, I found myself standing in the midst of a group of colleagues, glued to the ground. I could not lift my legs. They were incredibly rigid. Externally I may have appeared calm and fully engaged in the proceedings, but internally, my heart was racing and my mind in panic. How on earth would I be able to pry myself from the spot in which I stood? Miraculously, when I was called to receive my present, a spike in adrenalin maybe contributing to my sudden agility, I found myself walking, rather woodenly, forward. I received my recognition and managed a few words of gratitude and some amusing comments regarding my years at the university; at any rate, my colleagues laughed. Seemingly, I appeared fine.

For the remainder of the party, I was once more stuck in one spot, never able to circulate with the other partygoers, unable to enjoy this occasion. That saddened me greatly. My colleagues expressed their excitement about my life in retirement and all the pleasures it would bring, some even sounding envious of my future freedom. I found myself mouthing hollow words of enthusiasm about my new life and the treasure chest waiting to be unlocked, while inwardly voicing pitiful groans: "Not true. Doubt it." I was frightened, dreading what might be looming on the horizon. I knew something was amiss.

When I had my appointment with the rheumatologist at the end of June, I showed him my x-ray and explained my diagnosis. His immediate reaction was, "You need an MRI." I was also asked to demonstrate my walking. According to the rheumatologist, my right leg was shorter than my left, so it could affect my gait. I was tested for nerve responses on various parts of my body. Some were ultra-sensitive, indicating damage had occurred. I was surprised to receive a booking for July 14, the usual wait time being much longer. I took a taxi to the MRI because by now I was loath to drive; I couldn't trust my flexibility. My feet were also becoming harder to manipulate.

Immediately following this MRI, I sought further advice from an ER doctor, so worried had I become about the incredibly quick deterioration in my mobility. The doctor ordered a further lower back MRI for the following week: Wednesday at 9:00 pm. In the meantime I had had a recurring UTI and had been prescribed my regular antibiotics. Towards the end of the weekend prior to my second MRI, I began to feel unwell. By early Wednesday evening I was beginning to feel nauseated, with a bad taste in my mouth and overall malaise. Knowing I needed extra help getting to the hospital, I called Christopher, a strange choice perhaps, but he had been with me during my previous crisis many years before and had been very support-ive. I felt he would understand now. Christopher kindly agreed to come "at once" and accompany me to hospital, He in fact remained by my side throughout, during what turned out to be a long evening.

After my second MRI, we once more went to the ER department. As we were walking, me pushing a walker, he alongside, I asked, "Do you think I should tell the doctors how ill I am feeling?"

"I would never hold anything back as far as doctors are concerned," he said.

The doctor ordered a full panel of blood tests. The results showed a con-siderable increase in my creatinine levels. They were in the mid 300s, much, much higher than my usual reading of 250 micromoles per litre (µmol/L). No wonder I was feeling the way I was. The results showed a significant drop in my glomerular filtration rate (GFR), one of the tests used to deter-mine the level of kidney function. My kidney was definitely in jeopardy. This was not good news. The doctor's consolation message was, "Your liver is functioning well."

"Some consolation at least," I thought. He also prescribed a new antibiotic to help alleviate some soreness related to the UTI.

In spite of my compromised mobility and pain in my arms and hands, I had still been trying to maintain my fitness level by cycling on a stationary bicycle in my condo's sports room. Returning to my condo after my work-out on Friday morning around 11:00, I noticed a message from the rheuma-tologist's office on my answering machine. I had an emergency appointment with a neurosurgeon across the bridge at 12:00. I was the surgeon's only appointment. He would be coming directly from surgery. I needed to get there urgently. Since I didn't feel comfortable navigating the streets on my own, I called my friend Penny. She normally leads an active social life, but happened to be home. I asked her if she could she drive me to the doctor's office if I got myself to her place. "No problem," she said.

The cause of the pothole revealed

Once we found the doctor's office, in we went. The doctor arrived still in full surgical garb. I was about to sit down when the doctor asked me to have my companion come too. I said that really I was fine, and that she was a friend. Undeterred, the doctor repeated that it was important for someone else to hear what I was going to be told. I called Penny in and learned the truth. My vertebrae were sitting on my spinal cord. The doctor asked me what symptoms I had been experiencing. I explained about the tingling, numbness and pain in various parts of my arms and hands. "Do your legs felt like wood?" he asked.

The coin dropped. "Yes, that is exactly what they feel like," I told him. I realized I must have incurred this injury when I had tripped in the gas station in 2009. For three years, I had walked around and lived with a compromised spinal cord. The doctor's analysis was simple: "That was then. This is now. We take it from here." I would need immediate surgery. I had already sustained some permanent damage, so the purpose of the surgery was to prevent me from incurring any further damage. It would not fix what was already damaged, but it would alleviate whatever had been affected. My walking would improve but never be perfect. The symptoms I had were typical of spinal cord damage, and had they been picked up sooner, intervention could well have mitigated some of the effects I was now suffering.

I was to have cervical discs 5, 6 and 7 fused, with the possibility of further surgery to fuse other discs if necessary. I told the neurosurgeon about the one glitch: "I may be having kidney failure." That did delay the surgery but only briefly. The neurosurgeon needed assurances I was fine to have surgery. The hospital where my surgery was to be performed had no dialysis facility. As soon as I arrived home, I called the transplant nurse, explained to her what was going on and that I needed to see a nephrologist. She made an appointment for me to attend the Monday clinic, have a blood test and discuss my situation with a nephrologist.

That weekend was one of the worst weekends of my life. I felt unwell, nauseated and in considerable pain. I was terrified of what might be coming next. A friend, Anne-Marie, whom I had met through my book club, came to visit on Saturday. She has a wonderful ability to simply be present for another person, neither offering unwanted advice nor imposing her opinions. I told her I was not doing well. Anne-Marie was very conciliatory and did her best to pacify me. Sometime later when we were reminiscing about this time, she did confide to me that she knew I was uncomfortable and felt distressed but helpless as to how to assist me. This led me to reflect on how hard it is for a person to fully understand how another feels. We share commonalities such as birth, death, pain and grieving, but none of us can really, fully enter into someone else's suffering or pleasure. Each of us, and each experience, is so individual.

I finished the antibiotics on Saturday and spent Sunday at home, clearing my work files. Since I was now retired, I didn't require the information. It was a long and boring task, not helped by my feeling unwell and the horrid pain in my arms and hands. I really thought I was going to die. I wasn't worried about the possibility of death; that seemed quite reasonable and easy to accept. The discomfort, pain and continual feelings of being unwell are ones I had never experienced before, nor have I ever again known anything close to how I felt that weekend.

I called Roland to let him know what was happening with the surgery and my kidney. He told me later that he had thought I was teasing him at first, because he just couldn't imagine me having sustained a spinal cord injury. We also talked bluntly about what he should do should something go wrong. I assured him, though, that I did not feel the need for him to come home and suggested he stay where he was.

Needless to say, I survived the night and began to feel better on the Monday. I saw the nephrologist I had last seen in September. I couldn't resist telling the doctor that I had felt deserted in my time of need, after having been encouraged to make sure we were to meet again. We shared a laugh. Surprisingly, my blood test showed my creatinine levels had dropped significantly and were now in my usual range. Panic over. I was okay. I explained about the surgery I needed and asked if one of the doctors could talk to the neurosurgeon. There must have been some conversation between the doctors because I received a call mid-week from the neurosurgeon's office asking me to attend a pre-op appointment that Friday. Surgery was to be performed on the following Monday.

On the Friday, a nurse asked me a number of questions, checked my blood pressure and ordered a blood test. I next saw the anaesthetist, who told me, "You are a mess on paper." He had been worried about how I would do in surgery but after having met me he felt relieved. Paper tells the theory; only human contact can verify the reality. I am stronger than my records report. Then I met with an occupational therapist, who supplied me with a hard collar that I was to bring with me to the surgery, and I watched a video previewing hospital routine. I would next return on Monday, as scheduled, two days from my official retirement.

The surgery entailed the neurosurgeon cutting into the front of my neck. The neurosurgeon had explained to me that it was necessary to perform the surgery from the front rather than from the rear because it was impossible to cut through the discs, due to their hardness. The operation was executed by first lifting my vertebrae off my spine then fusing the vertebrae with plastic plates, rather like a bonding glue. The entire surgery was performed using a laparoscope, a device consisting of long, fiber-optic cables with pincers attached to the ends. One of the pincers lifted the vertebrae while the other pincers attached the plates. The neurosurgeon facilitated the operation through a camera. My airways were intubated to keep them open. When I awoke from the operation, hard collar in place, the neurosurgeon informed me everything had gone as planned. I would be kept in overnight. Before being discharged the next day, I had another blood test. The neurosurgeon returned with the results: "No dialysis for you. Your creatinine is good."

Home I went to recuperate. I had to wear the collar for two weeks and do neck exercises. I was pretty much grounded for some time. I had an extremely sore throat, resulting from having been intubated for a long period of time. The surgery had taken several hours to complete. My sore throat seemed to continue for longer. I often felt feverish with a chill coursing through my body. I had contracted an infection from the intubation. I also found it difficult to talk, as though something were blocking my throat. I constantly needed to clear my throat. At first I thought it might be a blood clot, but the blockage continued ceaselessly, changing from a nuisance to an affliction. Already compromised by scleroderma, my swallowing had worsened too. Often when I talked I would gag and stumble on my words, creating awkward moments for me.

Two years later, in January 2014, following a swallowing test that uncovered no evident cause for my difficulty, my GP referred me to an ear, nose and throat (ENT) specialist. He diagnosed a cyst in my throat. It had definitely impacted impaired vocal cords already affected by my surgery. He ordered surgery for that summer. That surgery finally took place in April 2015, delayed because other conditions and situations had taken precedence.

In August, a few weeks following my surgery, I had two medical check-ups. One was my yearly consultation with the gynecologist, and the other my six-monthly appointment with the infectious disease doctor. Interestingly, the first thing both asked me was, "How is your walking?" My lameness had obviously been noticed! I let each of them know about my emergency surgery and the effects of my sustained damage. I cannot remember what the gynecologist said, but my infectious disease doctor was very sympathetic and prescribed some pain medication that I had already tried but had proven unhelpful. As we talked, I uncharacteristically felt emotional and shed a few tears. My doctor was most solicitous. I asked if there could have been any correlation between my UTIs, intestinal problems and spinal injury. The doctor certainly felt there was a strong possibility of it being so.

I chastised myself for being so stupid in failing to connect my two symptoms. The doctor kindly responded, "You were not to know that." I feel this was said to mollify me while in reality I felt like Winnie the Pooh, the bear "of very little brain." So I am the human "of very little brain!"

The consequences of the pothole

In early fall of 2012, I received an unexpected visit from Roland. I had not anticipated this visit, because I was doing as well as I could and he had already been back twice that year. His travel costs were mounting; however, he assured me he had obtained an outrageously economical flight since it was between seasons. When his arrival date came, Christopher collected him from the airport and brought him to me. First, there was a knock on the door, then it opened and in walked the most elegant, smiling European-looking young man I had ever seen. Incredible the transformation he had gone through since his last visit. How to explain the difference in appearance between North Americans and Europeans? Something in the cut, colour and style of apparel, as well as the manner of presentation seems to set us apart.

Roland attended to all the household tasks for me and became, once more, my chef, chauffeur and chief bottle washer. I was able, for the first time in weeks, to venture out. This was heaven! I also had some delicious meals even though Roland was not a cook. We dined on simple fare, but the artist in him shone when it came to food presentation. I was astonished by what he did. With a quick flick of the fork, something ordinary had been transformed into a work of art. Much as I loved cooking and entertaining, no matter how hard I tried, my meals always appeared to resemble slop.

Despite the thrill of having Roland home, I realized the pain in my elbows, arms and hands was not disappearing and was often becoming unbearable. Medications were to no avail. To this point, I had never fully believed in the notion of chronic pain. I had experienced scleroderma-associated pain that I had been able to handle, so assumed that my current pain would be alleviated by surgery and eventually subside. How wrong I was! My intense pain was here to stay. I had become initiated into the world of chronic pain. It was horrendous. As I write this, it remains so. It varies in degrees and type, from tingling, itchy, plain sore to dreadfully sore. It varies from cold chills to burning and intense tightness gripping me in a vice-like hold, always changing, but everlasting in its intensity. Often, my fingers, thumb and parts of my hands twitch. Furthermore, my fingers are numb and my coordination is imperilled. I drop things easily, or should I say, things fall easily from my hands. These are classic symptoms of neuropathic nerve damage. Once during Roland's visit, uncharacteristically unable to contain my despair, I broke down into inconsolable tears wailing, "It is absolutely horrible." That's all I could say.

Roland rushed to my side, saying, "Oh, mum," and hugged me most dearly. That, of course, reduced me to even more tears. His kind act did help, however. I obviously recovered. Needless to say, Roland's visit soon came to an end. Once again, he returned to Belgium.

In spite of feeling moments of real despair, I understood that most likely there were others who were equally affected by chronic nerve pain. I was encouraged to join Pain BC, a wonderful organization created to support people living with chronic pain and raise awareness of this condition. Pain BC offers online seminars and sponsors a monthly newsletter containing the latest research, relevant research information and news about forthcoming events. That autumn I spent many afternoons participating in numerous online pain workshops to learn strategies to cope with my condition.

At its second Provincial Summit, held in February 2017, Pain BC outlined ten key actions to move toward a provincial pain strategy. Among these are plans to create a Vancouver Coastal Health Pain Program and a BC Pain Agency and to enable early intervention beginning in the community. All will help in raising public awareness of chronic pain issues, as well as leading towards developing more effective treatments for those suffering from chronic pain.

My three-month visits to the transplant clinic continued. No change showed in my kidney function—it remained static. The nephrologists tried to prescribe medication to ease my pain, but either I related badly or else found little relief. In November I received a telephone call from the hospital giving me a date to see a neurologist. I can only imagine the referral must have come through the transplant doctors. They are a most thoughtful and caring team and really want to assist us, their patients.

The neurologist inserted electronic needles in various parts of my right arm, the one most affected by my injury. The tests were uncomfortable, similar to being given mild electric shocks, but the evidence pointed to me recovering considerably. It would be a slow, painful process but the future was promising. As both my neurosurgeon and the neurologist had predicted, my walking would gradually improve. I would benefit from "lots of massage, acupuncture sessions and physiotherapy." I remarked to the neurologist how amazed I had been by the body's ability to withstand tremendous assault, and yet still function adequately. I believe the neurologist concurred with me.

In November, on the advice of the neurologist, I contacted my previous physiotherapist, Dee, who agreed to treat me at home. Dee came weekly and massaged my neck, back, legs and arms, as well as giving me acupuncture. She also prescribed numerous exercises to help me gain strength, flexibility and hopefully increase my mobility. Dee became my constant in-house companion for virtually a year and discontinued only when she was due to have her baby.

I approached the remainder of the winter full of hope. However, as time progressed I began to realize I had actually sustained far greater spinal cord injuries than I had originally thought. Not only were my hands and arms affected, but also my neck, shoulders, back and feet. My right side had atrophied; my arm was reduced in size, as was my right leg. Both my shoulder muscles had sustained damage and were exceptionally weak, as were my upper back muscles. I could neither lift my arms nor pick up anything easily. Everything I tried to move, from the lightest towel to a chair, was an effort. I had simply lost strength.

I tried to compensate and develop upper arm strength by daily lifting of small cans for fifteen reps each. Although I acquired muscle in my upper arms, I could never increase my overall strength. Likewise, my feet and my right big toe, in particular, remained flat and inflexible. Again I worked valiantly, trying the numerous feet and toe exercises Dee had suggested. While I experienced some improvement, full mobility never returned. I also had difficulty bending over to pick up anything that had fallen to the ground. I could do it, but only with supreme effort and much patience. Often, where something fell, it stayed. I was not the housekeeper I had once been. I could move, but rigidly. My legs were still fairly inflexible. I could only stand for brief periods of time. I could not talk and walk at the same time.

Towards the end of November I felt confident enough to start driving. My first attempts were very short journeys, driving around the block and returning home. Although my right hand hurt incessantly, I could drive fairly easily. It was my gateway. However, I was limited to nearby destinations and venues with parking facilities since I could not walk long distances. I did not possess the confidence to venture farther afield. To do that, I needed to use HandyDART, a provincially sponsored, locally run transport facility, designed to assist mobility-challenged people with access to medical, educational, work or social activities. The cost is affordable, the service beyond compare. HandyDART is deemed an essential service. The drivers are personable and kind, sometimes providing the main social interaction in many riders' lives.

Sometime during the early spring, I was referred to a hospital specializing in spinal cord injuries and invited to attend a number of informative sessions pertaining to the spine and the effects of spinal cord injuries. During one of these sessions, I learned I had what is called an "incomplete" spinal cord injury. Not every part of my body had been affected. I could walk, move my head, neck, arms and other parts of my body, perhaps not as easily as non-injured people, but I had agility compared to others who had sustained more severe injuries.

My ability to drive appears to suggest that my life had resumed some form of normalcy. This was, in actual fact, far from the truth. Yes, I had some access to the wider world, but I also had some severe incapacities. I told one of my nephrologists that I was much more incapacitated than I seemed. The nephrologist agreed. My walking never improved beyond a shuffle. Every step I took felt as though I were carrying a one-hundred-pound weight on my back while climbing a steep hill. I needed a cane to support myself. I was also frequently consumed with horrendous pain. Incessant, intense pain, whether emotional or physical, can be exhausting. It is the single, most challenging aspect of my spinal cord injury and hangs on me like a mantle, sapping my energy and spirit. It requires effort to shift feelings of despair into positive feelings of hope and well-being. I believe we can survive and even overcome most tragedies, but chronic pain—that's different. I struggle daily to keep my energy and optimism up.

Its subsequent effects

So how did all this affect me? My world had been turned upside down overnight by my fall. I needed a paradigm shift if I were to progress. I had already experienced three other such shifts: first with the scleroderma diagnosis, second with kidney failure and third, living with a transplant. Intellectually, I could understand the importance of having to readjust my thinking and actions, but emotionally I was stuck. I would sit for days staring into oblivion, or if I could muster the energy, out the window. Although I would not admit to it, I was suffering from the characteristic symptoms of loss: grief, disbelief and shock. My one relief was that if a friend visited or called, I could immediately present a cheery presence. I also knew that I needed and craved human contact, and therefore, it was essential for me to appear positive, full of life, energetic and happy. I knew that my friends did not want to hear sordid details of my injuries. Of course, if I could smile and laugh, my mood would be elevated and I would actually feel happy. But my underlying grief prevailed, as it does today, somewhat dimmed by time and easier to accommodate. At least I no longer sit for days staring into nothing.

My social life took a hit. At the beginning of my recovery from surgery, I was awash with visitors and calls from friends offering help, but as the days grew into months and autumn into winter, my recovery showing little progress, the calls decreased. One friend asked, "Are you better yet?" We can cope with temporary illnesses or injuries, knowing recovery is inevitable, but chronic conditions are different. They are complicated. There is no fixed date of recovery. It's hard to know how to respond or what to say or do. I have had phone calls, texts or emails from friends saying they will drop by for a visit or go to lunch with me in the next few days or so, but that seldom happens. It's not that they don't care, but more that they are caught up in their own activities.

To maintain contact with someone who has a limitation requires commitment and empathy. Not everyone can or wants to make such a commitment. Because of this, I experienced a downward spiral. The less I socialized, the fewer things I did. I became a forgotten member of society. Fewer interactions with others and fewer experiences of new things lead to dull, uninspiring conversation. Now, I find it hard to share things of interest with others because of my limited horizon. I hope, though, I have become a better listener.

I recall meeting a parent and a child at one of the specialist hospital's sessions. The young person, a really bright student soon to graduate from high school with a promising future, had been involved in a horrific car accident one wintery evening. No one could work out how the accident had happened or what had caused it, but the young person had received terrible injuries and had virtually lost the ability to talk. Home was a wheelchair. The parent confided that socializing with friends and hearing the latest exciting things their children were doing was painful. This parent said, "I feel absolutely isolated. I cannot join their conversation and share exciting stories about my child. I just feel left out."

Being incapacitated can result in isolation. Often people assume an isolated person must be lonely. This is not so. Loneliness, I believe, is a state of mind. We can feel lonely in the midst of a crowd. Christopher Hadfield, in his memoir *An Astronaut's Guide to Life on Earth*,[1] said that he never felt lonely while isolated in space. Isolation is different from loneliness. It means being secluded, often feeling secluded, lacking contact with people, left out. Seniors may experience isolation as a result of aging or health issues. Equally so, dialysis patients may feel isolated as a result of their need for constant treatment and the challenges accompanying dialysis itself, as indeed does anyone whose situation or circumstances prevent them from accessing educational, work or social pursuits.

At this point in my life, I often felt isolated because I simply could not do the things I used to: join groups for spontaneous outings or easily cross town to visit friends, especially if these involved walking distances. I needed to rely on someone else, a taxi or HandyDART (which requires booking a week in advance) to drive me. If no one was available, then I was left out. Further challenges occurred when walking with friends: I am slow. Invariably I would be trailing several feet behind as my friends, keen to reach a destination, barrelled ahead, leaving me in their wake. I am also a member of a group that has made it clear only able-bodied people can be accommodated, since the group's preferred meeting locations require the ability to climb stairs. I clung on to my limited mobility as a button does to a disintegrating thread, fearing if it worsened I would no longer be able to participate, isolating me further. One of my fellow patients told me isolation was not a problem but having to be dependent on others was. Independence can be our last bastion of freedom, our precious ability to navigate our own course on our own terms.

When our physical condition changes drastically, so does our self-esteem. We are not who we were. Our personalities may remain intact but our ability to live as we wish has been compromised. We want to be like we used to be, the same as others, but can't be. I kept wanting to say, "I am not really like this. You should have seen me a few years ago." I really wanted to be on an equal plane. I soon realized that no one was really listening, nor was there much interest in what used to be. People want to live in the present and look to the future. In frustration, I said to one of my doctors, "Life is for the living, not the dead." My forced isolation made me feel as though I were among the dead. It took me a very long time to adjust.

My friends would say, "If you need something, just call." I am sure they would have been only too happy to oblige. I could always use some help or some shopping but several things prevented me from taking up their offer. First, my pain was endless. Picking up the phone required me to engage in friendly banter, meaning I was with it and able to happily converse. Inevitably, at the beginning of a conversation I would cheerily be asked: "How are you?" I just couldn't bring myself to sound bright and cheerful on some occasions. I could manage if I received a call, but to make one myself was too much for me. Secondly, with my self-esteem plummeting, I felt as though I were pleading for help. I loathed this feeling. Lack of self-esteem can lead to an imbalance in thought. Thirdly, my injuries were not temporary. I wondered just how many times I could call a friend for help before their generosity was tried.

I have probably made the same offer—"If you need something, just call,"—to others. I wonder whether my friends may well have been experiencing the same emotions as I have. Now I realize that I would have appreciated friends calling to say, "I am doing something. Would you like anything or would you like to join me?" This would have been absolutely wonderful.

In addition to practical aid, I yearned for the kind of empathy only friends can provide. Family support, while essential to our well-being, is often disrupted by the routine business of family life. Family members don't always have time to simply sit and stay by our side. Friends can sometimes do this. After my first kidney failure, my good friend, Jane, was staying with us. She would sit by my bedside for a few hours every day as she worked on her needlepoint project. We didn't speak. We didn't need to. The silent comfort of her companionship was enough. She exuded a gentle spirituality, the energy of her simply sitting with me. Friends may feel they need to distract or entertain us, when really the greatest support they can provide is to be in the moment with us.

Patching the pothole

Two new developments on the pain-management front came at the beginning of 2013. At my six-month appointment with the neurosurgeon in January, the results of a November MRI revealed the need for further surgery. This time my cervical discs 3 and 4 would be fused during surgery in May. At my session with the neurosurgeon, I was shown the MRI results and the place on my spine where the damage had occurred. It appeared like a little black pinprick in one small area. I was amazed that this tiny dot, such a small hole, could be the cause of my subsequent impediments. Also, I had my GP refer me to the pain clinic. It would be six months before I saw a pain specialist.

Meanwhile, in March, I had a follow-up appointment with my infectious disease doctor, who asked if I would consider trying marijuana. It had proven very effective with HIV and cancer patients, I was told. This doctor would give me the required referral. I did not want to smoke it since I liked neither the smell nor taste. But I gathered that marijuana existed in other forms, so agreed to try it. I had endless forms to fill in both for local dispensaries and for federal approval. I was also required to have two photos taken, one for each application. My first acceptance came from the local agency. I could now join the band of medical marijuana users.

The dispensary recommended by my doctor was only a short distance from the hospital. I asked a friend if she would be willing to come with me in case I found walking difficult. So, here we were—two fairly nondescript, middle-aged women entering an unexplored world. We had no idea what items were available to me or what I should request. Fortunately, our ignorance was short-lived. There was a young person in the waiting room—an experienced customer, ashen-faced, sitting hunched over, arms held tight to the body, obviously suffering from an adverse condition—who, lifted from her stupor, happily showed us a vast menu of goods ranging from different varieties of marijuana to a plethora of smoking equipment to an assortment of edible items. Our experienced customer recommended some edible items for me to try. We learned our young guide was on dialysis and used marijuana to stave off the effects of both kidney failure and treatment, explaining the cause of her suffering. Two things crossed my mind. One, I wanted to say, "I may well be joining you soon." The other, I thought how much better quality of life this young person would have were a kidney transplant offered! With so few donors available, though, the likelihood of this happening could be slim. It upset me greatly.

My turn to be served soon came. Protocol was rigid: only one person at a time was admitted into the dispensing room. My friend had to stay in the waiting room. I was required to show my ID, first to the receptionist before entering the incredibly small dispensing room, and again every time I inched along the counter. Each tiny step required evidence of my legal right to buy marijuana. The counter, fortuitously, was only a few feet long. I chose a small jar of honey and a cream chocolate. Then, showing my ID once again, I paid for my purchases, all cash transactions, and was directed to another exit. One of the assistants had informed me that, should I find I had taken too much marijuana, the effects would wear off within two hours with no residual effects. I was asked not to smoke marijuana in front of the dispensary, never draw attention to myself, always carry my ID and promise not to share my supplies. I signed a paper declaring my good intentions. My friend and I left the dispensary, now so much wiser in the world of medicinal marijuana.

It took me a long time to use the honey, but eventually I did. The chocolate sat untouched for weeks in my fridge because I was worried about what kind of reaction I might have. Modern marijuana is infinitely stronger than what I had known in the 1960s. By the time I cut the chocolate in half, the outside had hardened and its cream filling was dry. I don't remember if it had much effect or not. But, in due time I needed to replace my honey and made another trip to the dispensary. This time, I felt more confident. I chose a larger jar of honey and some hand cream that I could rub on my arm and hand to lessen the pain. While at the till, I noticed a basket filled with bags of what resembled Bits and Bites, a popular snack. Emboldened with my greater knowledge, I purchased one. The assistant advised me to use a small quantity at a time, around a quarter of a cup. The snacks would last a long time. I hoped so, because this small bag cost me eight bucks!

I put a teaspoon of honey in a cup of hot water just before bedtime. I had no idea if it helped or not. I would like to think I felt a little lighter headed but it could have been my imagination. I certainly had no trouble sleeping. The Bits and Bites, like the chocolate, sat untouched for a long time until the Thursday evening before my pre-op appointment. My pain seemed particularly bad so I thought, "What the heck! I'll try some of the marijuana snacks before dinner." I retrieved the snacks from the back recess of a cupboard, poured a tiny amount—well under ¼ cup—into a little dish and went into my den where I had been watching the news on TV. How delicious they tasted! I couldn't wait to devour every last one of the morsels.

About fifteen minutes later, I suddenly realized the landscape in front of me had changed. Nothing was as it had been. I was stoned, absolutely pie-eyed. I could not move and struggled to organize my thoughts. Whatever was on TV was like a blur. I did grasp my need to eat, because I had to take some of my regular medication with food. That required a two-hour gap before my immunosuppressant. However, I would fall if I stood up. I couldn't stand up. I knew if I could get myself into the high-backed office chair that I had kept in my den to support my neck after surgery, I could wheel myself to the kitchen. Very slowly, after inching my way along the sofa, I grabbed one of the chair's arms and pulled it towards me. Holding the arm as tightly as I could, I elevated myself off the sofa and clumsily fell onto the seat. Then using my legs and feet, I propelled myself towards the kitchen. It was a slow process.

Once there I could open the fridge and help myself to food. But, there was a glitch. Fearing I would fall if I stood up, I could only select items that were within eyesight and within reach. I recall picking out a tomato. The rest was a mishmash of anything within easy reach. Fortunately, I could grab a plate and some cutlery from the draining board by the sink. At least I think I did that. Luckily I had already prepared my medication. With supplies in my lap, I made the slow return journey to the den. I must have eaten the food but my memory is hazy.

Still in no shape to do anything other than sit, my anxiety level, already high, edged higher. The pain I had hoped to ease was in fact stronger. I was living in a surreal world, an extremely painful one at that. None of the objects around me seemed to be where I thought they belonged. Should I call an ambulance? I reasoned that I wouldn't be able to get to the phone on the far side of the room, and what's more, even if I could, I would probably only be able to mouth gibberish. Besides, I could envisage the paramedics having a field day with me in my present state. As well, the hospital couldn't do anything, only time could. At least, I hoped it could! In spite of my panic-ridden state, I could appreciate the humour of my situation. Here I was, a bland, middle-aged woman, no risk-taking revolutionary, doped to the gills. I recalled the dispensary assistant's words: "…two hours, all will be fine." My new mantra.

I sat, staring at the dial on my wristwatch. The watch itself appeared miles from my eyes, located somewhere in space, and my wrist appeared completely detached from my body. I peered at the dial, watching every foggy second of its hand creep around the watch's face for the required two hours. Nothing happened. No relief. Now I was really worried. Would I ever regain my composure? I had no control over my thoughts or movement because I seemed to be in a spatial void. I simply continued to stare at my watch.

Finally, around 11:00 pm, some six hours after I had first realized I was stoned, I began to see objects a little more clearly. My arm had reattached itself to my body. This was comforting. I could get up and move around more naturally. I could relate to real time. Since I had a 9:00 am appointment for my pre-op the next day, I felt I should go to bed, foregoing my usual honey mixture. Once in bed, however, I was terrified of closing my eyes in case I passed out, overslept and missed my date with the anaesthetist, causing me to lose out on the surgery. I stayed awake the entire night, counting hours instead of hands. By morning's light, my stoned state had been replaced with a washed-out, bleary feeling, but I had survived. I would not miss my appointment. Now I was worried in case the night's episode would rule me inadmissible for surgery. I had visions of the doctor pointing to the exit door and warning me to clean up my act.

When my companion driver collected me at our prearranged time, I explained my bedraggled appearance and confessed my worry about having to admit my sad tale and the possible consequences of my having been stoned. "Should I be worried?" I asked.

"Who knows?" was the response. I fussed all the way to the hospital. In the pre-op waiting room I continued to feel uneasy. I knew that I needed to admit to having been stoned the previous evening. My first hurdle was the nurse. When I met with her, I hesitated but couldn't let time lapse too long because I knew I would be having a blood test, so I blurted out my sorry story. The nurse laughed loudly. Instead of scolding me, she asked if I had enjoyed it and continued with her routine tasks. Well, so much for that, I thought, but I had a further hurdle to contend with: the anaesthetist.

This time, pleasantries exchanged, I immediately confessed my previous night's lack of judgement. Like the nurse, the anaesthetist burst into hoots of laughter and asked if I had enjoyed my experience. "I don't care how much marijuana you use, as long as you don't turn up for surgery stoned," he said. So much for all my anxieties and pitiful worries, deflated like a balloon! My surgery was on schedule.

The result of my escapade was that I relegated the honey to the farthest corner of my spice shelf, never to be used again, and the Bits and Bites likewise to some dark recess from which they eventually found their way to the garbage. Poor slugs! I continued to use the marijuana cream and do so today because it does seem to provide me with a little comfort.

A few weeks previously, Roland had phoned to let me know he was coming once again to help me. He was able to stay for a month. However, he could only book a flight that would arrive the Saturday before my surgery. My newly minted European son duly arrived on the Saturday full of smiles and youthful energy, replete with Belgian goodies for friends and family. His bag was a treasure chest crammed with delights that magically materialized every time his hand dipped into his suitcase. Somewhere in the depths were his clothes, too. Each item came with a story. We spent the entire Saturday watching the spectacle of him producing goods from his suitcase, hearing their stories.

Monday came. Roland drove me to the hospital, remaining with me until I was called into the operating waiting area. Having being gowned and prepped, I waited and waited before being called to the OR. It felt peculiar to experience the OR as a walk-in patient, off the street and into surgery. The room itself seemed cavernous with only one very narrow gurney in the middle. I wondered how I was going to fit on it, so narrow did it seem. But I did, comfortably. Then began the process of receiving the anaesthetic, of course, but not before I loudly rambled on about some trivial drivel.

No sooner were my eyes open after being awakened by the anaesthetist and nurse than I burst into floods of tears, crying out, "No more pain!" My two attendants probably thought I was issuing a demand, referring to the surgery itself so they may have upped the pain killer meds. I was, in reality, thinking about my chronic pain. I regained my composure and called Roland to inform him the surgery had gone as planned. He took me home the next day. I wore my collar for two weeks, and Roland resumed his customary role, helping me through the initial stages of recovery.

This visit was different from his previous one eight months ago. Not only had his cooking skills improved, so had his interest in food. Here was my son, who a few years ago couldn't even differentiate between pork and beef. Now he was showing me how to use a knife, slice onions, mince herbs and prepare dishes without using a recipe. I was impressed. We even entertained several times during his stay, Roland preparing and serving three- to four-course fancy fare as I stared in awe.

All too soon the month came to an end. This time I felt capable of accompanying him to the airport. Christopher collected us. We escorted him to the check-in and departure. I pushed the trolley for support. We might have raised a few eyebrows as people watched me pushing a laden trolley with two tall, strapping men walking one on either side of me. I wondered if anyone "tsk-tsked'" as they saw us, thinking, "Isn't that typical. A woman doing all the work."

Not too long after Roland's departure, I had my first visit with the social worker from the spinal cord hospital. I knew that pain following surgery is at its worst. Mine, already bad, had increased. The numbness in my hands was even more evident. I was hurting! When I met with the social worker, I was emotionally distraught. I remember her saying to me, "You're depressed. I am going to be keeping in contact with you to see how you are doing." This the social worker did for several weeks until I saw the physiotherapist. When the social worker asked me about my goals, I told her I wanted to be able to walk better and to swim.

Thus prepared, the physiotherapist spent time massaging me and getting me to practice walking, first using walking poles and then having me concentrate on how I walked. I had already been using a cane. I learned to walk more consciously with it. I also tried increasing my leg strength while lying on my back by pushing on a board. This was hard work, but beneficial. Two months later I was given an opportunity to try walking in the hospital pool. The occupational swimming instructor joined my social worker and me in the pool.

I had a one-piece, skirted bathing suit that I had hardly worn for three years. Dressing and undressing was difficult for me, not only because my hands were compromised but also my movements were stiff and inflexible. Because my swimsuit was new, it was a tight fit. I struggled getting into it. Then when I was finally in, it didn't feel quite right. My assistants took one look at me and burst into fits of laughter. I had put my bathing suit on backwards! Duly rearranged, into the pool we went. It felt wonderful, walking from side to side, supported by the water's buoyancy. In the water my legs were supple. This was true therapy. I joined the hospital swimming group that met one evening a week, and practised water Tai Chi in another local hospital pool. So began my water therapy.

In September, I finally met with a doctor who specialized in treating chronic pain sufferers. This took place at a teaching hospital so I entered a roomful of students, the doctor and another person who was introduced as a physiatrist, someone who specializes in nerve assessment damage. My doctor was a happy optimist who exuded warmth, humour and good-naturedness. Pain seemed to evaporate as we talked about my condition, its root cause and my ability to cope. Having recovered from my earlier depression, I felt I was managing my pain well so didn't need follow-up treatment. The doctor gave me a card and said I would be more than welcome to come for a further session should I need it. I could also attend pain management sessions for additional support. The doctor further suggested that I try a marijuana-based pill, but one that would not cause me to feel any abnormal side effects. My GP could prescribe it for me. I chatted briefly with the physiatrist who provided me with further information about my neuropathic pain.

Meanwhile, I continued with the swimming group, improving in my balance ability as a result of learning how to move and stand from the Tai Chi exercises. In January I joined a new group session, an open one in which we could do whatever we found helpful. I am a swimmer but found I could not lie on my back or try traditional swimming strokes. My neck fusion made it impossible to actually swim. I could, however, walk, run, jump and kick my legs lying on the poolside railing and practice standing still on one leg at a time. The water enabled me to do things I could not do on land. It was absolutely wonderful to feel the real freedom of unencumbered agility once again. I loved my weekly, hour-long sessions and really worked hard to increase my stamina, walking ability and general strength. For the first time in years, I felt more human and in control of my physical ability.

Each time I left the pool, though, reality returned. Walking slowly up the wheelchair-accessible ramp, with the water level gradually receding behind me, my stumbling movement returned and with it a sense of disappointment. The freedom provided by the water's buoyancy felt like a short-lived mirage.

Chapter 4 | Second Kidney Failure

Que Sera, Sera
—Jay Livingston and Ray Evans, *Whatever Will Be, Will Be*

Blue skies

In late August 2013, Roland returned for a three-week visit; this time his girlfriend, Veerle, was able to accompany him. While some of their time was spent camping in Banff, a fair bit was with me. We had a number of lovely dinners with family and friends. Summer dining seems to revel in its own special essence, the warm evenings lending themselves to casual, long, languid suppers with a veritable cornucopia of summer flavours and aromas tantalizing our palates. Conversation feels more relaxed and laughter more uproarious. Our time together much reflected our leisurely meals and was a superb way to watch the sun fade into the evening shadows as days turned into autumn haze. All too soon, Roland and Veerle's holiday came to an end. Another very sad farewell to attend to. I wasn't sure when we would meet again. It had been a blissful time for me, not only seeing Roland and Veerle, but also managing my pain well and coping with my mobility issues. Furthermore, my kidney seemed to be holding up well.

I had been continuing with my swimming sessions. At the end of my time in the pool, I needed to rush to the washroom where I flowed like a burst pipe. When I remarked on this to the swimming therapist, the response was that it was a sign of excellent kidney function. For some reason, being in water appeared to affect my bladder. How I clung onto these words! They were my respite from anguish, and a propitious sign, I hoped.

Warning of storm clouds

The writing, however, was on the wall. Surgery often results in lowering our hemoglobin level, most likely from blood loss during the operation. Mine had dropped considerably following my second cervical fusion procedure. The transplant clinic nurse had told me not to worry, that it would improve in time. In September, during a clinic visit, one of the nephrologists drew my attention to my hemoglobin count. Four months after my surgery, my hemoglobin had not risen. This required close monitoring. It was slightly worrying news and, I guess, in retrospect, could be considered as warning number two, the previously one having been delivered in 2007, six years before. My other results had been in my customary norm.

The third warning bell rang in October. My potassium level had risen beyond the acceptable range. I explained its rise as a consequence of having indulged in a potassium-rich Thanksgiving feast, including comfort food such as, squash, various types of potatoes, Brussels sprouts, stuffing, gravy and pumpkin pie, all saturated with potassium. I was worried until I had talked with a former colleague, Annie, whose husband, Allan, had also had a transplant at exactly the same time as I had had mine, although in different places—Allan's in Vancouver, mine in England. We were twins, so to speak, and attended the same transplant clinic, though not at the same time. Allan apparently had received a comparable potassium result and had also brushed it off as the result of having consumed a potassium-laden meal. This information was an antidote for my concerns. I relaxed. Next month's results would no doubt be better. They were not. Further bad news was to follow.

The final warning bell rang in November when my blood test results showed an increased level of phosphorus from foods like dairy, cheese, chocolate and beans—all high sources. My results also showed a really sudden spike in my creatinine. Previous readings, in the 200s, though already high, had climbed to about 300 micromoles per litre (μmol/L).

Definite signs of a fading kidney. The dietician recommended, no, instructed me to start eating a kidney-friendly diet, one more restricting than any I had previously known. I could, for example, have a two-finger-thick piece of cheese once a week, two tablespoons of peanut butter once a week, and no beans, avocados, grains or winter comfort foods. Gone were high-fibre cereals, whole grains, brown rice and similar foods. The very things all nutritionists recommended were banished from my diet. This news was hard to accept. But I needed to adhere to it if I were to salvage the remnants of my failing kidney.

In November, too, I tried taking one tablet of the pain medication suggested by the pain specialist—to disastrous effects. I felt both drunk and hungover until it had finally cleared from my system. Upon reflection, I wonder if my bad reaction to the various pain medications had been connected to a considerable drop in the level of my glomerular filtration rate (GFR). The lower our GFR level, the harder it is to absorb or rid our body of the effects of medication.

Christmas was particularly challenging. I could only sit and watch enviously as my fellow revellers gorged themselves on cheese-filled appetizers, various tempting nuts, turkey stuffing, gravy, roasted yams, sweet potatoes, chocolates, mince pies and other succulent goodies, while I could only try smidgens of them. I was also beginning to feel the effects of my low hemoglobin. I seemed to exist in a fog. It felt as though the lights were on but no one was home.

My discombobulated state was apparent to me too when members of the book club I had joined years ago met in my building's lounge for our December 2013 meeting. Barely able to focus on the discussion, I sat between a new member whom I didn't know well and one I did. During our tea break, the new member began to chat with me. I couldn't concentrate on anything she said and turned my attention to the person I knew well, who, thankfully, kept the conversation afloat. I was terribly embarrassed. When our book club next met, I apologized to the snubbed member for my inattentiveness. It turned out that my friend had noticed nothing amiss. Worry and guilt had caused me to presume the worst.

A similar incident occurred later, in January. A group of my friends and I were having dinner together, sitting at a large round table. The restaurant was packed and noisy so we needed to raise our voices. I could hardly raise mine, let alone keep up with the repartee. I drifted in and out of a stupor with no idea what I said or how coherently I spoke. Spring seemed to pass with me blurring in and out of being present. I felt slightly tilted, walking on an angle. Sometimes I was perfectly fine and totally ordinary, but I could not predict when a blur would occur. The nephrologist prescribed a special medication for me called EPO that I self-injected subcutaneously. Its purpose was to stimulate red blood cell production. As well, I was given a number of iron infusions.

More evidence of looming storm clouds

In January my blood work again showed further rising creatinine levels and decreases in GFR level. There was no denying the obvious: my kidney was failing. The transplant nephrologists had no choice but to refer me to the dialysis nurses. Things moved quickly. I was still part of the transplant clinic because I retained my transplant and continued to need immuno-suppressants, and yet I was going to need dialysis. It was like living in the shadows.

The renal nurse spoke bluntly: "Your kidney will fail. It is just a matter of time—a month, a year. What kind of dialysis would you like to do?"

I did not want to do hemodialysis, so automatically and affirmatively replied, "Peritoneal dialysis." The nurse showed me the latest technique, a cycler, introduced after my first kidney failure. Much had changed in the twenty-two years since my last kidney failure. The machine is designed to automatically perform dialysis while we sleep. The time, length and num-ber of dialysis treatments performed can be pre-programmed. The cycler needs to be set up with at least three bags per night, and the dialysis solution drains in and out on schedule. Used solution is drained either into a sink, toilet or bath. In the morning, a lesser amount of fluid is drained in and left *in situ* all day.

The solution had changed, too. It varied in strength depending on the amount of fluid or toxins needing to be removed. Dietary restrictions were eased slightly. Peritoneal dialysis users could consume as much water as they wished, since any excess could be removed through dialysis by using one of the stronger solutions.

At some stage, I met with the peritoneal dialysis nephrologist, who exam-ined my abdomen to clear me for having a peritoneal tube inserted. Then I met with the peritoneal dialysis link nurse who arranged to come to my home to discuss the dialysis process and bring a cycler. We arranged to meet towards the end of January.

It sounds as though I had readily accepted my altered status. To be clear: I had not! I found the whole thing horrifying. I could not imagine having kidney failure again. I was living in a dream. However, the process contin-ued.

As arranged, I had my appointment with the link nurse. What an incred-ibly upbeat, jolly, friendly and compassionate person this nurse was. The perfect personality for the role as an intermediary between one world and the next. I thoroughly enjoyed our visit and general conversation, but not the topic. During the demonstration of how the cycler worked, I appeared interested and compliant, but underneath I was repulsed by the thought of what the machine represented and my pending status change.

Then the nurse examined my legs for fluid retention. Kidney failure can cause water retention and increase swelling in legs, feet and hands. I had none. The nurse also pressed my fingernails to show me how to see the effects of low hemoglobin. As he pressed mine, I could see the slowness with which the red tinge returned. In contrast, when his nails were pressed, they turned red immediately. Low hemoglobin manifests itself in how quickly blood appears on the surface of various parts of our anatomy. Hemoglobin is basically a protein of red blood cells that contains iron and carries oxygen from the lungs to the tissues and carbon dioxide from the tissues to the lungs.

We also discussed where and how I would store the dialysis solution boxes. My condo was small, but I had an office that could be used. Delivery could be every two weeks so I would not be inundated with masses of boxes filled with solution. I learned that my kidney would likely fail within the next six to eight months. Hearing these words, I almost wanted to cover my ears, so horrible was the whole idea of being reminded about eventually failed kidneys. One of the last things the nurse said to me was: "Dialysis won't kill you."

I had to have the last word, "No, but kidney failure will." Our meeting came to an end and none too soon. So much for my gratitude. At a follow-up conversation with the link nurse I confessed my concealed feelings. We laughed together about them. The nurse said they were not a surprise: many patients have the same sentiments.

In the following months, some of my results were more positive, suggesting that actual kidney failure could still be a long way off. This, I later learned, frequently happened as kidney failure occurred. Sometimes I even felt really, incredibly well. A tease, if you like. During this time, however, I kept visualizing me performing dialysis at home. I could envisage me using the cycler but, for some reason, I simply could not see my office filled with boxes. This puzzled me because I am actually quite good at visualizing things.

My emotions varied enormously between pure disbelief, utter denial and real dread. Nothing seemed real. It was like living in a dream world. I kept hoping it would all go away. If I could do something else—try a different therapy—things might change. I carried on with my usual activities, and to all outward appearances everything was the same, other than my diet. Except that it wasn't a dream, and it wouldn't go away. My worsening condition was here to stay.

In March, as recommended by the pain specialist, I did attend a six-week pain management course. It was most useful. The facilitators themselves had chronic pain. Apparently this was mandatory. It meant that the facilitators could more easily empathize with us, the participants. Our first session was most enlightening. We were all asked to introduce ourselves and talk a bit about our pain and what the word "pain" signified for us. It was a round-table format. The first person selected to speak was sitting about four seats away from me, and the pattern would be to carry on with the next person after this person, in an anti-clockwise motion. I would speak near the end of the group. I had plenty of time to hear the others' stories before I would give mine.

The first speaker set the tone. It was clear pain had been a nightmare. Pent-up emotions poured forth like a burst dam. I felt tremendous empathy. The next person also expressed strong emotions, as did everyone else. What struck me was not so much the hidden world of pain, but rather more the hidden grief, even though it is one of the most common effects of a change in a person's circumstances, regardless of cause. Yet, very little seems to be done by the medical community to address it. I realize that doctors' primary roles are to provide symptom treatment so it is not an easy provision to offer. I also understand that grief counsellors exist, but often they are privately separated from the medical services and can be costly. It is sad to me that somehow this therapy cannot be provided as a natural part of medical treatment. Our quality of life might improve more quickly and we may not require as much anti-depressant medication to cope with our losses.

The course made me think about how the grief that accompanies pain and illness could be better handled. When we are in the midst of a crisis, we are often the most perceptive but the least receptive. I wonder whether people or patients who have had a trauma or loss could automatically receive some kind of gentle, preliminary counselling concerning the ways a trauma or loss affects people and the different feelings experienced during grieving. I'm suggesting an acknowledgement that the effects of trauma are understood, that a mixture of emotions during grief is normal, that grief follows no predictable course and that follow-up resources and support are available.

Families could also benefit from receiving information about the effects of grief on their family life. Often, it is the caregivers who bear the brunt of another's illness and incapacity. Focus is mostly placed upon the affected individual's circumstances, and families' or caregivers' needs are lost. If family support groups exist, information or resources regarding their existence would be helpful.

At the same time I was mulling this over, I was still suffering the effects of having an intestinal bowel prolapse, possibly exacerbated by my spinal cord injury, since my affected cervical vertebrae controlled my bladder and bowels. I had an appointment with a surgeon whose prognosis was that my prolapse was not sufficient to require surgery. Later, it would be a different story.

As spring turned to summer, so my creatinine levels once more resumed their upward rise. The nephrologists began to talk about booking surgery for the insertion of my peritoneal tube. This was scheduled for mid-August before the nephrologist who performed the surgery went on holidays. The peritoneal dialysis would commence about four weeks later when my site had healed. I was fully confident that, if the worst came to the worst and my kidney failed, I would not be laid low, as I had been previously. I had plenty of warning this time and would ease my way into dialysis. Everything would run smoothly.

With my impending kidney failure a foregone conclusion, I informed my friends and former colleagues. Some of my friends found the concept difficult to digest and didn't know what to say. Many seemed confused about the treatment I would receive as well as its effects. A number of them would tell me, "Oh, you will feel better once you are on dialysis. Your life will be like new." Not so. Any form of dialysis is challenging and has a huge impact on our lives. I often felt as though I were talking gobbledygook when I explained how treatment worked and the downside of kidney failure.

Others would say, "You'll get a transplant," without understanding that this was easier said than done. To receive a transplant, another person, living or deceased, needs to be involved as a donor. Kidneys do not materialize on their own, nor do hearts, lungs, pancreases or livers, for that matter. Our welfare relies on the goodwill of benevolent individuals, friends and families.

The storm is here

In spite of the increase in my creatinine levels, I was able to continue socializing with my mah-jong group, with whom I had been playing since spring 2013, and with other friends. I carried on with my physio, swimming and exercise sessions, praying all the while that I might continue to do so. Towards the end of June, however, a change occurred. I started to feel unwell, tired and weaker. My walking that I had worked so hard to improve began to deteriorate. I had difficulty maneuvering from one end of my living room to the other. It was not a long room. Simply getting up from a sitting position was hard. On one occasion, I almost fell down doing this. My spinal cord pain amplified. My intestinal issues seemed likewise to intensify. All this frightened me. Things were not progressing as planned.

Furthermore, I seemed to be in constant contact with my transplant nurse. My original transplant nurse had retired, and I was in good hands under the care of a new one. By the second week in July, I was in a bad way, so bad now I was in daily contact with my transplant nurse. We had been discussing moving my peritoneal tube insertion surgery date forward to mid-July. As the days passed, my situation worsened, so much so that one evening I called the on-call nephrologist, whom I knew well from my transplant clinic visits. The nephrologist suggested that I have the surgery even sooner, in the next few days.

The next day the nurse called, directing me to come to the hospital twenty-four hours later, at 9:00 am. The nurse would meet me in the lobby with a wheelchair and transport me to the surgery room. I managed to get there and was met by my newly named angel of mercy, who escorted me to the designated room. There, I was instructed to remove all clothing except my underwear, don a gown and lie on the bed. A blood pressure cuff was placed on my arm. I was to await the nephrologist's arrival.

Being on my own, I concentrated on my thoughts. Such a mixture! They ranged from hopeless resignation that my life would again be forever altered to an abhorrence of the notion of kidney failure and all that it entailed. The nephrologist whom I had known close to twenty years duly arrived, accompanied by a resident nephrologist. As the nephrologist carefully explained the procedure, my thoughts turned to the last seven years. It had taken this long for my kidney to fail, one year short of the time I had visualized in December 2007. The nephrologist, in introducing me to the resident, said that I had been coming to the transplant clinic for a considerable length of time and we had long been acquainted.

Having arrived in their civvies, the nephrologist and resident proceeded to prepare themselves and then the surrounding area for the surgery. As I watched the nephrologist's transformation from ordinary doctor to surgeon, dressing in surgical garb—gown, mask and head cap—I noted the meticulous, hygienic precautions and rashly wanted to proclaim, "Oh, you really are a doctor!" as though I had been treated by a charlatan all these years. Fortunately good sense prevailed. I remained silent. We forget that many of our GPs and clinical doctors are also trained surgeons, since we usually see them in less surgical settings.

I was given a local anaesthetic, ordered to remain as still as possible for my own safety and then operated on. I couldn't see what the nephrologist was doing but could hear scissors cutting a tube, and I felt an odd sense of pulling as the tube was inserted and sewn in place in my abdomen. Upon conclusion of the procedure, which probably took no more than half an hour, my new wound was covered with a surgical bandage, and I was moved to a ward. Although this was a preliminary surgery, necessary if I wanted to dialyze using peritoneal dialysis, I kept thinking I would feel better. However, I did not feel better; in fact, I felt worse.

My wound irritated me. I could feel that something had been inserted and was rubbing next to my stomach. I knew the irritation would pass in time as my body adjusted to this new attachment. Currently, though, it was an unpleasant feeling. Sometime during the day, my angel of mercy visited me, although no longer responsible for me. I was extremely moved by this gesture of goodwill, and my unbridled emotions—so much was happening to my body, my future life and my environment—flowed to the surface. The excellent care, attention and empathy I received from this nurse certainly helped me through the next twenty-four hours.

Prior to my surgery, my friend and former colleague, Kathy, had insisted on taking me home. No matter how much I protested I would be fine, she would come anyway. Kathy is "personality gal" personified, full of lively spirits and incredibly upbeat, and she possesses a fabulous sense of humour. I cannot recount the number of times our conversations have led to tears streaming down our faces as we rocked with laughter over some inanity. She was the perfect person to temper my emotional state. When the time for my discharge arrived, I could hear her distinctive, tromping footsteps coming down the hallway. There she was, full of life and merriment, equipped with the ubiquitous hospital wheelchair. Together we rolled off to the outside, her dab hands wheeling me. While I waited on the pavement for Kathy to retrieve her car, one of my nephrologists happened to walk by me. We exchanged greetings. When he expressed some sympathy for my situation, I said, "It is what it is." I wished to appear upbeat and accepting of my circumstances; inwardly, though, I felt awful. I also complimented the transplant nurse for the care and support I had received; the nephrologist concurred. Kathy drove up, helped me transfer into her car, took me home, stayed briefly and left, both of us thinking all would be fine.

As the day progressed, so did my symptoms. By the next morning, I was feeling terrible. I couldn't eat anything and had begun to retch uncontrollably. I referred to the binder I had been given while in hospital, detailing the peritoneal treatment process and telephone numbers in case I needed to contact the clinic, a nurse or the social worker. I called at once, explained my situation and was told to return to the hospital. Once again I collected my overnight bag, called a taxi and made my way to the unit. Admitted, I found myself in the same bed that I had vacated only the day before, still almost warm from my exit.

Despite the fact that my wound had not yet healed, I would receive seven hours of continuous dialysis to remove the effects of toxins built up in my system. After seven hours of dialysis, I did feel somewhat better. The following day I was to receive ten hours of continuous dialysis. My friend Elizabeth had called and said she would visit me. When she saw me, I was sitting up almost cross-legged, looking a little healthier and definitely perkier. She commented on how well I looked. I had begun to show the benefits of dialysis. I was to stay until Sunday and then be discharged. Elizabeth, although she lived some distance, said it would be no problem to drive me home. She is another former colleague and friend, one of those rare people who, once having accepted you as a friend, becomes one for life, regardless of circumstances or her busyness. The kind of friend who fills our dreams.

The continuous dialysis, although beneficial, had a downside. Draining the solution in was fine but draining out was slow, often requiring a nurse's intervention. The peritoneal dialysis nephrologist assessed my situation. "We'll make it work one way or another," the doctor said. This calmed my worries but unfortunately, about a quarter way through my second marathon dialysis session, I noticed a wet patch on my bed. My wound was leaking! My dialysis session was aborted. Normal practice was to wait four to six weeks for the site to heal prior to dialyzing full-time. I would definitely be discharged on Sunday, but not before a reminder of my pitiful state. For my final breakfast, I received a hard-boiled egg, cream of wheat, limp toast and a smattering of jam. On the other hand, my ward mate, whose kidneys had not failed, was given sausages, pancakes with butter and syrup and hash brown potatoes.

Elizabeth called on Sunday to let me know she had some unexpected papers to mark, the bane of all teachers. Her husband, Witold, would be dispatched to pick me up. I had known him for some years, but not as well as I knew Elizabeth, so I was worried about asking him to do some grocery shopping for me on the way home. It was no problem, though. "Easy to do. I shop all the time and know where everything is," he said. True to his word, in a flash, he had completed the task. "See, I know all the prices and exactly where everything is. I have it down to an art form." I was suitably impressed. He was jolly company and a good companion.

I later remarked to Elizabeth, "How lucky you are!"

Having brought me home, Witold stayed briefly, then left. Any of the well-being I had gained from my brief dialysis session quickly faded. As the evening progressed, I began to feel exceedingly unwell. The next day, as soon as I woke up, I rushed to the bathroom where once again I started retching badly. I could not eat anything and ended up lying in bed feeling worse and worse. Not only was I suffering from kidney failure but I was also experiencing increased discomfort from my intestinal prolapse.

Extremely distressed and emotionally fragile, I called my newly assigned social worker. I explained that I felt my entire situation to be hopeless. The social worker's suggestion that I might have to start with a short session on hemodialysis was like a red flag to a bull. "I would rather die than have to do hemodialysis," I responded. I must have sounded most rude and ungracious, when in reality, the social worker was only trying to help me. I also asked if I could speak to the peritoneal nephrologist, from whom I later received a call.

"See how you are feeling tomorrow. If your symptoms continue, then it might be necessary to return to hospital," the nephrologist said.

The following day, I continued to retch, couldn't eat and felt terrible. I called my social worker again. I would return to hospital on the Wednesday. I could not travel by taxi, so called an ambulance. By this time I was functioning on autopilot. I had sufficient energy and presence of mind to collect an overnight bag, dress myself and hold off retching while waiting for the ambulance. I couldn't walk and had to be taken to the ambulance in a chair. I almost completed the entire journey before being ill. I then retched almost persistently while being transferred from the ambulance to the ER.

Living in a storm

One of the first things the paramedics do at the hospital is to take a blood pressure reading. This they did and found that my heart rate was elevated. I was experiencing atrial fibrillation. My heart beat erratically for a while and then settled down on its own. Safely in an ER bed, I waited for the nephrologists to assess me. Some hours later, a decision having been made, I was sent to the kidney unit.

I was placed in a two-bed ward but was the sole occupant. I was given a bed by the window. It was wonderful to have a view, and the light streaming in ameliorated the bleakness of my clinical surroundings. I had a daily peritoneal flushing to keep my tubes lubricated, but the draining-out still proved to be a slow process. For peritoneal dialysis to be effective, our intestines need to be clear; otherwise dialysis doesn't work. (Forgive my base subject matter, but it is an essential part of peritoneal dialysis.) Since a renal diet does not include a great deal of fibre, because of the high potassium and phosphorus levels, we frequently need a "booster" to regulate us. I was given such a "'booster" to see if it might speed up the draining. It didn't seem to make much difference.

About four days later, I was moved back into my original ward. My room was needed for a more serious case. Once again I had a bed with a million-dollar view. I loved being able to watch people in the street below. One afternoon, I was gazing out of the window, observing a crowd of people in the cafeteria courtyard several floors below me. Commonly, seagulls swoop down, steal an errant crumb and swoop off. One brazen and curious seagull meandering through the various groups, oblivious to any of its surroundings and appearing to be on a definite mission, caught my attention. Back and forth it went, when it spied the cafeteria entrance ramp, and without giving it a second thought proceeded to toddle up the ramp into the cafeteria proper.

"Good foraging here," it must have conjectured. And good foraging it must have been, too, because it was some time before the seagull re-emerged, presumably belly full, unhurriedly waddling back down the ramp. So successful was this venture that, after strutting around the courtyard a little while more, it returned to the ramp and into the cafeteria for dessert. Again it reappeared many minutes later. Not a single person had noticed. I couldn't wait to share my amusement with a nurse who came by to give me some medication.

This experience of kidney failure differed from my previous one. Although unwell and in a weakened state, I was more mobile and not as seriously ill as I had been then, apart from my challenges with slow dialysis drainage, resulting in a large volume of fluid accumulating in my hands, feet and legs so that I waddled like my seagull. It was uncomfortable and caused me much fussing and anxiety even though the doctors kept reassuring me all would be well.

What really affected me was my prolapse's worsening condition. The doctors told me that it wasn't uncommon to experience a number of other physiological occurrences at the onset of kidney failure because it is a total-body involvement. Initially, the doctors felt my prolapse would be manageable, but as it deteriorated, they referred me to the surgery team. Some of the doctors were in favour of surgery, others weren't. It became pretty obvious that something needed to be done. The main surgeon was hesitant, particularly because of the kind of dialysis I was doing. Considerable discussion between the link nurse, social worker and me continued for several days. They, likewise, were concerned about me continuing with peritoneal dialysis because of the effect it might have on my wound. Finally, one of my nephrologists told me, "I really went to bat for you and persuaded the surgeon the surgery was necessary. But on one condition: that you switch to hemodialysis until your wound has healed."

This was a blow. With Robert Burns's lines, "The best-laid schemes o' mice and men…Gang aft agley" resounding in my brain, I reluctantly agreed to have a catheter inserted in my lower neck. I had no other option, bearing in mind my abdomen was going to be in a compromised situation. "This is only for six weeks, until your surgery heals." These words eased my decision.

Radiologists performed the insertion two days prior to my surgery. The operation itself was not particularly uncomfortable, but the resultant wound was itchy and somewhat tender. I now had two tubes inserted in my body: one in my abdomen and the other in my neck, not to forget the customary intravenous needle in my wrist. I couldn't shower, anyway, because of my tube and now could only carefully sponge bathe my neck and face. I could, however, wash my hair in a sink.

The following day I had my first introduction to hemodialysis. The hospital provides four carefully scheduled hemodialysis sessions each day, serving around three hundred people a week. This number includes those attending community facilities, as well. To be effective, dialysis needs to be done three times a week, usually with a two-day break in between. In-patients are slotted into the schedule depending on the availability of a bed, a machine and a nurse.

My first session was scheduled for 7:30 am. I was helped into a wheelchair and covered in blankets before being wheeled to the dialysis unit. My porter tapped a button and two very large doors opened into my new morning quarters. The morning group had been settled. Everything was quiet and peaceful. The lights were dim. The room lay in a muted, summer shadow, the only sound a gentle click, click, clicking. Acclimatizing to my new environment, I noticed pods of people, only their faces showing above white blankets. They appeared to be attached to tubes hooked up to machines, the apparent source of the clicking sound. The entire room looked like a scene from a science fiction movie in which people were being cloned or having their brains reprogrammed. I fully expected Tom Cruise to appear from nowhere—white-coated, computerized clipboard in hand, scurrying from patient to patient, fiddling with the machines, while talking into his earpiece. I commented to my nurse about my observation. My nurse said, "I have been here far too long to notice my surroundings." Strangely my subsequent visit to the hemodialysis unit provided an entirely different sight: lights blazing, bustling activity, some patients conversing, a perfectly ordinary ward except for the number of machines and nurses at work.

When the nurse removed the bandage from my new catheter site and cleaned it, I felt relief, pure solace from the itching I had endured. Each bed was equipped with an overhead TV to help pass time. I certainly understood why the other patients were draped in blankets, because I froze during my session and had to ask for more and more blankets so that instead of lying like the princess on the bed of mattresses covering the pea, I was the pea covered by mattresses. I must have eaten some breakfast after I had been attached to the dialysis machine. For the most part, my session passed in a daze. At the end, I was unhooked by whatever means the nurses did, transferred to the wheelchair, fully covered in blankets and returned to my own in-patient's bed.

I had been warned by the doctors that it would take me a while to become adjusted to hemodialysis. That was an understatement! After the porter had helped me move from wheelchair to bed, I sat on the side of my bed in a petrified state, stone-like, motionless with my hands folded on my lap. I simply sat and stared into space, seeing nothing, thinking nothing and feeling nothing. It felt as though every ounce of my lifeblood had been drained. I was conscious of only two things: being spaced out and having a horrible taste in my mouth. I remained in this position and in this state for several hours. Gradually, I felt my blood begin to flow again, and some energy return. I was then able to get up and walk around. I experienced the same sensations for many dialysis sessions. It took me a long time to rebound from each session.

The principle of the electronic hemodialysis machine is to cleanse the toxins from the blood. It has a monitor on which weight, running temperature, amount of fluid and time for the session is recorded. Other information is routinely checked to ensure everything is working effectively. Two lines, one of which has first been attached to a saline drip, are connected once our sites have been thoroughly cleaned. There are a plethora of lines connecting to a jug of potassium mixture and bag of calcium that are connected to our main lines. They resemble a jumble of interweaving lines. The two lines attached to our fistulas work in sync: one to remove our blood to be cleansed and the other to return our clean blood. The artificial kidney looks like an elongated tube hanging attached to the side of the dialysis machine, resembling nothing remotely human. My lines are connected to my catheter that flows directly to my heart. The entire dialysis process takes about four hours to complete.

The routine starts with a weighing-in to determine the amount of fluid needing to be removed. We have a goal weight, the amount we should weigh at the end of our session, when we weigh ourselves again. The nurse calculates the amount of fluid to be removed based on our current weight and our goal weight then records both our present weight and the amount of fluid to be removed on the computer. We have our temperature taken to ensure we don't have a fever, and are well. As with weight, our temperature is taken both at the beginning and ending of each session. Next, we have a blood pressure cuff that is connected to the dialysis machine attached to one of our arms and are tested twice, once standing and once sitting before being hooked up to the machine. Our blood pressure is continually monitored throughout the dialysis process. A sudden change in blood pressure could affect the efficacy of the dialysis itself and indicate a change in our well-being. Although hemodialysis machines are computerized and easily programed to meet our individual needs, they are intricate and require considerable scrutiny. The nurses need to constantly check that everything is running smoothly and that the machine is doing what it should be doing. We either lie in a bed or sit in a specially designed chair. Patients usually sleep or watch TV; some may read. It is difficult for us to move, much due to our lines being attached to the hemodialysis machine.

The day after my introductory session, I had the prolapse repair surgery. The surgeon visited me the eve of my surgery to prepare me, forewarning me that it would be a painful procedure, although straightforward. Around midday, shortly before my surgery, I was given a sedative and carted off to the OR. Following a short wait, most likely chatting aimlessly while the anaesthetic took effect, the surgery was performed. Without a doubt, the pain was intense when I awoke. Even though I have been warned about the pain to come, I am never prepared for surgery's full impact. I lay in a fetal position on my right side, my left hand grabbing the bedside frame in a vice grip while I whispered plaintively to the recovery nurse beside me, "More painkiller, please, and please stay with me, holding my hand." The nurses couldn't have been kinder and more solicitous and did indeed remain by my side, taking turns to tenderly hold my hand. That in itself comforted me for what seemed hours. I believe I stayed in the recovery room well into the night.

Then the pain mysteriously subsided, and I was returned to my own bed. Hunger now replaced pain; I craved a piece of cheese. The night nurse obliged. I slept well that night and woke to one fleeting hope. A post-surgery blood test showed a tremendous drop in my creatinine level. Was I going to be all right, after all? "Not so fast," said the nurse. "Probably only a result of pre-surgery fasting." And so it was.

Members of the surgery team checked me the next day, pronounced all was well, recommended a soft diet and suggested I get up. I shuffled and hobbled more, but the excruciating pain had disappeared. Fortunately, I could walk. As long as I remained bedridden, I would receive two daily Heparin injections to prevent my blood from clotting. The injections themselves were painless but the after-effect was not. It felt as though I had been stabbed by a sharp knife, a sensation unpleasant enough for me to raise myself Lazarus-like from my bed. Because I was weak, I asked if I could have a physiotherapist help me in my early attempts. I would hold the physiotherapist's arm with one hand, cane in the other, while my physiotherapist maneuvered my intravenous pole as I stumbled down the corridor. I was surprised by my stamina. I attributed it to the year I had spent working hard on my fitness level. Gradually I was able to walk on my own and spent as much time as I could walking up and down the corridors, determined to sidestep "those injections." I began to meet other patients who were sitting in the patients' lounge—a social life was unfolding before me.

Kidney patients are among the most conversationally prone and sociable people I have ever met in hospital. We are only too willing to share our stories and involve each other in conversations with families and friends. We were part of a club, so to speak, brought together by our mutual bond of kidney disease. During one long weekend, I met four patients who were recovering from having received transplants. Greeting some of them effusively in the lounge, I said, "Well, you must feel absolutely fabulous," remembering how I had felt after my transplant surgery. My enthusiasm was met with perplexed looks.

"I am feeling a little better," one of them weakly said. I learned that not everyone feels an instantaneous sense of well-being. For some, kidney transplants take a while to work effectively. These are called "sleepy" kidneys. Some recipients require top-up dialysis. One patient had a biopsy during the week to assess the kidney's status. All ended up working well, and fingers crossed, I hope continues to do so.

One of the recipients, John, was helpful to me regarding my new status as a hemodialysis patient, and told me, "Hemodialysis is what it is. You just have to embrace it and accept that this is what you need to do." He also explained to me, "You won't understand this now, but I always ask the nurses to run the machine at 350. I tell them, too, you need to remove such and such amount of fluid *this* time." His advice helped me because hemodialysis was an enigma to me.

When I told my new friend that my kidney had lasted twenty-two years, his response was astounding. "Well, if mine lasts half that long, I'll be happy." Every time a visitor came, John would say, "You have to meet her. Her kidney lasted twenty-two years. Isn't that something? Just think about mine." I hope that my words gave him some degree of optimism for the future.

John also gave me this warning: "Kidney failure carries with it the possibility of side effects. You need to prepare yourself for losing people you get to know. It has happened to me several times during the years I have been on dialysis. One time the fellow who was receiving dialysis beside me suffered a heart attack." I held onto these words. It is not common for people to die during dialysis but some patients do have crises and need to be sent to the ER or even the ICU.

My bed with the million-dollar view was in a four-patient ward. One day, a fairly ill individual was admitted to the bed opposite me. My new roommate, who had had a kidney transplant that had unfortunately failed after only a few years, was on peritoneal dialysis. The patient had acquired an internal infection. The doctors weren't sure what had caused the infection and wanted to find its source.

What impressed me were the efforts they put into their search. As with me during my prolapse surgery, the patient was visited by a variety of specialists. Doctors are, at root, scientists. They are researchers and explorers who possess an abundance of curiosity. Their scientific minds tell them that for every problem, there must be a solution, as with Spock, who, given the same circumstances, could have said, "It is illogical not to have a logical answer." They were persistent in their quest to find the answer.

To this end, my ward mate was probed and prodded, tested and retested by various specialists. I only know this from observing numerous white-coated medical staff entering the closed curtains and from the number of times the patient was wheeled off for further examinations. As patients or everyday folk, we do not always see doctors in action. We know they are strenuously trained, have an enormous amount of medical knowledge and seem to either know instantly what is wrong with us or vaguely offer us some kind of haphazard guess. We rarely see them in full investigative mode. It was most enlightening and heartening to know that really they do have a vested interest in healing us, their patients.

Unfortunately, my ward mate's condition started deteriorating. I was again reminded of my previous kidney failure and how I had declined. I think at this time there were only two of us occupying the ward. On a return from one of the tests, the patient had lapsed into a semi-conscious state. The doctor on duty, seeing the patient in this condition, immediately pushed the emergency button, sounding the alarm. A nurse appeared from nowhere and summarily closed my curtains. Seconds later, the corridor was abuzz with sound and activity. I could hear the clomping of feet and noise of equipment thumping towards the ward. What sounded like an army of doctors suddenly bolted into the ward.

A large light was lit and voices everywhere began to call out. Then a male voice called out, "Only one person speak at a time." Someone obviously had taken charge and proceeded to decide what to do next. Fortunately, the problem seemed to be resolved fairly quickly. The patient must have been revived and was duly transported to ICU. All was quiet again. From my perspective behind the curtain, it was like being on a movie set in an episode of an ER type of program. I fully expected to hear the words, "Cut. That's a wrap," as the doctors and patient trundled off down the hallway. In actuality, the way in which the emergency team responded was overwhelmingly astounding. When the alarm rings, the doctors are right there. I really felt in good hands.

I had no idea if I would ever see my ward mate again. I was very surprised to see the patient return to the ward about four days later, looking so much better. The cause of the infection had been found, and the patient was on the mend. It was miraculous to see the change in this person who was now alert, talking, laughing and visiting with friends and family. The patient was then moved to a different ward, and when I next saw the patient, it was in the lounge, an infinitely healthier-looking person, waiting to be discharged.

It caused me to think how doctors, who live with life and death on an everyday basis and witness the frailties of illness, are humans, too. They undoubtedly feel emotions as we do, but are maybe just a little better at masking them. They must live on a roller coaster of feelings as they watch patients falter and survive. I can only imagine how disappointing it could be to work on a treatment or cure only to have it fail. Similarly so, how rewarded they must feel when a treatment is successful. I can only compare this to how my colleagues and I felt when our students struggled. We would agonize with them, and when they did well, we would celebrate their successes as though they were our own. Or how parents anguish over their children's well-being. I recalled the many years ago when I had regained my strength, having been so ill prior to receiving my kidney transplant, and on a follow-up hospital appointment happened to meet one of the doctors who had cared for me in the months when I was hospitalized. Seeing me in better health, he seemed to be delighted.

Weighing on my mind was my renal diet, itself not improved by the hospital meals. The hospital menu planners tried to vary our diet and attempted to whet our appetite with fancy-sounding entree choices, but the end product always resembled something less than its name suggested. I dreamt of forbidden pleasures such as the soothing comfort of a baked potato stuffed with butter, sour cream and chives, the appetizing, thirst-quenching taste of a cold lager on a hot day, the sensual succulence of a chocolate as it gradually melts and slides down the throat, the crisp, snapping, salty crunch of potato chips, the aroma of freshly made French fries and their piquant flavour, and the luxurious, velvety lick of a tasty ice-cream cone, made even more glorious on a sunny day. And to this day, as I nibble on my plain crackers or digestive biscuits, I dream of these pleasures.

All was not lost, however. The dietician who paid me frequent visits asked me if I liked cooking. I said, "Oh, yes, absolutely." For the next visit, my dietician came with two small booklets in hand. They were two copies of a publication called *Spice It Up*,[1] containing recipes tailor-made for renal patients. My dietician is among a group of national dieticians who work with a chef to create an assortment of recipes ranging from appetizers, soups, salads and sandwiches to entrees and desserts. My two copies consisted of a variety of summer and general recipes. The first recipe that caught my eye: mushroom pasta. Mushrooms had been eliminated from my renal diet but here was one in full view! I was astounded by this, but the dietician reassured me all the recipes had been adapted to our needs.

I pored over these booklets for the remainder of my time in hospital, reading and rereading them, thinking of the culinary delights I could make once home. Anyone who lives with a renal diet will relate to my rapture. Having a varied and interesting diet makes all the difference. I have since received a number of copies of *Spice It Up* and have used many recipes when entertaining my non-renal-diet friends.

During my time in hospital, I did not have many visitors for two reasons. First of all, not many people knew I was in hospital, and second, I actually suggested that friends not come because of my dialysis schedule, surgery and various tests I underwent. I did not feel alone or forgotten, because in hospital there is always something happening and someone to talk to. My emotions sat close to the surface, too. I varied between considerable optimism and lassitude. So much seemed to have happened to me over a fairly short space of time. I was in a shambles of feelings for a while. The nurses helped, and I was visited frequently by the renal social worker. I can imagine my state was probably like many other patients who are affected by dramatic changes in lifestyle and find the transition from one situation to another more complex than imagined. Ironically, the endless pain I had been suffering didn't bother me much during my hospital stay. Why, I have no idea.

Three people did visit me, though. My old school friend, Rosemary, whom I had known since grade six until we graduated in grade twelve and then had reconnected at a class reunion some years ago. It was a joy for me to see her and a wonderfully spirit-lifting visit. Old friends are like gold to us, especially as we age. My good friend, Elizabeth, and my brother, Robert, whose busy schedule frequently meant having to make arrangements long in advance but who happened to be available now, were my two others. Robert acted as my liaison between home and hospital. My recent in-and-out-of-hospital experience had left me either with a fridge full of food or an empty pantry. Robert could restore the balance by removing the surplus and filling the gap. As well, he could bring me needed things. On one such visit, Robert, not known for his housekeeping skills—home to him representing simply a place in which to lay his head—rather cheekily said to me, "When you get home, you'll need to do some tidying up." In other words, I must have left a considerable mess behind when I unexpectedly ended up in hospital. He was right. When I finally did return home, I was amazed to see the chaos. I must have been in a very disordered state the last few days of my kidney failure.

I also had a number of calls from Roland, who told me he could visit me for three weeks at the end of August. This was unexpected, fabulous news. Prior to being discharged towards the middle of August, I met with the discharge social worker who organized Meals-on-Wheels and a shop-by-phone grocery service for me. Robert collected me from hospital and took me home. I tried to tidy my condo as best I could, and excitedly awaited Roland's arrival.

I was to attend hemodialysis sessions three times a week for four hours each time, on Mondays and Fridays for the evening sessions and on Wednesdays for the afternoon session. My weekends were free. I would travel there and back by HandyDART. There was one complication, though. My hemoglobin level had dropped significantly. The doctors were concerned in case I had some internal bleeding. They stopped adding heparin into my dialysis machine, which in turn caused the dialysis machine to beep because my blood consistently clotted. This required the session to be restarted, adding time to my sessions. The solution was for me to have an already scheduled colonoscopy appointment moved forward to early September, coinciding with Roland's visit.

New storm clouds

A few days following my discharge, I experienced further intestinal discomfort and began retching. It couldn't have been kidney failure because I was receiving treatment. My recent surgery had been successful. It had to be from another cause. I was quite alarmed. The symptoms did not improve, so early one evening I went to the emergency department. The examining doctor decided I should have an abdominal scan using a highlighting dye. I had the scan around 11:00 in the evening. As I was being wheeled back to the emergency waiting room, the porter began chatting, "I really understand what you are going through with hemodialysis. I know how terrible you all feel. Okay for a short while afterwards, then bad again before your next session. I have been working with hemodialysis patients for a long time. Dialysis is not a pleasant thing to have to do."

Then he assured me, "You should have the results in half an hour." Half hour came and went: no results. An hour lapsed; still no results. By 12:30 am, I had yet to see a doctor. By 1:30, with a steadily emptying waiting room, no doctor had appeared. Well after 2:00, the doctor finally returned to my side. "I am really sorry to have been so long," the doctor said. "But I wanted to check with a nephrologist first and then with other colleagues. You have diverticulosis, small pouches in the colon where food can become trapped, but the good news is it is not diverticulitis, a more serious condition."

> Diverticulitis occurs when the colon pouches become infected, resulting in pain and sometimes fever. Antibiotic treatment is required to treat it.

Before I had time to respond, the doctor continued, "Has anyone ever mentioned cancer to you?"

"No."

"The radiologist is pretty certain you have cancer in one of your native kidneys. There is a mass in your right kidney that looks suspiciously like cancer."

I knew I had had cysts in my native kidneys but never expected a diagnosis of cancer. These words shocked me. I explained to the doctor about my cysts but didn't believe I had cancer.

The doctor replied, "The radiologist really feels it is cancer. I am sorry to be giving you this news quite like this, and at this time in the morning." That sounded humorous; such information would have been hard to digest at any time. Since I was to return for midday dialysis, the doctor suggested I stay the night in the emergency ward. I agreed, never thinking I would sleep. Surprisingly, I did and woke around 6:00 am to bright lights, scurrying activity and loud voices. The ER was once more in full swing.

My reaction to this latest news? Learning I had diverticulosis was certainly unwelcome information. It would be an added complication, but I knew it was a fairly common occurrence. Kidney cancer, on the other hand, was a shock. I think I entered a kind of suspended consciousness. I could hear myself repeat the information to my nephrologists but the words I spoke were merely empty echoes from my mouth. I must have remained in this kind of sub-world until my nephrectomy later in the autumn. Life carried on, just slightly off-kilter.

Roland arrived, and such pleasure it was to have him by my side once more. It so happened that on the weekend of his arrival, my cousin from Seattle, Deborah, also arrived for a short visit. I have one small bedroom, a den—in this case my second bedroom—and a large office space, but the three of us muddled along well together. We even managed to host a dinner party for a number of other friends, with Roland, the major chef, taking charge of the meal. It was great fun and definitely a marvellous remedy for my continuous challenges. Roland and Deborah took turns driving me to and from my dialysis sessions. Having a break from HandyDART was a welcome respite, too.

The scheduled colonoscopy required the removal of only a few small polyps, and it confirmed the diverticulosis diagnosis but showed nothing more serious. I could be given heparin freely. No more clotting while receiving dialysis. The kidney cyst was a different matter. Roland accompanied me for my appointment with the kidney surgeon, who showed us evidence of the cyst. We could both see the size and shape of it. It was large, flowing into the gap between my kidney and liver. "I am 85 percent certain it is cancer. I expect to perform the surgery either later in October or early in November," the surgeon said. I was assured that receiving a future transplant should not be a problem, providing the cancerous kidney and cyst could be fully removed. It did, however, necessitate further delaying my return to peritoneal dialysis. All would be fine eventually, though, as long as my peritoneal membrane remained intact during surgery. There was a risk that in the course of removing the kidney my peritoneal membrane could be cut. We both left the surgeon's office stunned but didn't discuss the prognosis. Somehow, deep inside, I felt positive that everything would be all right in the end.

That early fall was lovely and warm. Roland and I decided to spend the afternoon at the neighbourhood beach. It was mostly deserted. We chose a patio seat near a food kiosk that afforded us a panoramic view of the water and land. We had a simple junk-food meal that to most people would have been everyday fare, but for me, I was savouring forbidden pleasures, a moment of ecstasy and relief from my renal diet. Sitting together on a sundrenched deck, watching the swath of water glistening brightly under a cloudless sky, listening to the waves gently lapping against the shoreline—this was sublime. We didn't need to talk. Being together was enough. In my dark hours, I cherish this memory.

Roland's presence rekindled a longing for entertaining and socializing once more. My dialysis schedule had curtailed my mah-jong playing days, but the recipe books revived my interest in cooking. After Roland had returned to Belgium, my health permitted me to keep the social flames alive. I had a dinner party pretty much every weekend that autumn. I scoured recipes, both renal and non-renal, planning menus and dishes. I was determined to make up for lost time and see as many of my friends as I could. One afternoon I even managed to have a traditional tea party, with fancy handcrafted sandwiches, scones and pastries, for eight of my friends. The previous day I had been feeling really rough, hardly able to move, but the next day I somehow recovered sufficient strength to make the sandwiches and assemble the food. My tea party was a success, the novelty of it alone creating a merry atmosphere.

Late in September I received a date for my nephrectomy surgery: Thursday, October 30. I would be in hospital for only four days. I knew the routine. Arrive at the hospital in the early morning, meet with the anaesthetist, be prepped and taken to the surgical pre-room, chattering inanities in the intervening time, wait briefly before being moved to the OR, wake up in intense pain in the recovery ward and receive medication to ease it.

This time I woke to hear a number of voices by my bedside engaged in fervent conversation: I had begun to have atrial fibrillation—my heart was beating far too fast. I was constantly monitored throughout the rest of the day and overnight. The next day it continued. I stayed in the recovery ward, a nurse keeping vigilance by my side, only leaving while the hemodialysis nurse sat with me for the entire four hours of my dialysis session. I have never felt so well cared for. When I became well enough for the regular hospital ward, the reality of normal nursing care was a letdown.

While I was still in the recovery ward, the surgeon visited me to let me know that everything had been removed successfully and that I should receive the biopsy results in about ten days. However, in the process of removing my kidney, the surgeon had nicked my peritoneal membrane, thus further delaying my return to peritoneal dialysis. The surgeon told me, "Unfortunately, you have a very thin peritoneal membrane and I could not help snipping it when I removed your kidney." My promised six weeks had now been extended a further six weeks.

I also had a brief consultation with a cardiologist who had been called for advice regarding my atrial fibrillation. The cardiologist prescribed medication to prevent a stroke. This was equally unpalatable news. I would need to see the cardiologist again in a month's time. Finally, the following day, my heart rate returned to normal, and I was sent to the surgery ward later that afternoon. I had been in the recovery ward for almost three days. Later it was confirmed that I have episodic atrial fibrillation. I take a baby aspirin every other day as a preventative measure against a stroke.

My home for the next three days was another hospital bed with a million-dollar view in a four-bed ward. A public ward can result in an interesting mix of people, often a combination of very ill and less ill patients, irrespective of gender or age. An understanding of both openness and privacy exists. Because only thin curtains separate us from one another, there exists an unwritten code of etiquette. While we might be extremely open and chummy when we are alone, our behaviour changes when visitors arrive. Then, we become invisible to each other.

Those of us who live with chronic illness are more likely to encounter others similarly affected within the medical community. The grisly face of illness is never far from our domain. However, no matter how badly we might feel, there is always someone who feels worse. This time, I was relatively unscathed compared with my roommates. We were four—three women and one man who had either had, or were going to have, intestinal surgery as a result of cancer. I saw first-hand the brutal effects of colorectal cancer. It was not a benign sight. All the patients had had colon surgery and now needed colostomy bags. The courage, optimism and good humour of my fellow patients made a huge impression on me.

One of my roommates had wonderful artistic skills. I saw pictures of pieces of art that had been in a number of exhibitions. I also met the patient's spouse, an avid chef who visited daily, bringing tasty, home-cooked meals. Having undergone colorectal surgery a year ago, the patient had been in hospital for some time, being treated for a bladder tear. The treatment, in itself most unpleasant, was not proving to be effective. The patient confided, "It just feels never ending." It was an ordeal; however, the patient's fortitude was remarkable, brave and courageous.

One night, however, the stoicism broke. I could hear the muffled tears, almost concealed by a pillow, expressing feelings of frustration and despair. These are the private moments we keep hidden from public view, because we understand the need to retain a sense of dignity in the face of real personal battles. My heart wept in empathy. My fellow patients were still in hospital when I was discharged.

As far as my own cancer biopsy was concerned, about two weeks after my surgery I received a phone call from the surgeon. It was good news: my cyst was not cancerous. I was in the clear.

My unwelcome forecast

During the six weeks following prolapse surgery and subsequent nephrectomy, I had been having weekly peritoneal dialysis flushes. The results were always the same: easy in but slow out, irrespective of the volume. One of the nephrologists finally called a halt: "We have tried successive times to use this method. It clearly isn't working. I am afraid you are going to have to continue with hemodialysis." Not words I wanted to hear, but inevitable. Obviously I was absorbing more liquid than I could drain out. I think I knew this from the beginning, even before I started, when I couldn't visualize the boxes of dialysis solution in my office.

This heralded yet another paradigm shift. An aversion to doing hemodialysis had blocked my thoughts. It meant having to attend dialysis sessions three times a week, having a permanent fistula inserted somewhere in my body, living with a restricted diet and fluid intake and accepting the probability of feeling consistently fatigued. Now, there was no option. The same doctor who had inserted my peritoneal dialysis tube removed it in mid-November, using local anaesthetic. For some reason I developed a large hematoma or blood clot that persisted for months. Fortunately, the bruise that spread from my stomach down to my thighs was not painful; it looked worse than it was. Having accepted my new life, I began my regularly scheduled hemodialysis sessions.

Towards the end of November, though, my neuropathic pain increased. I started experiencing severe—really severe—neck and head pain. St. Augustine of Hippo, a philosopher in the fourth century, said, "There is no evil like pain." He was right. All intense pain is horrid, but pain associated with the back, neck and head seems even more terrible. It made my dialysis sessions a torture because I could never find a comfortable position. I tried using the hemodialysis-designed chair to no avail. It only seemed to exacerbate my back discomfort. I tried sitting on the side of the bed, but this caused the machines to beep and require constant rejigging by the nurses. Lying down was equally painful because it heightened the tension in my neck. Some of the nurses nimbly massaged my neck. How I revelled in their tender touch as they tried to gently ease my pain or kindly laid ice packs on my neck. I lived on hydromorphone during my dialysis sessions, every one of which I dreaded.

One of the nephrologists re-referred me to the pain doctor, and in January I resumed physiotherapy, as well as acupuncture and massage therapy. As the months passed, some of the pain's intensity abated. I still require physiotherapy, acupuncture and massage therapy just to maintain equilibrium. My pain doctor has prescribed a new medication, but I used it sparingly, because it made me feel nauseated. To lessen the nausea, I used Gravol.

I wanted to start swimming again, and the physiotherapist agreed that I could have water therapy in conjunction with regular physio. I had to check with the nurses if I could safely cover my catheter, which the doctors had decided I should keep instead of replacing it with a fistula. They thought my veins had most likely collapsed due to the effects of scleroderma. With excited thoughts and visions floating through my head of once again returning to water, I asked one of the nurses. "No," the nurse said and explained that my catheter was in essence open to my heart. An infection would be lethal. There was no safe way of covering my catheter to keep water from entering my system. This was devastating news to me. I had been a serious swimmer, a water baby, and had just been reacquainted with my love of water through my swimming classes. The effects of kidney failure can be extensive.

Routine weather

I had been having dialysis for over six months by this time. Many of the mysteries of the hemodialysis process have become clear. I understand how the nurses connect my catheter lines to the dialysis machine. Their carefully trained hands caringly perform their important tasks. They begin with removing my covering bandage, then cleanse the wound with a swab, which in my case contains no alcohol since I proved sensitive to it, and put on two new small Mepore bandages before cleaning the lines themselves with gauze soaked in antiseptic solution. Prior to attaching my catheter lines to the dialyzing lines, they use small syringes to flush my catheter lines, first to check the blood flow and then to ensure my entryway is clear.

During the cleansing stage, both the nurses and I wear a mask to ensure no bacteria contaminate the open site. At the end of my dialysis session, the nurses replace the blood removed during dialysis, then once again clean the catheter lines and inject a further saline flush before injecting a citrate compound to prevent blood clots forming in the catheter tubes. Finally they wrap my entire catheter lines with a bandage and tape the wrapped lines with a signed label indicating I have been given the citrate fluid. I can taste both the saline and the citrate fluid. The saline flush feels as though I have swallowed a giant mouthful of salt water. The citrate fluid has a paint-like taste. Both tastes linger and never really dissipate. I soon learned that I could ask for half a vial of saline to reduce the aftertaste but could not do the same with the citrate fluid.

Also I now understand the number "350" mentioned by John many months ago. It means 350 ml per minute and refers to the speed at which the blood is circulated through the system. It is the rate at which all the blood gets pumped through the artificial kidney so that it circulates about twenty times during a four-hour session. The higher the rate, the faster the blood is pumped through our system and the better toxin clearance; similarly, the slower the speed, the slower the blood is pumped through and the fewer toxins are removed. The nurses prefer to run the dialysis machine at 350, but it is not always possible. For me, the speed has frequently needed to be lowered because for some reason I seem to be sensitive to movement and other unknown variables.

I have also become conversant with the amount of fluid removed. The doctors give me a goal weight to attain at the end of dialyzing. After I have weighed myself prior to dialysis and reported my weight to the nurse, the nurse calculates the amount of fluid that needs to be removed in order to achieve my goal weight. It is a tricky calculation, one that doesn't always work out correctly, depending on the machine used. All machines have one thing in common, namely their ability to work according to plan. I have, on a number of occasions, gone home being what is referred to as "on the wet side," meaning heavier than intended, as well as on other occasions "on the dry side," meaning being lower in weight than intended. If too much fluid is removed, two things can happen. I can experience terrible cramps in my legs and feet, or I can crash, which means my blood pressure drops dramatically and I feel extremely ill and nauseated. Both can be easily rectified, the former by adding saline and the latter by reducing the machine's speed to minimum or by ending the dialysis session. Some of my fellow patients have blood pressure crashes easily, not necessarily related to fluid removal.

The machine temperature is kept on the cool side so that the blood flows easily through my veins. Research has recently shown that the lower temperature better protects us from having strokes. The nurse programs the temperature on the machine. It is most commonly kept at 36°C. This explains why we feel terribly cold throughout dialysis and need many blankets to keep warm. I have had as many as six blankets covering me, this on a warm day. I also wear gloves because my hands freeze, in part due to poor circulation caused by my Raynaud's disease, and in part because of my spinal cord injury. Many patients bring their own pillows, duvets and blankets, preferring their home comforts to the hospital's provisions.

Every three months or so, I have my lines checked to assess the efficacy of blood clearance. This procedure is performed using a Transonic machine. The machine has two lines with clamps on it that are connected to my two dialysis lines. Once connected and turned on, the machine reads the amount of blood flow. A low number is good. So far, my results have been fine. I also have yearly TB checks and other tests to find out if I have contracted any infections. I have also had jaundice and pneumonia vaccinations as an extra protection.

One of the downsides of the dialysis process, whether peritoneal or hemodialysis, is the removal of proteins from our bodies. All dialysis recipients require extra amounts of protein. This must be done while maintaining potassium and phosphorus levels. I have tried drinking supplements, but prefer using powdered protein supplements mixed in my food. I take calcium pills, called binders, prior to eating in order to bind uncaptured phosphorus.

Hygiene plays an important role in the dialysis ward. We are constantly reminded to wash our hands whenever we eat or touch any equipment, machines or scales. At the end of every session, the beds are stripped and thoroughly disinfected, as are the equipment, machinery and TV monitors. Anything that drops on the floor receives equal cleansing. I am required to wipe the scales each time I use them so they are clean for the next person. I cannot count the number of times my cane has been cleaned because it is forever falling down.

Living with new weather patterns

How has dialysis affected me? It is a peculiar state. There is no doubt that I feel infinitely better than I did a couple of years ago, but the effects are evident. I have experienced the frightening and helpless state of crashing while on dialysis. The symptoms usually start with a sudden spike in body temperature, followed by a weird feeling of uncontrollable disconnection and waves of nausea, as one experiences with seasickness, although at sea we feel dreadful but once on land fine. As soon as the nurses adjust our temperature by either raising or lowering it on the machine, or discontinue dialysis, we return to normal. My most recent experience occurred towards the last half hour of one of my dialysis sessions. I crashed, was sick and felt awful. The nurse immediately stopped the dialysis, but it took me ages to recover. Even after I had arrived home, I still felt the scary, unpleasant effects of the crash.

I have also found out what it is like to have low calcium levels. Too much calcium has a detrimental effect on the heart, as does too little calcium. It is important to keep levels balanced, hence the need to include a calcium solution in the dialysis treatment. For some reason, my calcium levels started falling. This happened over a period of time. I began to notice an increase in leg twitching at home. As I have restless legs, I was not overly concerned, but during my dialysis sessions the twitching increased in both strength and duration. A nurse who watched me as I twitched said, "I can only imagine how uncomfortable you must feel. I can hardly bear to watch you in this state." The twitching continued and then manifested itself elsewhere on my body. I lost control over my limbs. They would jerk uncontrollably. Then my entire body was affected.

I must have looked incredibly odd, even comical. During one of my more robotic moments, a doctor who happened to be doing the rounds watched me. I had been standing even though it caused the machine to beep, because the twitching and constant robotic spasms prevented me from sitting or lying down. The doctor said, "It is as though your whole body is contorting. I am going to check your calcium levels," and went off to do so. Minutes later, the doctor told me my calcium levels were slightly below the appropriate level and ordered an increase in the calcium fluid. In the next session my equilibrium returned to normal, and calcium levels no longer cause me to behave in a robotic fashion.

Restless legs are a common byproduct of kidney failure, resulting from an imbalance in electrolyte levels. In my case, restless legs have had a major impact on my well-being and social life. I have sometimes had to forego socializing because of having lain awake the entire night, suffering the effects of restless leg symptoms. Because of the syndrome, I have been put on a different dialysis program, one called hemodiafiltration, which removes larger toxin molecules from the blood.

I also take a special medication to remediate the extra effects of restless legs. Both have helped. Not only do I feel better, but I also have reduced symptoms. I feel almost human again.

Still, because of the effects of both kidney failure and hemodialysis, I live with constant, extreme fatigue, and I often feel nauseated and always unwell. I spend an inordinate part of each day just lying down. Since my activity is limited, I am alone much of the time. It is hard to gauge how I will feel, so it is difficult to plan for things or follow through with plans. After hemodialysis, I am subject to greater spinal cord pain. My hands burn and pulsate and my arms throb severely. I often wake up at night in severe pain and find it hard to resettle comfortably. Lack of sleep affects my mobility. My flexibility and walking have deteriorated so my movements become laboured and clumsy. Fortunately, the pain abates slightly the following day.

Prior to a dialysis session, I can feel the fluid retention in my hands and feet. My hands swell and hurt. My toes, already compromised by my spinal cord injury, feel like wooden pegs. This is particularly evident on the second day of the weekend and is more noticeable on the Monday of dialysis. Ideally, those of us who do hemodialysis really need to dialyze every other day in order to maintain a greater sense of wellness. I doubt that any patient would wish to do so, though, because we all need a break from the rigours of dialysis. Also, scheduling would be difficult.

Many kidney patients experience what is called "peripheral numbness." Kidney failure somehow seems to affect our nerve responses. I have been told by the doctors that even with a kidney transplant, the peripheral numbness may never improve. I am fortunate in that I have not been so affected.

The diet is also antisocial. Restricted foods make it hard to dine out. I know for sure that I would never be able to work were I still of working age. I spend about twenty-one hours a week either on dialysis or waiting for dialysis. It is comparable to a full-time job and requires a commitment. Whatever form of dialysis we do, it only serves to maintain our lives. It is not a cure for kidney failure and can never remove all the accumulated toxins.

The entire dialysis process is wearing. When waiting for HandyDART with my fellow dialysis patients, I can see the result of the four hours of continual blood re-circulation. Everybody looks drained and exhausted and either shuffles to a seat or is too weak to stand so is wheeled by a porter to the waiting area. The agony is frequently prolonged as HandyDART is timed for regulated pick-ups. Dialysis patients are transported in groups, so if a patient finishes earlier, the added waiting time increases fatigue levels.

Once the HandyDART driver has arrived and we have joined the regular passengers for our homeward journeys, our moods, spirits and conviviality return. We forget our dialysis session as we engage in lively and animated conversation. We are returned to our previous, happy state of mind. We live with the knowledge that while we may be experiencing trying times, we are not alone. We share a common bond. Life presents obstacles but our approach is *"Que sera, sera."*

Chapter 5 | Friends along the Way

Each friend represents a world in us, a world not born until they arrive, and it is only by this meeting that a new world is born.

—Anaïs Nin, *The Diary of Anaïs Nin, 1931–1934*

New connections

"How long have you been coming to hemodialysis?"

"This will be my third time," was the response. "I am finding it hard to adjust to the changes in my life. Kidney failure is new to me."

"Don't worry. It will get easier each time you come. It just takes time. None of us want to be here. But we are in this together."

I overheard this conversation between two strangers continue as each one shared mutual concerns and expressed otherwise private feelings.

Life is unpredictable. We are not immune to its quixotic nature. Changes in circumstances take us on different paths and can bring us into contact with those whom we would never have met had it not been for our new situation. My current lifestyle is very much a product of a change in circumstances.

Because of my time in hospital and my hemodialysis sessions, and because kidney failure is a long-term condition remedied only by possibly receiving a transplant or by death, I could spend years together with other kidney patients and am therefore more likely to form lasting friendships with them. Consequently, I have begun to make a whole set of new friends, friends who have influenced me greatly for their courage, strength and resilience during difficult times. My life has indeed been made richer through my varied personal experiences. It is almost as though I have had to endure the trials and tribulations in order to appreciate the valiant champions living amongst us.

When I had my first kidney failure, I was like a lone wolf in the wilderness. I had never met anyone else with kidney failure or kidney disease. Following my transplant, my initial contact with other kidney patients was in the transplant clinics both in England and Vancouver. Over the years I met others who had had their second transplants. Although the other patients and I would engage in conversation, the chances of our meeting regularly were rare because of everyone's different clinic appointments. We did not necessarily form lasting ties, not from disinterest but rather as a result of our differing schedules.

Through work connections I met three other transplant recipients, the first a colleague who taught in another department. When we would see each other on occasion at faculty meetings or workshops, our conversation circled around our kidneys' well-being and our health in general. My colleague retired a few years earlier than me. Since we both live in the same neighbourhood, I have on occasion met her while shopping or doing errands. Her kidney transplant, now more than fifteen years old, continues to function well.

The second transplant recipient I met through work connections is the partner of a close colleague, someone whom I have known for almost twenty years. My twin—as I refer to him, because we received transplants the same year but in different locations—continues to do very well, his creatinine levels within the normal range.

The third transplant recipient happened to be a student of mine. We would occasionally compare notes about how our kidneys were doing. My student had had two transplants, one lasting seven years and the other ten years, as I later learned through a chance meeting following the end of our time together.

During my swimming days, I met another transplant recipient who worked in commercial sales, and whose kidney was functioning well after twenty-six years. When I told my fellow-swimmer I was in the throes of kidney failure, the response to me was, "Well, I look at it this way. I already died when my kidney failed twenty-six years ago so everything else is a bonus." I also learned that it was a struggle to keep working while on hemodialysis because of the schedule and its after-effects. "It was taxing," I was told. "My quality of life has been improved enormously as a result of my transplant."

Kidney disease and kidney failure have pervasive effects on all aspects of a person's life. Kidney failure, in particular, affects an individual's emotional, physical, financial and social well-being. It leaves no stone unturned in its wake. Families often bear the brunt of having to care for a loved one and share the enormous burden of the disease themselves. Not everyone has the same experiences. Each person tells a unique story. But there is one commonality in all their stories: endurance.

"I will never, ever quit. No matter what, I am going to go on to the end."
This comment absolutely typifies the fortitude of the patients I have met in
the past year.

One of the nephrologists explained the ethos of treating patients with kidney disease. "We work with the patient from the outset of the disease all the
way through. We understand that this is a continuous-care situation. Unlike
other medical doctors, we have a long-term relationship with our patients.
During my career as a nephrologist, I have had the privilege of meeting and
working with some of the most remarkable individuals I could have ever
wished to meet. Remarkable because of their courage, dignity and spirit of
determination."

This resolve to survive against all odds has influenced me greatly. Those
whom I have met are only a small smattering of dialysis patients. Many
more of them remain unknown to me. I have met my fellow patients on
HandyDART, in hospital lobbies, in the waiting room before going into the
hemodialysis unit and while on dialysis itself. Some of the encounters have
resulted in only short conversations, others in longer discourse, and some
patients have joined me for meals and other social occasions. Most of my
fellow dialysis patients have more than one health issue. Many continue
to be beset with frequent health complications causing added worries for
them and creating more challenges for them to manage while maintaining
a positive and hopeful outlook.

The stories I wish to tell have particularly resonated with me for all the
reasons I have mentioned and deserve recounting. I have changed names
and sometimes gender to protect confidentiality. For some I have no names
because of the brevity of our time together.

Rebecca

I met Rebecca, a peritoneal dialysis user, while I was an in-patient. Rebecca, a tall woman with dark, curly hair and enormous congeniality and
dynamism, had broken her arm in a fall and could not perform the peritoneal dialysis exchanges on her own, so she had been admitted to hospital for support. I was immediately struck by her tremendous drive and
pluck. Had it not been for the consequences of kidney failure, she would
have been termed a mover and shaker. We had some lovely conversations,

during which I learned how life had presented her with many challenges. As is so often the case with all of us, one obstacle soon sets the tone for other obstacles. The expression "It never rains, but it pours" could not have been more accurate in its description of the difficulties Rebecca has faced.

She was a single parent, having recently gone through a very difficult divorce, one that had had an enormous toll on her financially and emotionally. Furthermore, her teenaged child had recently been diagnosed with diabetes. Rebecca herself had been living with diabetes for over forty years and had been previously diagnosed with an autoimmune disease called granulomatosis with polyangiitis.[1] This and her diabetes provided a double setup for kidney failure.

> Wegener's granulomatosis, now referred to as granulomatosis with polyangiitis, is a condition that causes inflammation of the veins and arteries of the nasal passages, lungs and kidneys.

Rebecca had been on dialysis for three years. A biopsy in her early stages of kidney failure had suggested that its cause was primarily from diabetes and less likely from Wegener's disease. Rebecca recounted her story to me: "Following my autoimmune disease diagnosis and prior to my kidney failure, I had had a number of health issues that had resulted in neuropathic complications. To counteract these, I was given a series of strong medications that may well have compromised my immune system. My initial symptom was difficulty walking. My knees felt as though I had been whacked with baseball bats, my feet were swollen and I was extremely fatigued. My blood count dropped significantly, requiring me to have several transfusions. Because my blood group is an uncommon type, I had not been on the transplant list but the doctors advised me to do so. Although I had been performing dialysis for a while, I was told this would not jeopardize my place on the wait list.

"To promote my own search for a transplant, I designed three different T-shirts to wear in public, each with a message, printed in capital letters on a black background. Message one: 'Gotta spare to share?' with a graphic of two kidneys. Another reads: 'Are you my type? I'm type B+.' The third reads: 'I need a kidney,' again with a graphic of two kidneys. I have also designed a number of pamphlets about kidney failure and the transplant process that I have distributed at fairs and in the local market. I happen to live in the same neighbourhood as the anchor newscaster for one of the main TV stations. I have been trying to contact the station in hopes that they will provide information about the donor process. I have also tried to contact the anchor."

Rebecca is an example of how kidney patients are leading the charge themselves in spreading the word about kidney failure and are having to advocate for themselves during very taxing times.

Rebecca also told me, "I have tried working while on dialysis but my fatigue was a hurdle. I couldn't do it. My finances are tight. I had to forego many things in order to ensure my son's needs are well cared for. I cannot afford a car and am living in a rented accommodation whose lease will soon expire."

When I met Rebecca in hospital, she and her son were living in a rented condo close to the hospital while the drains in her house were being repaired. A calamity with her dialysis solution had damaged the drainage system. For an unknown reason, some of the boxes containing the dialysis solution had come with improperly sealed bags that had leaked. As one box sitting on top of the other boxes caved in, so did the others; the result was catastrophic. Her basement drains overflowed, causing a massive flood that destroyed all the household items in its path. She has had other occasions where a solution bag has come with a fault in it but nothing quite like this one. Rebecca explained the downsides of dialysis for her: "I lack energy and feel unwell a good percentage of the time. I have frequent pain when I exchange fluids, a bad taste in my mouth and persistent itchy skin. I don't know how my future will unfold. My family lives some distance away, so I am pretty much on my own. My son is my rock and buttress in all of this. He gives me the courage and energy to carry on."

She has joined the paired-donor program, one of the ways in which an individual can be a living kidney donor. The way that it works is this: an individual, in this case Rebecca, who needs a kidney transplant can hook up with a willing donor who is not a blood match for her. That donor can donate their kidney to another individual who likewise has a non-matching donor. It is rather like an exchange of kidneys. Rebecca is still a relatively young woman who has many productive years ahead. Her life would be greatly enriched with a kidney transplant. This highlights the need for more donors.

HandyDART riders

Travelling by HandyDART has brought me into contact with a number of other kidney patients. Some I meet on a regular basis, others less frequently. We cannot design our own rides on HandyDART since the scheduling needs to accommodate many others, and journeys often are planned for convenience of time and locations. Sometimes we see our fellow riders for a period of time, then never again. These are serendipitous meetings.

Bill

I happened to ride with one particular fellow on a number of occasions and began what I call our quasi-friendship. I say quasi-friendship because it has been many months since I last saw him. My friend Bill was a fascinating person, short in stature and with a shock of black hair. He limped slowly with cane in hand and had a warm smile that suggested a gracious manner. His sweet nature rendered him an enjoyable companion. He had been a political activist in his earlier life and was a wonderful source of information, energy and optimism. He regaled me with many tales of his political involvement and years of fighting for people's rights. I could see, even now in his current state, that passion for justice burned deeply in his heart. Given different circumstances, I am sure he would have, banner in hand, joined many a crusade.

With arthritis in his legs and needing a cane to walk, Bill could no longer drive and therefore relied on HandyDART for transport. Born with genetic abnormalities, he had had kidney disease as a young child. Most of his youth had been spent on dialysis. When he was a young man, he had a transplant that had lasted thirty years but had failed in the last year, so he was back on hemodialysis in one of the local community dialysis units. There are a number of community units, in addition to the two local hospitals' provisions. The main differences are the presence of doctors and the independence of the patients. In hospitals, the doctors are on site, whereas in the community unit, the doctors are peripatetic. In community units, patients are able to perform their own connections to the dialysis machines, and they clean their own areas. I was most impressed to have met someone whose kidney had lasted as long as his had—even outshining mine! I am always hopeful of sharing rides with Bill again.

Doctor X

Doctor X, a small-framed man sitting either in a wheelchair or serenely in the recesses of the waiting room, accompanied by his care aid, is recognizable by his fondness for reading, always with a magazine or medical journal in hand. He is a retired physician and surgeon whose kidney failure was caused by unchecked high blood pressure. He has been dialyzing for three years. I first met Doctor X during my daytime ride to and from our dialysis sessions. We converse together a lot because he and I are the last two passengers to be dropped off on the way home. He would have happily continued practising medicine were it not for his kidney failure. He actually thought he could combine hemodialysis with his practice but found it to be an impossible undertaking. That was a great disappointment to him.

Doctor X is a wonderfully sociable and philosophical companion. Our conversations have ranged in topic from food to travel, philosophy and theology. He is a lifetime vegetarian, avoiding eggs, meat and seafood, something hard to do for renal patients because of the high level of potassium and phosphorus in the protein sources used to replace meat and seafood. We sometimes discuss medical matters but I am aware doctors are magnets for people wanting to query them about personal issues. Mostly our conversation relates to kidney subjects and hospital talk. The doctor practised medicine in the UK for a number of years prior to coming to Vancouver, so we have some shared hospital experiences.

As a young man, Doctor X was diagnosed with high blood pressure, a condition that is prevalent in his family. He said, "I completely ignored the warning signs. I worried more about my own patients than I did about myself. Also, when I was young I thought I was immortal. When I finally did see a cardiologist, it was too late; my high blood pressure had already caused kidney damage. The only recognizable aspect of my kidney failure was shortness of breath, and, of course, high blood pressure. I take a number of medications to control my blood pressure. I feel my story is a good lesson for young people to think about their long-term future and not exist just in the present. I believe a vegetarian diet or at least a reduction in meat is a smart option for maintaining good health."

Doctor X further told me, "I have some osteoarthritis in my knees and back but it does not prevent me from doing things. I find hemodialysis tiring, but the worst part of the treatment for me is the length of time it takes to perform. I can tolerate three hours but four begins to wear on me; I start getting anxious. To resist my anxiety, I practise meditation. I believe it is a useful tool to calm our emotions and to alter our thinking patterns, thereby acquiring a more positive outlook."

Age and a lack of appropriate donors have ruled him unlikely to receive a transplant, so he will probably remain on dialysis for the rest of his life.

Another comment Doctor X made was, "I feel weak following my sessions, but I lead a normal life on my non-dialysis days and still drive and travel." Recently, he has been away on a cruise and has also spent time in California visiting his sister and a week in Ottawa with one of his sons, also a doctor. It is absolutely possible to travel while dialyzing. Doctor X told me, "For some reason, I don't know why, but I actually feel better after my dialysis sessions when I am away than I do when I am here."

> There are cruises designated for people who dialyze, and hospitals around the world where visitors can dialyze. They can be costly, depending on where in the world they are. Our system in BC does provide reimbursement for some costs incurred, but not all.

Doctor X is an inspiration. "Kidney failure to me is more of a nuisance than a life sentence. I am an optimist," he told me. He exhibits a strong mind and continues to play an active role to play in his community. In his lifetime, he has organized a number of humanitarian projects and raised millions of dollars in charitable donations for his community. He played an instrumental role in building the first Hindu temple in Canada, in Vancouver. Doctor X explained his credo: "I consider helping others is of paramount importance. Money creates temporary excitement but helping and creating happiness will give permanent happiness no one can take away." He is a highly regarded and honoured member of many organizations having received several lifetime achievement awards from notables ranging from prime ministers to East Indian dignitaries. Most recently, in a major Hindu ceremony, he received his latest lifetime honour for services rendered.

I thoroughly enjoy our time together. What I am most in awe of is Doctor X's amazing humility and unaffected manner, considering his many accomplishments and his revered status among his community. He is congenial, possesses a good sense of humour—something not limited by his present condition—and is a fascinating font of knowledge. He is an optimist who serves as a fabulous role model.

Candy Man

One day as I got onto the HandyDART and sat down in a seat by a window, I noticed a fellow sitting across the aisle from me. He immediately turned to me and said, "Hello, Priscilla. What are you doing on the bus?" I looked at him quizzically and then recognized his face. Here was someone I had known about ten years ago when I was volunteering with a local symphony, and we had then lost touch. He still volunteers occasionally, and now we had been reunited by our mutual kidney failure.

Candy Man, his preferred name because he loves dolling out candies to nurses, staff and patients, explained, "It's something that fills me with pleasure when I see the smiles on people's faces. I know what candies each person prefers and give them out accordingly. I am such a regular customer that in one store the sales staff not only refer to me by name but also have my goodies packed and ready for me." Although of moderate height and small in girth, his bubbly, gregarious and happy disposition makes him large in spirit. Always smiling and grinning, Candy Man arrives replete with funny stories. He has a truly positive attitude and gets on well with all the nurses and staff. "I believe in the power of laughter. It keeps my spirits up. I also feel that a positive attitude wins the day, something I learned from my family that keeps me motivated, as does my partner, my bedrock."

When I met him, Candy Man had been dialyzing for just over a year since diabetes caused his kidney failure. He told me, "My only symptom prior to kidney failure was shortness of breath. I was surprised to discover I had kidney failure. I only take a small dose of medication for my diabetes, but like all dialysis patients, I take extra vitamins to replace chemicals lost through dialysis and kidney failure itself. The diet is not great, but I have become adapted to it as I have lived on a restrictive one for years." Laughingly, he added, "I have an insatiable appetite for ice cubes. I cannot quench my thirst enough so often end up needing to have more fluid removed than I should."

He went on to tell me, "I feel exceedingly tired and lack energy, although on non-dialysis days I work in my garden because I love gardening. When

I was a younger I worked in a garden centre. There I learned my love and knowledge of plants. Some days are harder for me than others. When my energy level is good, my partner and I enjoy the opportunities city living gives us."

Candy Man has begun to swim again, the cause of envy on my part.

He also told me, "Financially, having to do hemodialysis is hard for me, since we live on very little income."

Kidney recipients receive a tax credit, but with little income to start with, the credit does not make life much easier.

An ultrasound device the nurses use to pinpoint the position of the fistula on Candy Man's arm, where the nurses can insert the dialysis needles, fascinates him. He has awkward veins, and it takes the nurses awhile to hook him up to the dialysis machine. He added, "I believe I am in good hands with both the nurses and doctors and receiving quality care. Unfortunately I have recently been diagnosed as having weak heart muscles that will necessitate me having to take further medication to maintain a healthy heart.

"My advice for others is: If you need to go on dialysis, accept it; otherwise, you will only hurt your whole system and your mind. Trust the doctor. If you need to cry, do so, because it can relieve tension."

Candy Man is on the transplant list but is prepared for a long wait and is trying to make the most of what he has now. He is a pleasure to be with, and his infectious good humour interspersed with droll comments makes both our travelling time and our time spent in the waiting room fun and happy. While waiting our turns to be called into the unit, he and I share a playful little competition with Doctor X to see who will be called for dialysis first. Invariably, it's Doctor X, much to our amusement.

David

David, whom I call my party boy, greets everyone with a lovely, warm, "Hello, darling, how are you today?" He is a tall, extremely cheerful, gregarious person who exudes a natural amiability. He possesses deep spiritual beliefs, and as a result, feels things are meant to be. A dialysis patient for two years, he had been a major partygoer in his younger days, living on an unwholesome diet and drinking heavily. That most likely paved the way to his developing diabetes. Although he has been diabetes-free for many years, the lasting effects could have contributed to his present kidney failure.

He worked in a local hospital until his vision began to deteriorate, requiring him to be hospitalized. Suffering some loss of vision, he had to spend time convalescing. To read and write, he needs a magnifying glass. Although he travels to dialysis by HandyDART, he is able to use public transport to visit the love of his life, his young granddaughter. He uses a walker to stabilize his mobility, for carrying items and for a seat on which to rest when he feels the need to sit down.

He told me, "I had not been feeling too well and had lost a considerable amount of weight, so visited my GP who thought that my former diabetes and eye problems warranted a referral to a specialist. When the nephrologist diagnosed me with kidney failure, I had had no time to think. Everything moved quickly. I had a fistula for dialysis inserted into my groin immediately following my diagnosis.

"I was really frightened, terrified of what would happen to me, because I knew nothing about dialysis or how it worked. Once I started dialysis, I felt much more comfortable and my fears vanished. I also initially felt dreadfully cold throughout my dialysis sessions and could never get warm in spite of being covered by innumerable blankets. Today I don't feel quite as cold during dialysis. Dialysis really works for me. I always feel really well, wonderful, in fact, after my sessions. The downsides for me are the time spent waiting, the regularity of treatment and length of sessions, although I am extremely grateful to the nurses and doctors for their continuous diligent care."

David said, "In other ways I am fairly healthy. I don't worry about the diet restrictions because my blood levels are good, and I continue to use the bathroom. I keep fit by exercising prior to my dialysis session."

Maintaining physical fitness helps ward off the downsides of the dialysis process itself, although depending on their physical state, not everyone is able to follow a fitness regimen. Some patients use a cycle machine during dialysis so they can keep active and mitigate the effects of prolonged sitting. David, walker to the fore, walks for several hours on his non-dialysis days, rewarding himself at the end at a curry restaurant. "I love my curries," he told me.

Financially, David struggles because of not being able to work. He lives in a supported, church-run home. He is on the transplant list, hoping for a kidney that will give him greater freedom of movement, transforming his lifestyle. "I really want to do well, because I wish to be able to spend time with my delightful granddaughter and want to be with her for as long as I can."

David's advice: "People should be aware that we only really need one kidney to live full lives, so becoming a donor can provide enormous support to those whose organs have failed."

Waiting for HandyDART

The gloomy hospital lobby where I wait for my ride home after my late-evening sessions can be bleak and desolate. Fortunately, I have been joined by three cheery patients who have enlivened my sojourn. Our waiting time has become a time for socializing and sharing stories or tales of our evening dialysis sessions, a time for laughter and support. Two of the patients and I sometimes share rides home. The other travels separately because we live in different areas. These three are a great antidote to a tedious downtime.

Deborah

Deborah, an older senior confined to a wheelchair, has a warm, benevolent nature and a mass of greyish-white hair that has not thinned from the heparin, which is added to the solution to stop our blood from clotting. She has been a dialysis patient for nine years but has had diabetes for many years. She told me, "My original kidney failure symptoms manifested themselves in swelling and leg pain as well as an inability to pass urine. When I was diagnosed with kidney failure, I had been retired for a long time. My financial status has not been helped by my ongoing health challenges. I prefer to live independently in a rented studio apartment. I have a little help once a week with my cleaning that I pay for out of my own income. I have a wonderful daughter who takes me out to lunch every Sunday and who phones me frequently."

Diabetes can be a horribly pernicious disease and can contribute to many complications. Deborah explained some of her challenges to me: "A few years after I had been on hemodialysis, I developed painful blocked arteries in my legs. Walking for me was really hard. To treat the blocked arteries, I needed to have one leg amputated, although the doctors were able to save my other leg. To make matters worse, I contracted an infection and spent six months in a convalescent hospital. That's why I need to use a wheelchair to get around and rely on HandyDART. A downside is that occasionally taxis organized to pick me up have not turned up. I miss my session." A missed session is not good for a hemodialysis patient.

Deborah's eyesight has also been affected by her diabetes. She explained, "I cannot read or write easily and have trouble maneuvering." Adding her feelings about dialysis, she said, "I am exhausted all the time. I have trouble sleeping after my late-evening dialysis. So I spend a good part of my day sleeping." She manages all her own cooking, although she admits, "The diet is a problem for me. My blood results show raised potassium levels. I avoid tomatoes and as many high-level potassium foods as I can."

Recently Deborah has had difficulty with fluid removal. During a number of dialysis sessions, her blood pressure has dropped and a crash has occurred. To rectify this, the nurses tilt her chair as far back as it will go and raise her legs until her blood pressure rises. The effect: "I am weaker and more tired at the end of a session."

What strikes me most about Deborah is her enormously upbeat attitude and sense of fun. She is a happy person who has endured many trials, rising to them with a wonderful spirit and much cheerfulness. She shows genuine kindness towards all the patients, and will go out of her way to ensure others are given priority treatment over her. Her consideration for others has endeared her to the unit. I have been the beneficiary of Deborah's kindness. Whenever we travel home together late at night, the first thing she says is, "Will you please drop Priscilla off first." She has helped me tremendously with any questions or concerns I have had about hemodialysis.

Chatty Matty

My second evening companion is Chatty Matty, a lively, curious, youthful senior, who, though confined to a wheelchair, is not defined by her confinement. She leads a vibrant and energetic life away from dialysis. She is so named by personal consent because she is just that—a very willing conversationalist. It is a fabulous gift and one that instantly attracted my attention. If anyone ever wishes to talk to someone, Chatty Matty is the go-to person. She will enthusiastically converse with anyone, anywhere, at any time, on any subject, and is thoroughly interested in hearing about other people's lives and interests. I have often overheard her sharing stories with the refreshment volunteers. Our unit is particularly fortunate in having a number of volunteers who provide tea, coffee and biscuits to dialysis patients. They are often young students who generously give their time to assist others. Some are potential medical students; others are interested in being good citizens. It is a wonderful service for which we, the patients, are most grateful.

Chatty Matty has been on dialysis for twelve years, ever since the end of her working life. Her kidney failure is a result of diabetes, an illness that she has had for many years. Coincidentally, sometime after Chatty Matty had been on dialysis, her mother informed her she also had renal failure. A diagnosis was never confirmed but her mother died not too long after having learned her kidneys had failed. Diabetes can be inherited, but so far, none of Chatty Matty's own children or grandchildren have been affected, for which she is very thankful.

"Some years before my kidney failure," Chatty Matty told me, "I was referred to a nephrologist who told me I would never be on dialysis. I was really shocked to find myself needing it. I cannot recall having any particular symptoms that would suggest kidney failure. Today, I am fairly okay and only take medications to control my blood pressure and diabetes and ease my digestion.

"Because my blood results are good, I do not do the renal diet." This Chatty Matty stated loudly and clearly when I invited her to dinner, further adding, "I do not eat much red meat and potatoes. I mostly eat fish, chicken and vegetables. I don't eat bread and other starches and very little of anything in large quantities."

Socially, she is very active, and goes out most days with friends. "Sometimes dialysis interferes with my activities, but never on weekends!" she said most emphatically. "I have very close ties with my son, daughter and grandchildren who are supportive and helpful. Since I worked until I retired, having kidney failure has not affected me financially."

Physically, though, Chatty Matty has been affected by the side effects of diabetes. Some years following her kidney failure, she succumbed to an infection in her toes that did not clear up. Her symptoms were extreme pain in her legs. She explained, "I could not climb my stairs and had to sleep on a couch in my living room. When my son-in-law, a doctor, found out, I was rushed to hospital. I didn't realize how close to death I was, but the treatment proved successful, and I pulled through, but not before my left foot was amputated, and I lost my right leg below the knee. I spent eight months in hospital recovering. Now I use a motorized wheelchair to get around. I also have no feelings in my fingers and am constantly burning them when I cook. These are side effects of diabetes and kidney failure.

"I find the amount of time spent dialyzing difficult. An acquaintance of mine, when learning I attended a four-hour, three-days-a-week dialysis session, said to me, 'Oh, it's all right for you. You only just have to lie around for four hours doing nothing.' I was saddened to discover my friend could be so lacking in understanding and empathy. Indeed, I am frequently uncomfortable during sessions and find my neck and body gradually start aching as the hours pile up.

"Another challenge for me is that sometimes I have difficulty stopping the flow of blood when the needles are removed from my fistula at the end of the session. I need to press on my fistula site for up to fifteen minutes before the blood stops. I am sensitive to the needles. They need to be carefully positioned when I am hooked up to the dialysis lines."

Bleeding after the needles are removed is a common side effect of having a fistula. Many patients need to press on their site for some time before they can leave the unit.

Chatty Matty retains a very positive outlook, and although she has been ruled out for a transplant, she feels most optimistic about her future. Chatty Matty's hope and dream: "To continue to live a happy and loving life."

Bob

My third evening lobby companion is best described as a resolute fellow who has been on dialysis for eight years, also as a result of diabetes. Resolute because of his forbearance in the manner with which he has handled the numerous challenges confronting him. Bob, his pseudonym, is a short, middle-aged man with a receding hairline and deep brown eyes peeking from behind glasses. He walks slowly using a cane to support his unsteady gait. He told me, "My symptoms were swollen legs and fatigue. I worked as an airplane technician prior to my kidney failure and have not worked since. I need to rely on my wife for financial assistance. Our income has been slashed by my condition."

Bob's daughter and son, of whom he is very proud, are currently back in Vancouver after working in other provinces for many years.

Bob said, "It is really comforting to have all my family close at hand again. It is a wonderful feeling."

He shared with me the current status of his health. "I only take medication to control my blood pressure. I have chronic obstructive pulmonary disease but am managing it well. I find the diet very restricting and tough to follow, one of the more difficult sides of kidney failure for me to deal with.

"I believe my kidney failure has contributed to me experiencing greater physical weakness. One of my legs is very frail and can easily buckle under, so I rely on a cane for support and to help me walk."

More recently, after several falls, Deborah kindly gave him a walker she no longer uses to ease his struggles.

Bob continued, "In spite of frequent falls, I have not sustained a break or permanent damage. Some days I feel weaker than others but I carry on."

Bob lives some distance away from the hospital so, including travelling time, he probably spends well over twenty-four hours a week doing dialysis. Consequently, the amount of time for social activities is reduced. Bob said, "I have little opportunity to participate in other things while having to have dialysis. I am frustrated by my condition and am sometimes low-spirited, but I am determined to carry on as well as I can. I am on the transplant list and hope to receive a kidney transplant in the near future.

Bob's advice to others: "Always make sure you go for your yearly medical check-up. Don't overindulge."

I have been impressed by his resilience and his pure grit determination to endure the limitations imposed by having to do dialysis and its residual effects with grace, dignity and courage. Bob's forbearance is very motivating, and he is a good role model for others.

The waiting room

The waiting room can be a busy place between daily sessions. Our dialysis time is often determined by the readiness of the previous patient, the prepared bed and the cleaned machine. We can sometimes wait up to an hour before being called in.

We are creatures of habit. Just as my students liked to sit in the same seats, so do we dialysis patients. Usually patients who come in wheelchairs sit near the hemodialysis door, others seem to like to sit closer to the main corridor, and still others like me, towards the back of the waiting room.

A pleasant, supportive aura fills the waiting room, as we frequently chat in our code language. The word "crash" refers to a drop in blood pressure, and "dwell time" to the length of time between exchanging fluids in peritoneal dialysis. We wish each other a "good run" as one of us goes in for dialysis, just as thespians wish each other a successful performance by saying, "Break a leg." Following a session, we ask each other, "Did you have a good run?" We always hope to hear the answer, "Good, and I feel okay," as opposed to hearing, "I had a bad run. Things did not go well for me." We invariably respond empathetically and wish them well for their next run.

The kindliness of my fellow patients is much in evidence. Patients like to know how other patients are doing and will often enquire about their well-being if they haven't seen someone in a while. This happened to me one afternoon as I was exiting the elevator. Someone with whom I had never spoken stopped me to ask if I had seen a certain patient recently because they hadn't seen that person for a few days and were wondering whether I knew if the patient was okay. I could reassure my inquirer that indeed the patient was doing fine as I had been talking to the person only a few days before. My inquirer was instantly relieved upon hearing my response.

An older gentleman

An older gentleman who sits in a row of chairs across from me is distinguished by his willingness to engage in conversation with any of us and proffer sage words of advice if we are having a bad time. When his kidney diagnosis was confirmed, he was advised by his GP to keep active and not just sit around. Already a keen vegetable gardener and skilled cook, he decided to follow his doctor's advice. He brings samples from his garden and cuisine for patients, staff and nurses. He told me, "The sole purpose of my vegetable garden and results from my cooking are specifically to be given away." As an example of his generosity and care for others, I have received bay leaves, green peppers and fruit from this gentleman.

The four young men

Many young people have flourishing careers and are in the prime of their youth when their lives are changed dramatically from kidney failure. They will continue to be affected until they receive a transplant. While waiting my turn to be called in for dialysis, I have had the opportunity to converse with four young men. Our conversations were limited due to changes in scheduling or treatment.

The first young man, who appeared strong-willed and determined to survive his ordeals, explained to me, "I have to work because I do not receive any financial aid for living with kidney failure and have no additional support. I am working thirty-five hours a week just to cover my rent and food. And that is on top of having to attend dialysis sessions for four hours three times a week. I have little else to spend on entertainment or fun things. I continually feel drained of energy but I have to do what I have to do." Although the young man told me of his plight, I was moved by his pluck. It was particularly heart wrenching to hear of his struggles. This is often the unknown side of kidney failure: people having to cope with a very challenging illness while needing to provide for themselves.

The second young man worked in the scientific field. He was well-built, and would have been a strong looking young man were it not for his present condition. He had known for some time that his kidneys were failing and wearily told me, "I have gradually been feeling worse and worse over the years and now just want to get my old life back. A kidney would help me do that." He recently had had both kidneys removed because he had polycystic kidneys. Polycystic kidneys can be an inherited condition causing massive cyst formation in the kidneys.[2] His kidneys each weighed over eight pounds when they were removed. A normal kidney weighs about five ounces.

The third young man worked in the community. He left a strong impression on me for his vibrancy and zest for life. In spite of his compromised health, he appeared to have an abundance of enthusiasm and energy. I did not learn the cause of his kidney failure but his gratitude to the medical staff was very apparent. I only conversed with him briefly since he was transferring to an overnight session. I often wonder how he is doing. I do know that he was committed to his work and really wanted to continue with it.

The last young man was employed in customer service. From him, I learned his work required him to travel frequently. I never learned the cause of his kidney failure, but he seemed fairly healthy and was fortunately able to continue working and travelling between his hemodialysis sessions. He was switching to peritoneal dialysis in order to better accommodate his work schedule. He appeared to be adjusting to his new status with considerable good humour and optimism. I marvelled at his ability to combine such an active schedule with his treatment. The fatigue created by the combination of kidney failure and dialysis treatment may begin to take a toll on his life. These young men are all examples of why we urgently need more donors.

A young woman

Recently I met a young woman while she and I were the sole occupants in the waiting room. We had a short but light-hearted conversation. Diabetes had caused her kidneys to fail. Like me, she had a catheter in her neck because the doctors felt her veins could no longer accommodate a fistula. She confessed, "I need to dialyze four times a week in order to remove my fluid," laughingly adding, "I drink too much."

We enjoyed exchanging some of our funny moments about our dialysis sessions and talked about how our daily lives are so peculiar, split between the rigid routine of dialysis sessions and the absolute antithesis of non-dialysis days. We decided the best description was a cross between inflexibility and total flexibility. She continued laughing while saying, "I cannot understand why, when I am lying doing nothing for four hours, at the end I feel as though I have been running in a marathon."

Her infectious sense of humour enlightened our wait, and was very uplifting, causing me to admire her positive outlook.

Mischievous Marty

Mischievous Marty, so named because, "I was a naughty child. I was the youngest of five and grew up on a farm in a three-story house. I thoroughly enjoyed climbing up on the roof to sit by the chimney where I could watch my mother searching the yard looking for me."

The family grew up in a fun-filled environment, but also one filled with sorrow. He had four siblings, three of whom died from diabetes. He was the only one to have polycystic kidneys, which he knew about from the age of seven. His mother died when he was sixteen years old.

Marty told me, "My kidneys failed four years ago. I had experienced the common symptoms of back pain from my polycystic kidneys, nausea and problems peeing. I also suffer from angina, controlled by blood pressure pills."

Like me, he has experienced restless legs at night, explaining, "Sometimes I found myself waking my wife as I unconsciously kicked her. I take medication to control my symptoms. This has worked. Both my wife and I now enjoy a peaceful sleep."

Kidney failure has contributed to a major loss of income for the couple. "We live in a single-room suite with only a one-ring burner on which to cook and a sink and toilet. I used to work in construction, but can now only do light work such as dishwashing, and that only when I feel strong enough. I tire easily, use a cane for support and need frequent rest stops. We don't have much money. Mostly we stay home. My wife loves to sew. I didn't think the diet would be a challenge until my blood results made me think again. I make lots of sacrifices, especially on little money. I am always wishing for forbidden pleasures."

He said that following dialysis, "I am tired and nauseated. The hardest thing for me is to not be able to come and go as freely as I would like or do the things for more than three days at a time. I used to enjoy spending many weeks camping." Mischievous Marty sadly confessed, "I sometimes feel as though I have been a failure because kidney disease has impacted my life to such a great extent, but in reality I know there is nothing I can do to alter my situation."

He added, "My wise grandmother, whom I remember only as a very old woman, gave me the stamina and resilience to carry on. I recall her telling me, 'Never forget, we'll be together again but only with those who endure life to the end.' I am determined to last to the end so I can be with my grandmother again."

Mischievous Marty and his wife, his constant companion, inspire me with their sense of humour and good nature, despite their circumstances. He is on the transplant list, and there is no doubt a kidney would give him opportunities to do more than he can now.

Visitors from out of town

I shared a short exchange in the lobby with a very personable couple, who were from out of town. They had come for a family occasion and were using the dialysis unit at the hospital while here. I mostly spoke to the wife while her husband was dialyzing. She told me, "My husband has diabetes, and recently has had kidney cancer."

When I asked her if he was on the transplant list she explained, "My husband needs to be cancer-cleared for five years. I expect when that time comes he would defer receiving a kidney because he is doing fine on dialysis. His diabetes is well-controlled. Apart from the cancer he has no other medical issues."

She continued, "He is able to perform dialysis at home. Kidney failure has not stopped us from visiting friends in many parts of the country or leading an active life."

It was most heartening to hear their story and learn they were doing so well.

The hemodialysis unit

The dialysis unit is a series of rooms, each containing a number of chairs or beds. Some patients consistently use the same bed or chair; others, like me, vary. Conversation while on dialysis is limited because the beds are spread apart and it is difficult for us to move around. Because of the sensitivity of my catheter placement, even a simple movement triggers the machine's mechanization, causing it to beep, pausing the dialysis process and forcing the nurses to reprogram it, which adds extra dreaded time to my dialysis session.

Still, sometimes I have been placed beside the same patients, enabling me to get to know them, even if it is only to exchange greetings. I have been fortunate to meet family members, who, while accompanying their loved ones to dialysis, can walk to my bedside and talk. I have been moved by the care and attention given by family members—wives, husbands, sons, daughters and other relatives—who remain by their family member's side throughout the course of the dialysis session. It is a testament to families' devotion for one another that they are willing to give so much of their time to their family member. The phrase, "Love conquers all," is firmly evident and echoes resoundingly throughout the dialysis unit. The following stories illustrate the familial bond heightened by kidney failure.

Mr. Tims

Mr. Tims, a spirited, conversational fellow, accompanies his wife to dialysis, driving her three times a week to her sessions and remaining with her. He has spent time conversing with me. I learned their story. "We first went to our GP because my wife was suffering from the effects of constant nausea. Our GP referred us to the hospital, where, eight years ago, my wife was diagnosed with kidney failure. The cause of her kidney failure was never determined. Shortly after my wife began dialysis, she suffered a severe stroke, leaving her incapacitated, requiring constant care."

Mr. Tims proudly told me, "We have been married for over fifty-seven years. We still live independently because I am the primary caregiver. I complete all the household tasks myself with only occasional help from our grown children." He added, "I miss my wife's good cooking, but we muddle on."

He continued, "Kidney failure has not created a financial hardship for us since I have a very good pension, but it has absolutely affected our social life. We never go out other than to dialysis or for doctors' appointments and have not had a holiday in eight years. Because of my wife's condition, she is extremely fragile. I daren't leave her alone for even a brief moment. We are together pretty much twenty-four hours a day. Together—for better or worse—until the end. We make the most of what we have." Mr. Tims told me, "The only break I take is on my wife's dialysis days. I know I can leave her for an hour to go out to lunch because she is in good hands. This is my luxury."

He carried on explaining more in the process. "My wife needs to take blood pressure pills that I administer. Since she has had a heart condition for years, she is ineligible for a transplant."

A side effect of poor heart function can be circulatory problems leading, in Mr. Tims' wife's case, to a toe infection. I observed just how excruciatingly painful cleansing her toe and changing dressings was for her as Mr. Tims stood by her side, kindly uttering encouraging comments: "Oh, how well you are doing. So brave and courageous. I am proud of you. You can do it."

He ruefully and sadly said, "Whenever I tell friends that my wife requires dialysis, they look at me blankly, completely as though I am speaking a different language."

This is something others have confessed, too.

Gerri

I first learned about Gerri's kidney failure from his wife, who told me, "Gerri has had two kidney failures. His first kidney failure was caused by polycystic kidney disease. He was made aware of it by the common symptoms of high creatinine levels, extreme fatigue and high blood pressure. Gerri's kidneys had become engorged with cysts as a result of his disease. When surgically removed, they weighed 17 pounds. His sister-in-law kindly donated a kidney that lasted five years. Unfortunately that kidney failed. Gerri had become a victim of focal segmental glomerulosclerosis.[3] He had been dialyzing using peritoneal dialysis for a year prior to his transplant, but since his second kidney failure, for the past four years, he has been doing hemodialysis."

One of the nephrologists told me that it is not uncommon for a dialysis patient to switch from peritoneal dialysis to hemodialysis because of changes in physiology.

An instructor in a food science program at a technical institute, Gerri had to retire early when he suffered from kidney failure the second time. Having to retire has placed some constraints on the couple financially, but his wife said, "We have been able to adjust to the change in status. Emotionally, it has been hard for Gerri to accept his need to retire early, as it certainly wasn't something he had intended to do.

"We feel restricted by Gerri's dialysis schedule. The hardest part of kidney failure for us is the lack of freedom and spontaneity others enjoy. Our social life is limited; travel has been, too, because we can never rely on the state of Gerri's health."

Gerri, like most dialysis patients, requires blood pressure medication, vitamins and, like me, continues to take anti-rejection drugs because he has a transplanted kidney, even though, like me, it does not function properly. He is in the preparation stages for a second kidney transplant. His wife said, "I wanted to donate a kidney but could not because I am the wrong blood type. Something that really saddens me."

"The constant side effects are wearing," she continued, "However, what keeps our spirits up is that it is something you just have to do, and life is what you make it. I also believe everyone deals with diseases differently and everyone exhibits their symptoms differently."

Mrs. Serena

Sasha, a delightfully sunny person, brings her mother, Mrs. Serena, to her daytime dialysis sessions. Mrs. Serena had been admitted to hospital for a minor surgery in the early 1980s, given the wrong antibiotics and ended up spending a month in hospital. The medication caused her kidneys to fail gradually over the years until three and a half years ago when they completely failed. Sasha said, "It is difficult to define my mother's symptoms because when her kidneys finally failed, dialysis was started immediately so that whatever side effects she might have had were not evident."

Sasha added, "My mother has had a quadruple bypass surgery. She takes blood pressure and thyroid medication, as well as vitamins and sleeping pills because she experiences difficulty sleeping. The restrictive diet is not a problem for my mother. She is able to prepare her meals and eats what she can."

After her mother's diagnosis, Sasha and her family welcomed her mother to live with them in their open-plan basement, which contains a suite where her mother lives independently but close enough so that the family can help her as needed. As Sasha explained, "She is my mother and I love her. Providing a home for her is something I can do to help her. I just help out with what I can and keep an eye out."

"My mother usually feels terribly cold and tired following her dialysis session. Her feeling of wellness varies on her off day. Sometimes she feels great, and other times not.

"We have definitely noticed a change in our lifestyle since my mother has needed our care. I can't go away for more than a week at a time because I don't want to leave my mum unattended. I need to escort her to her dialysis sessions. When I have to be away, my older brother or daughter take over. Our social life has been affected; we see less of our friends now, but it is what it is, and my mother's needs come first. My concern for her and my family is that my mother's quality of life has gone from a rating of ten to four.

"The hardest part for us is the countless appointments with a myriad of doctors. It is time consuming and means more time away from my family. I worry about the amount of time and attention I can give my teenaged daughter, too. I also feel family support is extremely important, and that kidney patients need extra help and someone to advocate on their behalf. I do not know how my mother would manage without our care."

Mrs. Serena is not eligible for a transplant because of her multiple health issues and age. Sasha further added, "I am on the organ donor list for everything but my kidneys, because I have two children and my husband is also not too well. I would prefer to donate a kidney to my family, should the need arise."

Dan

Leah and her husband Dan are a lovely, sociable couple. Dan has multiple myeloma, a blood disorder form of cancer that can contribute to kidney failure. That is what happened to Dan. Leah said, "Because the multiple myeloma caused his kidney failure, it is difficult to determine his symptoms of kidney failure. Extreme confusion was one symptom prior to diagnosis. Also, unusual behaviour possibly attributed to the multiple myeloma was another symptom, as were extreme sleepiness and an inability to walk. Dan's multiple myeloma had advanced before his admission to hospital, as had his kidney failure. He has been dialyzing for two years.

"In addition to attending dialysis sessions three times a week, Dan undergoes chemotherapy treatment once a week as an in-patient. The combination of the two treatments takes its toll. Dan is tired a good deal of the time. My main concern for him is keeping the cancer under control." She said, "Because of the cancer, everything is a day-to-day process."

There is no cure for multiple myeloma. It is an emotional roller coaster during Dan's extremely tired times. Leah said, "I have to step back and allow him to rest when he needs it. At first it was very difficult, but as time goes on, it gets easier. Dan and I spend a considerable amount of time together and are happy to do so."

In spite of his fatigue, he has continued to work in the consulting field. This is a huge undertaking and really highlights his enormous courage in wanting to carry on with his customary tasks. Work is demanding even at the best of times, let alone when someone is coping with a serious illness. His fortitude is exemplary.

"At first," Leah said, "the diet restrictions were problematic; however, I have found lots of good recipes through *Spice It Up*,[4] a specially-designed cookbook for dialysis patients." She also explained, "There is an American organization called DaVita[5] that has a good recipe selection. Mealtimes are now infinitely more interesting with the help of these two resources.

"One of the downsides for us is the challenge of travelling. A great deal of pre-planning is required, and finding dialysis in another country can be an issue. The hardest thing for us is our anxiety about the unknown outcome of the multiple myeloma and the constant chemo." As she said, "All of these changes are our new reality. We try not to think about tomorrow but just get through one day at a time.

"We need to remember there are thousands of others in the same position and that each day is a gift. The worst part of kidney failure for us is knowing that kidney disease is a lifelong condition. I feel kidney disease is terrible on its own; however, when combined with cancer, it is devastating." Leah admitted, "I can't imagine what Dan is feeling on a day to day basis."

Leah said, "I have thought about being a kidney donor myself, especially when I see the numbers of people waiting for a kidney. It breaks my heart because their quality of life could be so improved with a donation."

Leah and Dan are a most remarkable, positive couple.

During my stay in hospital

Steve

When I was an in-patient, I happened to meet Steve whose story saddened me greatly. He had been in hospital for several weeks due to a number of health issues, during which time he had no visitors. This was unusual. Most patients have visitors, some more than others. I was interested to learn more. In one of our conversations, Steve confessed to me, "I have been having a bit of a rough time with my family. I don't feel they understand my kidney failure. I spend a great deal of time on my own and have been relegated to a small room at the top of the house. I am rarely invited to join family outings. I can't contribute to my family financially since I am unable to work." He added, "My illness makes it hard for me to help with chores."

It was apparent that because of his kidney failure and continued health problems he had become a burden to them. In spite of his family's neglect, Steve did not tell me this with rancor, nor was he expecting pity. He was a determined optimist, bearing his sadness with enormous resilience. He spoke highly of his family and of his love for them, praising his children for their successes. I thought about what an unkind race we are when things do not go according to plan. There was much to admire about his persistent graciousness. I am only sorry I could not do more. I have no idea what happened to him since my discharge from hospital, but his story is embedded in my heart.

Matthew

Matthew's family is in direct contrast to Steve's. His Fijian family was wonderfully kind and generous, constantly by his side. The family consisted of Matthew, his wife, Muskean, and his three-year-old son. Matthew had just received a kidney transplant from a deceased donor. His wife is an excellent cook who one day brought in a most succulent dinner for me. It was delicious and a welcome respite from the hospital fare. I thoroughly savoured every tasty mouthful.

Six months after arriving in Canada, a move made to afford the family new opportunities, Matthew suddenly fell ill. He explained, "I had previously been diagnosed with high blood pressure, but seemed to be doing well and had begun looking for work. I suddenly started feeling very weak, had difficulty seeing, and my optic nerves began bleeding. My already high blood pressure skyrocketed. My family was terrified. We were in new surroundings and on our own. Our next-door neighbour kindly drove me to hospital where I remained for well over a month."

"In hospital I was diagnosed with kidney failure. The doctors said it was due to my high blood pressure, but a later biopsy did not show this."

It is assumed he had a genetic predisposition to kidney disease. After having been hospitalized for several weeks, Matthew began hemodialysis. The family moved from the province in which they were living to Vancouver.

Once in Vancouver, Matthew tried working. He said, "I needed to work to support my family, but I found it required more energy than I could muster. Luckily my wife found work and could provide some needed resources. It was a lean time for us. We were able to find our own accommodation and a school for our son. Things were hard for all of us emotionally and socially."

Muskean told me, "It was a worrying situation."

Matthew said, "I continually felt dreadfully fatigued, could not sleep well and had limited movement. I lost considerable weight and was frequently short of breath. My interaction with my son suffered because I lacked energy to play with him or support him as I would have liked. We were all feeling drained by the struggles of having to deal with my kidney failure. Our lives were dramatically affected."

Muskean confessed, "Our marriage was heavily tried."

Two years later, Matthew received his transplant.

Matthew told me about a struggle on a trip to Fiji while he was still on hemodialysis: "I felt I couldn't tell my dad about my kidney failure because he would find it hard to accept."

It was a cat and mouse situation, Matthew dialyzing one day and visiting his father the next, with never a word spoken about his illness. Later, having recovered from the transplant surgery, the family returned to Fiji. This time he told his father what had happened to him.

Following his transplant surgery, Matthew's kidney took a while to function effectively. Much to his family's delight, Matthew was discharged almost a week after his transplant and spent a number of months recuperating. When her husband was in hospital for his kidney transplant, Muskean admitted, "I never slept the entire time Matthew was in hospital. I was so worried about the outcome especially since Matthew's kidney took many days to start working and Matthew needed a biopsy to make sure everything was okay. The doctors told him it was a good kidney and would work well."

Today, he has resumed full time work; he and his family are doing well. Their quality of life has vastly improved, and the future looks bright for them. This is a happy story and a wonderful ending to several years of prolonged hardship.

The effects

Kidney failure and its treatment can be brutal. It is definitely not for the faint of heart. Dialysis requires commitment. My fellow patients are indeed warriors of a different kind. I feel honoured to have been able to share their stories of courage, optimism, perseverance and endurance in the face of horrendous challenges.

Chapter 6 | Kidney Failure Explained

For the secret of the care of the patient is in caring for the patient.
—Dr. Francis W. Peabody

An overview of kidney disease through a story

I never met Art. He was no longer with us when his daughter, a good friend of mine, recounted his experiences with kidney disease. His story, although not current, is nevertheless a good example of what can be the turgid underbelly of kidney failure. Art, promoted to the less-active position of Assistant Fire Chief, developed high blood pressure, became overweight, exercised little, didn't follow a healthy diet and had been advised by his GP to change his habits to stave off a heart attack, a condition to which firefighters are particularly vulnerable. Why this is so is currently being researched by the British Heart Foundation.[1] It is thought that the stress of the job, along with constant exposure to extreme heat and smoke, contributes to a heightened propensity for heart attacks. Art had tried over the years to adhere to his doctor's advice but, like so many of us, had started well only to lapse. Still, he led a full life.

While working full time, and in the process of completing construction on his family's new home, Art noticed his legs were swollen and covered with a rash. He was perturbed by this because he avoided doctors whenever he could. My friend said, "He was not a guy who ever believed in mortality or gave in to an illness." This time was different. He begrudgingly sought medical advice. Test results indicated these were the first signs of kidney disease. This was the last thing on his or his family's mind. However, Art began living with the knowledge he had kidney disease but continued working until his retirement was due. Gradually his condition worsened, and the inevitable happened: full renal failure.

He began hemodialysis, attending morning sessions at a community dialysis unit. He found the treatment not only exhausting but also painful and debilitating. Upon his return home after his morning session, he would be fine for an hour but then would need to lie down. He spent much of the remainder of the day recovering. He would revive the next day only to have to return the following day for further dialysis. The family felt a sense of loss and uncertainty as they stood by helplessly while Art struggled to maintain a physical equilibrium. Art's dreams of travelling during retirement were abandoned.

While Art was still on dialysis, his brother from Alberta visited the family. Wanting to take his brother sightseeing, Art decided they should to go to Whistler but the only way Art could go was to have his daughter drive them. During their visit to Whistler, Art's daughter and her uncle did the sightseeing while Art and his wife sat on the benches, Art depleted in energy by renal failure and subsequent hemodialysis.

Renal dysfunction is a complex, challenging illness that courts additional health complications. There can be neurological, cardiovascular, respiratory, gastrointestinal, integument (skin) and reproductive complications. Kidney patients are more likely to have high blood pressure, anemia, edema (swelling in feet, legs and hands), poor appetite and cardiovascular issues. Excessive calcium or phosphate levels in the blood can cause stiffening and narrowing of blood vessels.[2] Prolonged anemia can cause the heart to develop a left ventricular hypertrophy, meaning thickening of heart muscle, leading to congestive heart failure. Even a minor loss of kidney function can dramatically increase the risk of damaging the cardiovascular system. There is a high incidence of heart attacks among renal patients. Low hemoglobin contributes to a reduction in red blood cells. To combat this, most renal patients receive regular EPO injections to stimulate red blood cell production. EPO is short for erythropoietin, a hormone that in a healthy kidney activates red blood cell production. For kidney patients, a lack of iron leads to fatigue and subsequent low energy, for which iron supplements are often required.

Art was not spared. He had a heart attack. He developed swollen feet, skin rashes, bruising and dark blotches on both his arms and face. He often complained his dry skin seemed endlessly itchy and bothersome. He endured sleep disturbances and stomach issues. It was hard to know whether his heart attack was related to his kidney failure or vice versa. A cause for his kidney failure was never confirmed. It may have been exposure to the insulation he was using when building his family's new home. He may have had kidney disease long before he had been diagnosed and simply had not experienced any particular symptoms.

Art had been proud of his mass of wavy hair, but after his kidney failure, it soon became limp and thin. This is not uncommon for patients on dialysis, since heparin, a blood thinner used to prevent blood clotting while on dialysis, can affect hair quality. His personality also began to change. Formerly a vivacious person who loved socializing, he began to withdraw and become isolated. His family watched as he dropped out of social activities. Feeling perpetually drained, he had neither the energy nor the inclination to do much. Eating, once a pleasure, became a routine act of putting something into his mouth. Not long after he began dialysis, he lost the taste for food, probably because of toxin build up from renal failure. He employed an ingenious method to combat his fluid restrictions: he drilled some holes in a spoon, poured milk in his morning cereal bowl and ate his cereal using the spoon so that he could at least taste an essence of the milk. Renal patients are creative and versatile when it comes to working around obstacles.

Art's hope and optimism were strong, because he knew he was on the transplant list and was medically cleared for the procedure. His hope became reality two years later. Once he recovered from the transplant surgery, his life changed dramatically. His hair, while never returning to its former glory, improved in thickness and waviness. He began enjoying food again, and he soon regained his zest. After his reclusive existence, he couldn't wait to get out for his coffee sessions. He was forever going out for coffee, conversation and socialization. Now it was his turn to visit his brother in Alberta. He not only drove there but then, sufficiently re-energized, he was able to ride his brother's horses during his visit. His life had improved beyond expectations.

Here's an odd part of Art's story. Years prior to his diagnosed kidney disease and renal failure, he had been found to be sensitive to eggs. Art's wife had been diagnosed with Parkinson's disease, and her doctors wanted to test her sensitivity to food as a way of treating it. They decided to test Art's, too, and so discovered his egg intolerance. The amazing thing is that once he had received a transplant, his egg sensitivity disappeared. Why? That's an unresolved mystery.

Art did, however, have a bout of skin cancer similar to mine. It was not life threatening and easily dealt with. And, like me, he also experienced renal bone disease, sustaining a couple of fractures, one of which was a broken wrist when he fell after a visit to the transplant clinic. Later in life he suffered from dementia, but his kidney transplant lasted the remainder of his life.

Kidney disease

Kidney disease has no favourites, recognizing neither gender, nor age, nor culture, nor economic status. It is at one multicultural and egalitarian in all the wrong ways. It can strike suddenly like a curled snake hidden in the grass, injecting its poison into an unsuspecting individual and immediately cause havoc. Or it can slither languidly over time through the body, gradually shutting down a person's life force. It can take a short while or years to fester. I think of my hallucinatory snakes lying sleepily entwined at the foot of my bed during my first kidney failure. These snakes, having devastated my body with their venom, were feeling well sated and effectual. Their purpose accomplished, they could rest easily. I had felt their sting. There was no going back. As one renal nurse said, "Once your kidneys fail, it is irreversible." Fortunately that is not always true. Kidney failure can occur as a result of an acute illness or trauma to the body. This is referred to as acute kidney failure and can sometimes be reversed.

My HandyDART driver, one of the unfailingly reliable drivers whose duty is to get us dialysis patients who aren't mobile to our treatment sessions, told me of another snake attack. The drivers are well acquainted with us, as we are with them, so I was interested when he told me about another driver's sudden kidney failure diagnosis. Mel, a relatively healthy fifty-five-year-old, had begun to feel unwell, so unwell that he bypassed seeing his own GP and rushed to an emergency department instead. Following blood tests, he learned he had kidney failure and was immediately started on hemodialysis. No cause for his kidney failure was ever explained.

My driver, the informant, sadly shook his head, "Oh, kidney failure is an epidemic. It is absolutely an epidemic." That's a bit of a hyperbole, but the Kidney Foundation of Canada estimates that during their lifetime one in ten Canadians will have kidney disease—an umbrella term covering a number of conditions—and may be unaware of it.[3] Currently there are approximately 1,500 patients attending the kidney care clinic just in my local hospital. While the statistics are high, most people do not progress to total kidney failure and may require only medical monitoring of their condition.[4] Kidney disease is considered the ninth leading cause of deaths in the United States, ahead of breast and prostate cancers.[5] The statistics suggest more men than women will succumb to kidney disease.[6] First Nations people in

Canada, because of their increased prevalence to diabetes and hypertension, are twice as likely to be affected by kidney disease as the general population.[7]

The kidneys' function is to clear extra water and waste products from the body. They also produce hormones that create red blood cells and control blood pressure. The term *chronic kidney disease* is used to refer to the condition in which kidneys are damaged and have lost the ability to function adequately for more than three months. End-stage renal failure occurs when the kidneys are no longer able to clear water and clean waste products from blood at all.

Causes

The causes of kidney disease are numerous and varied. Precisely how they contribute to kidney disease or failure has been determined as a result of years of study, research, statistics, knowledge and frequent occurrences. A young resident doctor explained to me, "We develop our knowledge over a period of time as we begin to see familiar patterns."

Not all of the following conditions necessarily end in renal failure. They depend on a number of factors being present, and an individual's own particular physiology.

Number 1: Diabetes

The most common cause of renal failure is diabetes. Unfortunately, the incidence of diabetes is increasing. In 2016, it was reported that approximately 29 percent of Canadians will have diabetes, with occurrences rising as the population ages, becomes less active and more obese.[8] Dr. David Davidicus Wong wrote in his weekly medical article in the *Vancouver Courier* newspaper on November 25, 2015, "The prevalence of diabetes in adults over 20 is one in eleven." Health Canada has recently issued a warning stating that we Canadians are not doing enough to prevent diabetes from happening,[9] and consistently advertises the need for people to change their habits, both dietary and physical. Diabetes occurs when the body's ability to produce or respond to the hormone insulin is impaired, resulting in abnormal metabolism of carbohydrates and elevated levels of glucose (sugar) in the blood and urine.[10]

Kidney failure in diabetes is related to a buildup over time of high blood sugars that damage the kidney filtration structures. Normally, proteins are retained in the blood rather than being excreted in the urine. When the kidneys are damaged, protein leaks into the urine. Doctors monitor this by measuring the amount of a common protein (albumin) in the urine. Tiny amounts are called microalbuminuria. As kidney disease progresses, more protein is found in the urine.[11]

Sain, a kind and warm-hearted man, typifies many whose kidney failure began with diabetes. Having just retired from teaching in 1994, he noticed he was terribly thirsty and could not satisfy his desire for fluid. He also became short of breath. He sought medical advice. The doctor informed him that he had diabetes, as well as high blood pressure, and prescribed blood pressure medication. He was able to control his diabetes for many years, but in 2006 he found he required insulin to manage his symptoms. A year earlier he had also been diagnosed with polycystic kidney disease, a condition that is normally inherited, but not so in his case. He has no idea how he acquired this disease.

In 2009 Sain's kidneys failed completely. He began hemodialysis treatment. Like others he felt exhausted after his dialysis sessions. Similarly to other renal patients, and those with diabetes in particular, the longer he remains on dialysis, the "more intense the symptoms become, the more tired I feel," he said. He has also experienced heart problems and suffers from terrible neuropathic pain in his feet and legs, a symptom of nerve damage from diabetes. Support from family, his wife, children and friends gives him the courage to carry on. He feels it is important not to complain to them about his situation. This is typical of the people I have met. Renal patients are not martyrs; we are simply realistic in acknowledging that it is really hard for others who are not so affected to understand the challenges besetting us.

Number 2: Hypertension

High blood pressure, often referred to as hypertension, is the second most common cause of kidney failure, according to the National Institute of Diabetic and Digestive Diseases in the United States.[12] The Kidney Foundation of Canada posits that one in five people has high blood pressure but remain unaware of it.[13] It has also been referred to as "the silent killer." High blood pressure can harm the blood vessels in the kidneys, reducing their ability to perform properly. With high blood pressure, the flow of blood is much stronger than it should be. Eventually this intensity causes damage to the blood vessels so that kidney function becomes further impaired and is no longer able to filter waste products effectively.

Wendy is an exuberant young woman who has been plagued with a number of health challenges. In 1980 she began to feel incredibly tired, was endlessly thirsty and constantly needed to use the washroom. She made an appointment to see her GP, who, after listening to her symptoms and performing some tests, diagnosed diabetes. She was initially prescribed pills to control her diabetes, but eventually needed to use insulin to control her blood sugar. Now, she is able to keep the diabetes in check through diet and exercise.

Her story does not end there, however. In 1983, she was diagnosed with hypertension, a common aspect of diabetes. Typically, she did not feel any symptoms. To treat it she was given further medication. Everything seemed to be under control for many years until she began to feel further bouts of low energy, fatigue, bloating and infrequent urination. A visit to her GP in 2010 confirmed a diagnosis of polycystic kidney disease, an inherited condition she shares with her brother.

Several years later, her kidneys failed. She believes her renal failure was directly caused by her high blood pressure. She began hemodialysis shortly thereafter and continues receiving treatment today. Wendy has realized that when our bodies are not functioning normally due to kidney failure, we often feel less well and are unable to overcome other ailments. She has experienced sleeplessness and continuous fatigue.

However, she continues to work as a stock assistant with a major retail company. She has the most incredible resilience and steadfastness. She tries to manage her stress level so she can stay relaxed. Additionally, she eats healthily, exercises and keeps a positive outlook. Her advice to others is "to watch both what we consume as well as the size of our portions, manage our fluid intake and, above all, keep exercising." To me, Wendy is a real life warrior.

While hypertension is more common in older people, it can affect young people. During my dialysis sessions I met Jade, a pleasant young woman who had been diagnosed with high blood pressure when she was on the verge of completing her high school education. One of her parents had died of complications from high blood pressure, indicating the possibility of a genetic tendency in her family. Her high blood pressure led to kidney failure, causing her to abandon further educational ambitions. She developed complications including a rare condition known as calciphylaxis. It is a disease in which calcium accumulates in small blood vessels of the fat and skin tissues. This contributes to extra vascular calcification, clotting (thrombosis) and tissue death (necrosis), resulting from blood vessel stiffening and reduced oxygen blood flow to tissues in the skin. Calciphylaxis is extremely painful and requires rigorous remedial intervention. Usually attacking the abdomen, legs and buttocks, it can lead to death. Treatment for this condition is intensive and involves hemodialysis since peritoneal dialysis cannot be used. Dialysis sessions are longer and more frequent than the usual regime. Sometimes patients are given hypobaric oxygen therapy, as well as concentrated wound care to remove dead skin and help open sores heal.

When I met Jade, ten years had passed since her kidney failure diagnosis. She is still in her twenties, her calciphylaxis sufficiently controlled for her to receive a kidney from one of her siblings. Life for her had been difficult because of her condition and constant need for dialysis. She had often found herself out on a limb as she recounted her friends' inability to understand the pressures her illness wrought or her need to have to undergo dialysis constantly. Doctors were monitoring her condition in preparation for her forthcoming transplant. Life will improve dramatically for her following her transplant but that will never erase the hardship of the past ten years, only dull its memory. Her story is a stark reminder of the challenges young people, in particular, experience as a result of kidney failure, and the tremendous impact it has on their lives.

Number 3: Polycystic kidney disease

Polycystic kidney disease (PKD) is the third most common cause of kidney failure and can also affect liver function. PKD is a gene mutation, a permanent change in the deoxyribonucleic acid (DNA) sequence that makes up a gene. In most cases, PKD is inherited. In the remaining cases, the gene mutation develops spontaneously. Once spontaneous gene mutation occurs, it can be passed on. Statistics tell us that from one in four hundred to one in a thousand will be affected. It is more likely for men to fall into this category than women.[14]

Autosomal dominant PKD is the most common form, with a child inheriting the gene from one parent. In many cases, PKD does not cause signs or symptoms until cysts on the kidneys are half an inch or larger. Common symptoms are pain in the back and sides between the ribs and hips, resulting from cyst rupture. As cysts grow, they curtail the kidney's ability to filter waste products effectively and consequently impair kidney function. In some cases, the kidneys may need to be removed.[15]

My longtime friend, Allan Wheeler, whom I earlier referred to as my twin, is an excellent illustration of the impact PKD has on kidney function. To begin with, a little background. Allan Wheeler is an alias, a name he gave me because it is associated with his youth. When he was in junior school in Toronto, the class mischief-maker was named Allan Wheeler. A few years later, after my friend and his family had moved to Acton, Ontario, he and his friends were caught misbehaving. While his friends gave the policeman their real names, when it was my friend's turn to be questioned, "Allan Wheeler" just popped out. Today, my friend is a most upstanding citizen.

He told me PKD runs in his family, although his sister has been spared. He said his father died at the age of forty-one due to a cerebral aneurysm associated with PKD. His father's younger brother also died at forty-one from complications of PKD. Allan's grandfather also died at forty-one. His death was attributed to being gassed during World War I. Since there was no autopsy, Allan suspects that he, too, died from PKD.

Because of this family history, Allan decided at the age of twenty-five to have himself checked for PKD. He had not experienced any symptoms but felt this was a wise and safe move. His doctor confirmed that indeed he did have PKD and said that, while there was no specific treatment to prevent progression of PKD, he still had "a few years" before he would succumb to kidney failure. Allan was advised to continue having his blood pressure and blood work monitored on a regular basis, which he did. The doctor also suggested he seek genetic counselling. Allan, at the time, thought this meant something to do with his having children. He explained to me, "The thought was enough for me. I didn't follow up."

By the time Allan was thirty-seven, he was taking blood pressure medications and continuing to have his blood work checked. He and his wife Annie, my former colleague, had moved to Whitehorse and were living in an isolated area. There, Allan informed his new GP about his PKD diagnosis, and the doctor kept a close watch on his blood pressure and blood test results. When he was forty-five, test results showed a gradual rise in his creatinine levels. At the hospital in Whitehorse, Allan's condition was monitored by a doctor who used to be head of the transplant department in the Vancouver hospital that Allan was eventually referred to. The doctor informed Allan he was near end-stage renal failure. His best option was a transplant.

Other than a metallic taste in his mouth and bouts of gout, Allan said he felt fine. One day he and Annie, both keen sailors, were driving home from a boat trip. Allan, in his words, began to feel really "shitty," exactly how his doctor had predicted he would feel when his kidneys had "more or less given up." He was immediately sent to the Vancouver hospital to be assessed for a transplant.

He needed to start dialysis before he received a transplant, because no one could predict how long the process would take. Only eight months later, he was offered a transplant. Never having met anyone who had received a transplant, Allan had never realized that he himself would. For most of his life, he was convinced he was going to die at forty-one, just as the other men in his family had. He thought keeping his blood pressure in check had given him a few years longer than his father, uncle and grandfather had had. Following the transplant, however, he was "faced with the unimagined rest of my life." Allan continues to experience his unimagined life, doing extremely well in the process. He and Annie are a warm and magnanimous couple with whom I have shared many enjoyable events and dinners.

Number 4: Autoimmune diseases

Autoimmune diseases, the fourth most common cause of kidney failure, are a condition in which the body's own immune system works against itself, like a civil war within the body. It is an interior rebellion as opposed to an exterior assault. The body attacks its own tissues, including the skin, joints, heart, lungs, blood and kidneys. Autoimmune diseases such as scleroderma, systemic lupus erythematosus and granulomatosis with polyangiitis, formerly known as Wegener's disease, can all cause the kidneys to fail. Additionally, focal segmental glomerulosclerosis is occasionally associated with autoimmune diseases.

Scleroderma

The word *scleroderma* is formed from the Greek words *sclera*, meaning hardening, and *derma* meaning skin. Scleroderma refers to a hardening and thickening of the skin, in which it loses its elasticity and is no longer pliable, like plastic that hardens over time. Skin thickening can occur both externally and internally, causing blood vessels to narrow and making it more difficult for blood to circulate. Renal involvement occurs when there is a sudden intense increase in high blood pressure. Left undiagnosed or untreated, the combination of narrow vessels and high blood pressure can cause kidneys to fail.[16] While scleroderma can contribute to kidney failure and patients are advised to have their condition monitored, renal involvement is most likely to occur within the first two years of having been diagnosed. Scleroderma renal crisis, as it is termed, can happen suddenly, within days of blood pressure escalating. My first kidney failure occurred almost a year after I had been diagnosed with scleroderma. I experienced exceptionally high blood pressure. While I don't remember the exact readings, I do recall nurses telling me it was around 250 over an equally high count. About two percent of people diagnosed with scleroderma are affected by total renal failure. For the remainder, after a short spell on dialysis, their kidneys begin functioning again. It is, therefore, a very small percentage whose kidneys fail entirely.

Systemic lupus erythematosus

Systemic lupus erythematosus (SLE) can affect the skin, joints, brain and kidneys. The word *lupus* is derived from the Latin word for wolf and *erythematosus* from the word for redness. In the 13th century, physicians thought the shape and the colour of the skin lesions resulting from lupus resembled wolf bites.[17] Lupus can damage the glomerulus, or tuft of capillaries, a funnel-like frame where the filtering of waste begins before the blood enters the main structure of a kidney, with its some one million nephrons that do the main work of filtering. The damage weakens kidney function. One third of lupus patients will have some kidney impairment, while only about two percent will require dialysis.[18]

Not long after I had written this section, I was waiting alone in the anteroom prior to being called in for my treatment. There I was joined by a young-looking woman, whose story I learned as we talked. Haida, who works for a financial institution, is married and has a seventeen-year-old daughter. One day in 1980, she noticed her entire body was swollen. She immediately went to her GP, who referred her to a specialist.

The specialist carried out a number of tests, including blood work that indicated the root cause was lupus. Only her kidneys had been affected. She was encouraged to watch her diet and was prescribed with prednisone, an immunosuppressant steroid, to control both the lupus and her kidney disease. Unfortunately, the prednisone increased her level of swelling. For the next decade, her kidney function gradually deteriorated until it failed entirely. Her symptoms were high blood pressure, swollen legs and extreme fatigue. High doses of prednisone not only contributed to her leg swelling but also to her experiencing dramatic mood swings. One day she would feel fine, the next, wretched. She also noticed that if she had been lax with her diet, the swelling in both legs increased drastically at night. When her kidneys failed, a vascular surgeon created a fistula in her arm. She remained on dialysis for five years until she received a transplant. Prior to the transplant, she needed to undergo the most uncomfortable and painful procedure of actually having her fistula changed four times.

Having a transplant meant she could finally have children. One of the complications of kidney failure is the effect it has on an individual's reproductive system. It can contribute to low sperm count in men and loss of menses in women.[19] After her transplant, Haida was able to give birth to her daughter.

> The impact of uremic syndrome on the reproductive system can be devastating for renal patients, particularly young people who are facing sexual dysfunction or infertility.

Haida's kidney continued to work well until 2008, when blood tests revealed an increase in creatinine levels and decrease in glomerular filtration rate reading. When she learned this, she became "scared and depressed." Two biopsies later confirmed progressive scar tissue in her kidney. The doctors revised her fistula in 2012 in case she needed dialysis; however, her kidney continued working until August 2015, at which time she resumed dialysis. Between 2008 and 2015 Haida and her family travelled as much as possible, because she knew that if she started dialysis again, holidays and her freedom to travel would be limited.

Extraordinarily, Haida has continued working full-time throughout her ordeals, only taking time off for the birth of her daughter. Her day begins at 7:00 am when she drives her daughter to school. Then she heads downtown for work and returns to the hospital in the evening for dialysis. She prefers to try and stay active and to work while waiting for a second kidney transplant. Dialysis has so far been manageable but she is tired "and the worst part is getting home around 11:15 pm when my daughter is already in bed, and my husband can't stay up too long, as he is tired too, so sometimes I feel slightly low spirited." Still, she is grateful that lupus has only affected her kidneys and that her transplant lasted twenty years. She is also appreciative of having a dialysis machine that keeps her alive and fortunate in having a lovely daughter and great family support. All of these things keep her positive. I am taken by her tremendous drive and thriving spirit. Yet another remarkable kidney patient!

Granulomatosis with polyangiitis

The third autoimmune disease was formerly called Wegener's granulomatosis after the German pathologist who described this rare disease. However, when it was discovered in 2000 that Wegener had served as a high-ranking German medical officer near Lodz Ghetto in Poland during World War II, the American College of Chest Physicians renamed the disease ANCA-associated granulomatosis vasculitis. Now it is known as granulomatosis with polyangiitis.[20]

It is a rare disease marked by an inflammation of the walls of the small and medium sized blood vessels. Like scleroderma and lupus, it can be potentially life threatening. The inflammation damages the walls of the small- and medium-sized blood vessels. This inflammation results in tissue damage, severely impairing normal function. The affected tissues contain islands of inflamed cells and are known as granulomas.[21] Most kidney involvement can be mild but in some cases it can lead to total kidney failure.

Rebecca, my friend of whom I wrote earlier, has this condition.

Focal segmental glomerulosclerosis

A lesser-known but equally significant condition is focal segmental glomerulosclerosis (FSGS), also known as focal glomerular sclerosis or focal nodular glomerulosclerosis. It accounts for about a sixth of the cases of nephrotic syndrome. It is a cause of kidney disease in children and adolescents, as well as a leading cause of kidney failure in adults. Males are affected by FSGS slightly more than females, as are African Americans.[22]

In this condition, the glomeruli—the cells at the entrance to the kidney—become scarred. The scarring of FSGS only takes place in small sections of each glomerulus, and only a limited number of glomeruli are damaged at first. FSGS can have many different causes. The scarring may happen because of an infection, or a drug or a disease that affects the entire body, like diabetes, HIV infection, sickle cell disease or lupus. FSGS can also be caused by another glomerular disease that a person had before getting FSGS. Different types of FSGS are based on the cause.

In its early stages, FSGS may not cause any symptoms, but it gradually becomes apparent as large amounts of protein leaking into the urine (proteinuria) cause swelling in the legs, ankles and eyes and weight gain from extra fluid in the body. It also results in high blood pressure, high cholesterol, low blood protein and a risk for infection and blood clots.[23]

One evening as I sat in the waiting room before my night's treatment, out of the corner of my eye I noticed a young man whom I briefly described earlier in the book. I had lost touch with him. There is nothing more satisfying than being able to tie loose ends together. Tall, lanky and sturdy looking, he swaggered elegantly towards the receptionist's office. "Fabulous," I thought. "Now is my chance to find out how he is doing and hear his story at last."

Having completed his conversation with the receptionist, he sauntered over to the chair beside mine. Thus began an enjoyable friendship with my Renaissance Man. I call him this because he is a poet, philosopher and musician. He possesses an insatiable curiosity, and he is free-spirited. Others refer to him as The Cowboy because of his lean physique, his long, flowing, beautifully coiffed hair and his denim apparel, cowboy boots and hat. His stride suggests he has just jumped from the saddle, having left his horse tethered outside. Renaissance Man, whom I also think of as "Easy Rider" because of his love of motorcycles, engaged me in wonderful conversations about philosophy, music, life's quirkiness and, of course, the effects of our mutual kidney disease.

As we talked, I learned his story. Some years earlier, after a lengthy period of inconclusive and frustrating testing, he had been diagnosed with FSGS. He had been constantly feeling ill and found it difficult to explain to his co-workers why he was below par and not effectively performing his tasks as a community worker with the homeless and people at risk. He takes his work seriously, cares deeply about his clients' well-being and wants to perform his duties to the best of his abilities. He worried that his co-workers often considered him disengaged, not shouldering his responsibilities. "This," he said, "was disturbing and far from the truth. I just felt really unwell and couldn't work out what was wrong." The diagnosis helped solve the mystery of his fatigue and low energy, but did not necessarily enable him to carry out his duties with greater ease. He struggled for years trying to maintain his equilibrium and deal with his co-workers' concerns.

Then one day he woke up feeling absolutely dreadful. He said he knew he needed to get to the hospital as soon as possible. He quickly (keeping to speed limits) rode his trusty motorcycle to the emergency department, where, upon reaching the main entrance, he collapsed, out cold. He awoke in a bed surrounded by medical staff. The prognosis this time was kidney failure. Renaissance Man spent two months in the ICU as the doctors worked on his recovery and started him on hemodialysis. His motorcycle? Friends retrieved it from the hospital. When I first met him a year ago, he appeared to be in fairly good condition and certainly strong enough to drive himself to and from his treatment. Little did I know that a mere two months previously, he had been on death's door. As it had been with me all those years ago when I too had suffered from my first kidney failure, and then my second, he found the recuperative effects of dialysis significant.

What of Renaissance Man today? Having tried nocturnal dialysis, he has found the evening session works best for him. He says life remains taxing; kidney failure has cost him leisure, social and work time. He only has energy to work part-time, doing weekend shifts, thereby losing income and personal freedom. He no longer has the stamina to ride his prized motorcycle or play his drums on a regular basis. He usually feels enervated. He has challenges with his diet: even a small amount of potassium will cause his fingers to tingle, so he needs to vigilantly control his food intake. Recently his hemoglobin levels have skyrocketed and his blood production increased so significantly that without dialysis he would perish from an accumulation of it. While blood removed during dialysis is cleaned and returned to our bodies, extra fluid such as water—in Renaissance Man's case this also includes his surplus blood—is permanently removed between treatment sessions. CT scans have shown the presence of a cyst in one of his kidneys may be the culprit. Currently the doctors are deciding how to treat this situation, wondering if a nephrectomy is the right solution.

A secondary concern for Renaissance Man is the location of his fistula. It is positioned very close to his wrist bone and can be exceptionally painful when the nurses insert the needles. To combat the excruciating pain he takes painkillers that not only provide him with some relief but also enable him to sleep through part of his treatment. His other worry is that anyone seeing his fistula site might assume he consumes drugs and is, therefore, an addict, so he keeps his wrist well hidden from view. One of the nephrologists told me that many patients are sensitive about their fistulas because they stand out, look obtrusive and can appear unsightly. They will go to great lengths to cover them, wearing coats or jackets even on warm days so no one can see their fistula sites.

In spite of the many challenges confronting Renaissance Man, he remains vibrant and lively. Although he is immensely private, his insatiable drive for learning and interacting with others means he is popular and held in high regard by the other patients and staff. His optimism brightens our sojourn while we await the call to treatment.

Number 5: Failed transplants

Failed transplants are the fifth leading cause of kidney failure. Transplant failure can be caused by a number of factors: recipient rejection, high blood pressure, immunosuppressant medication, scarring or other traumas. I and my friends Bill, Haida, Wendy and Gerri are examples of people who have been affected by failed transplants. A kidney can fail at any time following a transplant—a few weeks later, several years later, at the kidney's estimated life span (see the box), or even up to thirty years later, as in Bill's case.

Second and third kidney failures are not uncommon, either. This does not suggest transplants should not be considered. They are a necessity for an individual to improve quality of life. Researchers are working valiantly to find ways to resolve the issue of failed kidneys.

> The life span of a kidney from a living donor is greater than that of a kidney from a deceased donor. On average a kidney from a living donor functions from 12 to 20 years, while a kidney from a deceased donor functions from 10 to 15 years. These figures are estimates. Some transplants last well beyond their estimated years.[24]

Number 6: Congenital abnormalities

Other causes of kidney disease and failure are related to congenital abnormalities in children. Defects can occur in the womb. Boys can be affected by posterior urethral valve obstruction, caused by a narrowing or obstruction in the urethra. It can be treated with surgery. A second condition called fetal hydronephrosis is an enlargement of one or both kidneys, which is caused by an obstruction in the developing urinary tract. It is also related to vesicoureteral reflux, in which urine flows backwards into the ureter when the bladder contracts. It is primarily diagnosed at a young age and requires monitoring and sometimes surgery. As opposed to polycystic kidney disease, multicystic kidney disease is characterized by large cysts that grow in an underdeveloped kidney and usually affects only one kidney.

Glomerulonephritis is an inflammation of the glomeruli that can result in the leaking of red blood cells and protein into the urine. This can result in a reduction in kidney function. Glomerulonephritis is more common in adults than children. High blood pressure and kidney stones can affect the kidney's function. Nephritis or any inflammation of the kidney caused by an infection or an autoimmune disease like lupus can contribute to both kidney disease and failure in children. Urinary tract infections (UTIs) in babies are more common in boys than in girls, because boys are more affected by congenital kidney problems, thus increasing their risk of kidney infections. In girls, shorter urethras contribute to their experiencing UTIs.[25]

My HandyDART friend Bill and my former student are examples of people who had congenital abnormalities as children, as is Henry Uptown, a truly exceptional individual to whom I have recently been introduced. Henry has endured the tediousness of hemodialysis on and off for thirty-four years. The nurses tell him he is the longest surviving patient in the unit. During this time he has written a journal of his experiences, feelings and thoughts. He has given me permission to share his journey. Henry was diagnosed with Type 1 diabetes at the age of six. He learned many years later that the doctors had told his mother they hadn't expected him to live past twenty-one years of age. To date he has beaten all odds, and some!

It wasn't until his early twenties that Henry began to feel unwell. He made an appointment to see his GP, who ran a number of tests to see if he had suffered complications from diabetes. A few days after the tests, Henry received a telephone call at the dining room where he worked as a waiter. The doctor informed him that his kidneys were failing, and he was referring him to a nephrologist.

Henry thought the doctor was overreacting and asked him if he could write him a prescription to fix the problem. The GP said there was no drug that could heal him so it was necessary for Henry to discuss his situation with the nephrologist. The nephrologist confirmed that his kidneys were failing; the only option was to start dialysis. Since Henry had no idea what dialysis involved, the nephrologist arranged for him to visit the hemodialysis ward to meet the nurses and other patients. The idea of dialysis so revolted him, such was his denial, that he refused the invitation and instead arranged to meet with the nephrologist a few weeks later to discuss things further.

At the second meeting, the doctor boosted his spirits by telling him he would feel much better once he had begun treatment. The doctor said the nurses were "a great bunch," so Henry agreed to visit the hemodialysis unit. Henry thought the machines were odd-looking with numerous IV bags and two small wheels whirring away in front; their motion circulated blood in and out of tubes attached to the patients' arms.

The first patient Henry talked with, although very friendly and willing to chat, had difficulty explaining the procedure to him. Henry believed the patient's inability to explain how dialysis worked resulted from the effects of the dialysis itself. He envisaged the same thing happening to him. He panicked and felt his legs turning to rubber as he fought back light-headedness.

He almost passed out but was rescued by one of the nurses who took him to her station, gave him a glass of water and reassured him that nothing ill would happen to him while he was on dialysis.

The following weekend he was attending a party with his friends, who, like him, were in their twenties. He watched them playing volleyball, swimming and laughing merrily in the warm sun while he sat, emotionally drained and staring blankly, realizing life was never going to be the same. Following the party and as time passed, he began to feel increasingly nauseated and weak, becoming sicker and sicker. His brain bogged down by toxins and increasingly unable to think clearly, he realized, "It was time to head to the hospital and face the reality that waited."

A few weeks later, a vascular surgeon created a fistula for dialysis treatments, but before it could be used, Henry had a temporary catheter inserted near his neck vein. The first time he was connected to a dialysis machine, he was tense, unsure as to how the process would work but with time, he began to feel more comfortable. When his fistula was ready to be used, and the nurse showed him the needles she was going to insert into his arm, attaching to the fistula, Henry's "anxiety went off the charts." The needles "looked like they were for horses, not me," he wrote. As the nurse gently inserted the needles, he held his breath, wondering how he was going to endure the same procedure three times a week for four hours at a time.

That was in 1982. The dialysis unit he attended consisted of six beds. There were seventy patients dialyzing on alternate days. Because the unit was so small, the patients few in number, and everyone spent so much time together, they got to know each other very well. The nurses truly were a great bunch, as the doctor had assured him, joking with the patients and making tea and toast for them. They talked about anything and everything. He was even invited to retirement and Christmas parties and other social events. The staff gave him a sense of security and belonging. "To this day, I have warm and loving feelings for them all," he wrote.

After a while, it became clear to him this was going to be his existence, forever on a merry-go-round, his life revolving around treatment after treatment. To him, "enduring dialysis three times a week was not living, but existing." His food intake was constantly monitored by dieticians; for a long time, he adhered to his new renal diet. However, the temptations of working in the food service industry got the better of him, and he decided dialysis was not going to take away his enjoyment of food, even if what he ate made him feel awful. If he was going to exist, "it would be on my terms," he decided. He began eating and drinking what he liked.

About two years later Henry learned that another local hospital performed transplants, although the one Henry was attending was a year away from doing the same. Henry was referred to the other hospital but told not to get his hopes up. During his appointment there, Henry learned that statistically he could not expect to live for more than two years. Stunned, he asked, "You mean I have only two years left to live?"

"Don't blame me for your disease," the doctor snapped. The conversation stopped quickly. But the upshot was that following a meeting with the transplant coordinator, Henry learned he was on the transplant list. The information was hard for him to digest; he was still reeling from the prognosis of having only two years left to live. He began living in a constant state of fear, waiting for his imminent demise.

In 1985 Henry received a phone call; he was about to receive a transplant. Elated, he rushed to the hospital. The surgery was a success, and his recovery proceeded well for about two weeks. Then the first signs of rejection appeared. The doctors reassured him that rejection was not uncommon and tried valiantly to reverse it with drugs. Unfortunately, it was not to be. The kidney was removed, and Henry once more found himself on dialysis.

He was emotionally crushed; hope had vanished. Henry had grown up in a violent, alcoholic home, devoid of love and comfort, where feelings of hostility and rejection left their mark. Even when he left home at the age of twenty, those feelings remained etched in his psyche. He adopted a persona to hide his true feelings of unworthiness and lack of self-esteem. He became the life of the party, "complete with a sarcastic sense of humour." He wanted to be liked and became what he thought everyone wanted him to be: a "chameleon," an all-purpose guy to fit in with others. He laughed on the outside while living a life of despair on the inside.

Henry was preoccupied with thoughts of his death. He wondered whether there was a heaven, and if so, would he be good enough for it. He imagined a "darkness beyond black," and "felt a loneliness that shook me to my innermost core." He had struck bottom. Panicking, he wondered how he was going to escape the horror. Henry had not adhered to anything remotely religious, because he was inclined to feel those who did so lived a rule-bound life, judging others who did not abide by their beliefs. He was now determined to seek a way out of his hole. He wanted to find someone who could explain how a belief in Jesus Christ worked.

He was sitting on a bench in the hospital by the elevators, having just made this intention, when the elevator doors opened. A man emerged, approached him and asked if Henry recognized him. "Why should I?" Henry asked.

"Because I am your uncle," the man responded. He had heard Henry was ill and had come to find out if Henry would like him to pray for him. This was "a surreal moment" but not a coincidence. It had been ordained; it was Henry's epiphany. It is not uncommon for us renal patients to seek solace in whatever ways we can. We draw on whatever resources we have at hand to cope with our ordeals. There is a long-held belief in the ability of prayer to shape our outcomes, however they might unfold. What Henry experienced has enabled him to carry on and deal with a chronic condition. His life changed dramatically when he accepted Christ into his life. He contributes his continued well-being to the impact this belief has had on him.

He tried to return to work, but as with many renal patients, found the work too challenging. He had little choice but to apply for social assistance after his unemployment sick benefits had run out. He applied for disability assistance, because with it, he would receive $75 extra per month. The Ministry of Health worker rejected his application, explaining if he received any further transplants, he would no longer be eligible to receive the benefit. No further transplants were on the horizon at this point, so Henry, enraged, took his case public.

A leading local TV channel ran the story about his plight. His doctors were also interviewed, along with other patients. All agreed that there was no guarantee a subsequent transplant would work. Even the Minister of Health agreed the policy was erroneous, and renal patients would now be classified as disabled. The next day Henry had a phone call from the Human Resources Department letting him know he would receive the requested benefits. Henry's achievement is mammoth and miraculous, especially since bearing the burden of renal failure is huge in itself. We renal patients owe our benefits to Henry's strength of commitment to righting a wrong. He deserves a tremendous accolade.

A year later, Henry did receive a second kidney transplant. This time it lasted two years. After it failed, Henry returned to dialysis. During this time, he had the good fortune to meet the woman who is now his wife. She has given him stability, companionship and even more importantly, the love he had never had. Astonishingly, a year later, after his return to dialysis, Henry's sister gave him his third kidney. That kidney lasted ten years, giving him his long-desired quality of life. He was able to work and enjoy time with his wife without any major health issues due to the generosity of his sister.

However, in 1999, his third kidney began to fail. The doctors also informed him he was no longer a candidate for a fourth transplant because of the increased number of antibodies in his blood. These had been a result of a series of transfusions he had received while being on dialysis. In the early days of dialysis, before EPO injections and iron infusions, blood transfusions had been commonly used to replace diminishing red blood cells. Henry reluctantly returned to dialysis. This ushered in another low period in his life. He could feel himself physically deteriorating, his muscles weakening and beginning to atrophy. He returned to the grim renal diet, having to monitor his potassium and phosphate levels as well as his fluid intake. Even his belief system had been tested. Fortunately one of Henry's renal doctors noted his change in demeanour and told him about a program in Toronto that supplied home hemodialysis machines to patients.

> A Frenchman, Jean Baptiste Denis (1643–1704), personal physician to King Louis XIV, is credited with carrying out the first blood transfusion in 1667. It was done on a fifteen-year-old boy who had bled so profusely that he required an infusion of blood. Interestingly enough, the blood used was that of a sheep. The boy survived.

Inspired by this information, Henry felt new hope. He encouraged patients interested in this program to write letters to their doctors and politicians in the desire to jumpstart the program. He met the Toronto doctor who had been brought to Vancouver to look into the possibility of providing the same service in BC. Finally, in the fall of 2004, Henry was accepted into the new home hemodialysis program. He responded well to this kind of dialysis. Life changed considerably for him. He could return to work, holding down two part-time jobs at a major sports arena, and experiencing a much-improved quality of life. Home dialysis allowed him to work swing shifts because he could choose his own times to dialyze.

He learned through a chance meeting with one of his first renal social workers that his doctors had not been very optimistic regarding his survival chances, but they had never told him this. He feels that, in retrospect, theirs was the right decision because had he known, he probably would not have had the resolve to continue. Instead, he fought to remain active, involved and optimistic by compartmentalizing his illness. It existed, but he believed "life was for living without limitations." He rarely talked to anyone about his disease; it remained in the hospital. These sentiments are so often shared by other renal patients. "Looking back," he wrote, "even in my darkest moments, I knew I would survive." Other renal patients often express this powerful optimism.

Having reached sixty-one years of age, Henry has contracted Hepatitis C, developed atherosclerosis and has calcified veins that restrict his peripheral blood flow. He has retinopathy, possibly attributed to diabetes and hypertension, and is blind in one eye. He has scarred lobes in both lungs from pneumonia, and emphysema. Additionally, his pancreas does not produce insulin and his kidney function is nil. In spite of these conditions, Henry knows he is a walking miracle. He owes his endurance to his faith, his wife, his sister and the marvellous care of his nurses and doctors. He says, "My caregivers have treated me as if I were valued." When I read his story, I know that I have been in the company of an extraordinary individual who deserves an enormous amount of credit for both his verve and achievements. I am privileged.

Number 7: Urinary tract infections

According to the National Kidney Foundation, "Every year urinary tract infections account for 10 million doctor visits." UTIs are more common in women. It is estimated that one in five women will have one UTI in their lifetime.[26] People with diabetes are also more prone to UTIs. The source of UTIs is usually a stream of *E. coli*, bacteria found in the intestines of humans and animals. Most strains are harmless, but a virulent one called *E. coli 0157:H7*, occurring in uncooked beef or unwashed fruit and vegetables including sprouts and unpasteurized milk products, can contribute to a serious illness, resulting in severe stomach cramps, diarrhea and vomiting. In its extreme, it will lead to kidney failure.[27]

> A UTI left untreated can move towards the kidneys via the ureter and cause a more serious infection that can also lead to chronic kidney disease or kidney failure.[28]

A less common cause: Medication

Other lesser known causes of chronic kidney disease, but equally important, are those resulting from medications. A number of patients have told me their kidney failure was directly related to prescribed medications. Recently in the dialysis ward I observed a relatively young woman waiting in a wheelchair for the bed I was soon to vacate. While gathering my things, as the bed was being cleaned and prepared, she told me that she had just been diagnosed with kidney failure and explained wryly, "I brought it on myself through overdosing on Ibuprofen." That's a warning: prolonged use of nonsteroidal anti-inflammatory drugs (NSAIDs) to control pain can have a detrimental effect on kidney function.

One afternoon, while waiting my turn for hemodialysis in the very crowded anteroom, I noticed a new patient, a man, who, while exceedingly thin from the effects of kidney disease, projected authority. I had been talking about my book with another patient. The new patient, upon hearing this, asked, "Are you writing a book?"

"Yes," I said.

"I have a proposal for a TV documentary about transplants. I hope to raise awareness about the need to increase the number of transplants performed in Canada. It is going to be my contribution to helping people," he explained.

Will, it turned out, had been a TV producer for a major broadcasting company. He told me, "I am very keen to produce a documentary highlighting Spain's opt-out program referred to as the 'Spanish Model.'"

"What is that?" I asked.

He then told me: "It is an organ donation program in which every citizen is considered to be a potential donor unless they or a family member specify otherwise. The program was devised by a Dr. Rafael Matesanz when he was appointed head of the Spanish National Transplant Organization in 1989. My film director has had a number of conversations with him."

Should citizens wish to opt out of an organ donation program like the Spanish one, they need to apply in writing to the responsible government agency. The age of consent for most countries begins at twelve.

I further learned that in Spain every hospital has a specially trained team of transplant experts who are on 24-hour call so they can be present in an ICU whenever an individual has been pronounced brain dead. Although Spanish law presumes consent, in practice the specifically trained surgeon always seeks a family's permission first. The program's emphasis is on personal contact with families, with whom the surgeon discusses the benefits of having their loved one's organs donated to another person in need. In the case of a patient who has been pronounced dead, a sixteen-hour window of opportunity exists in which to retrieve their organs, and this enables families to have time to consider the donation. Most families agree. As a consequence of this program, the waiting time for any organ in Spain is eight months as opposed to years.

The program has been in operation for twenty-five years. During this time, the increase in donors has risen from fourteen donors in a million to thirty-five donors in a million.[29] Interestingly enough, the recent recession that caused tremendous hardship and upheaval in Spain does not appear to have affected the Spanish organ program. It has continued to produce effective results in spite of the expenses incurred to maintain it. But as with all countries, while attempting to address the needs, shortfalls in supply still prevail. In contrast to the deceased donor program, Spain's living donor program results fall behind other countries.

The first country to propose a law for opt-out donation and to pass it was Belgium. The law was proposed in 1986 and it passed in 1987.[30] Twenty-four countries have adopted the opt-out model for organ and tissue donation. Some of the participating countries include Belgium, Spain, Austria, Finland, Czech Republic, France, Greece, Hungary, Israel, Italy, Luxembourg, Norway, Poland, Slovenia, Wales, Singapore, Chile, Sweden and Turkey. Countries not participating are called "opt-in," meaning individuals need to actively consent to organ donation.

Opt-out programs in general remain controversial in terms of both economic maintenance and ethical considerations. In order for a program to be operational, it requires a tremendous amount of investment in healthcare infrastructure, including transplant centres, trained doctors, transplant nurses and aftercare. Ethical considerations factor into the equation since the establishment of a program of this nature falls within either federal/national or provincial law. The question, therefore, that needs to be asked is whether or not such a program affects an individual's civil rights. A number of countries have debated the pros and cons of adopting a similar program. Australia is currently considering whether or not to participate in the opt-out model.

Will had begun his career as a cameraman many years ago in Africa, eventually becoming a producer, producing numerous documentaries over the years. One of his jobs was working for the Canadian government on an environmentalist project in Brazil. While working on the documentary, he met and collaborated with Al Gore, who impressed him not only because of his dedication to environmental issues but also because of his vast knowledge of the subject.

Will and I have enjoyed many wonderful conversations. Will is a natural raconteur and full of enchanting stories both about his work and of the many renowned people he has met. I have found his company in the waiting room a delight and a good break from the dull routine of dialysis.

Will believes he succumbed to kidney failure as a result of a particularly strong medication, prescribed to deter the effects of atrial fibrillation, an abnormal heart rhythm characterized by rapid and irregular beating.[31] After having taken one dose, Will woke the next day to find he could not open his eyes. The specialist who prescribed the medication did not explain the reason for his difficulty in opening his eyes, but insisted this was the best medication for his condition. He suggested that Will use eye drops to alleviate his problem. He did, with little relief. He had a blood test taken some time afterwards that showed a sudden drop in his glomerular filtration rate (GFR) reading. GFR in a healthy individual usually registers at 60 millilitres/minute per 1.73 m^2 (ml/min/1.73 m^2). His had dropped to 45, an initial indication that his kidneys were not adequately filtering waste. He developed headaches, but otherwise seemed healthy. Another cardiologist recommended switching medications to control his atrial fibrillation. The switch proved effective, his atrial fibrillation controlled and his eyesight normal.

Some two years later, further blood tests showed an even greater drop in his GFR down to 35 ml/min/1.73 m^2. He was referred to the kidney care clinic at my hospital, and his condition and blood count were monitored every six months. Will did not receive any treatment other than being advised to carefully watch his diet. In other words, he was counselled to use a renal diet. Slowly his GFR levels deteriorated, as did his kidney function.

Six years later his kidneys finally failed. Six months before starting hemodialysis, he had a fistula created. Will also believes in taking more natural remedies and has been prescribed some medication by his naturopath, who, interestingly, has himself had two kidney transplants. (One was at sixteen, donated by one of his sisters, and lasted twenty years, and the second was donated by his other sister immediately upon failure of the first. Twenty-five years later, it continues to perform well.) Will trusts his naturopath's recommendations, knowing he has a good understanding of kidney disease. Although the cause of Will's kidney failure was never fully confirmed, he believes it was likely related to the strong medication he was initially prescribed.

Will has recently told me that after having eight months of hemodialysis treatment, first in the hospital unit, then in a community unit, he has found this type of dialysis treatment more draining than he had anticipated so is switching to peritoneal dialysis. He feels this is the preferred option for him.

Symptoms

Each of the contributing causes has its own symptoms. Here are a few. Diabetes often results in nerve damage, mostly felt in extremities such as feet and toes and, in some cases, blindness. High blood pressure in extreme readings can cause severe headaches and dizziness. In polycystic kidney disease there can be back pain. Autoimmune diseases often manifest themselves in muscle and joint pain, headaches, fatigue, tightened skin and rashes, and limb swelling, as well as the condition known as Raynaud's disease that is characterized by narrowing vascular channels leading to poor peripheral blood circulation affecting fingers, nose and toes. The appendages turn blue or white, even in warm temperatures. Focal segmental glomerulosclerosis can contribute to excessive swelling and weight gain. Kidney infections lead to lower back pain, nausea and increased temperatures. Cystitis or bladder infections result in fevers, as well as pain in the lower back and the urethra. Urinating is particularly painful. Each of these presents their own level of discomfort and a feeling of illness for the individual.

Kidney failure itself has a number of symptoms that may or may not be combined with the contributing cause. These are the classic symptoms of kidney failure: little or no urine; swelling, usually in the legs and feet, less often in the hands or face; disorientation, a lack of being connected to the world and trouble concentrating on tasks due to low hemoglobin or iron; feeling unwell or undue fatigue; generalized itchiness resulting from dry skin and an increase in creatinine levels; headaches, possibly due to high blood pressure; severe weight loss, often coupled with reduced appetite and nausea accompanied with vomiting; sleep disturbances or extreme sleepiness; skin discolouration; muscle cramps in legs; and shortness of breath. However, while there are common patterns and symptoms, a number of people with kidney disease never experience any symptoms at all, hence the name "the silent killer."

For my second kidney failure, I was alerted by a number of the symptoms. The first one that distressed me the most was a feeling of disorientation due to low hemoglobin and iron. It led to me feeling a sense of confusion that ebbed and flowed for some months without an ability on my part to counteract its effects. As my kidney failure became more obvious, my physical strength decreased. I had been working hard to develop muscle strength lost through my spinal cord injury and had really just begun to feel that I was gaining some ground when I began to suffer from physical weakness. I experienced overwhelming weakness along with loss of movement. While I never lost sleep or felt unduly sleepy, I certainly felt more tired than usual.

The second symptom I was most conscious of was an increase in the strength of my neuropathic pain. I experienced an intensity of burning in my fingers and muscles and sharpened aches in my limbs and neck. I understand that whenever one aspect of our physical being is under attack, our whole system suffers the effects. Just as a bout of flu can send us crashing, so can the effects of kidney failure.

My final symptom that confirmed my kidney failure was nausea. It was extreme and definitely affected my desire for food. It also limited my rational thought. I was a mess by the time I had been admitted to hospital.

The benefit of therapy has meant somewhat of a return to normal life. I say "somewhat" because there is always a residue of the kidney failure itself and the treatment.

Prevention

When I talked to others about my proposed book, I was asked if there was anything that could be done to prevent kidney disease and its subsequent kidney failure. I discussed prevention techniques with doctors, dieticians and nutritionists and did my own research. I learned that the standard good health strategies are as important in preventing serious illness as they are in maintaining our well-being. Good hygiene, frequent hand washing, thorough cleaning of fruit and vegetables, and proper handling and cooking of meat and poultry all rank high on the list. Eating nutritiously, avoiding both junk food and overly sugary foods, cooking what we eat as simply as possible, avoiding processed foods and cutting down on our salt intake are significant measures. A low-salt diet is a part of renal health and a necessity for those with high blood pressure, but even people whose systems are not compromised benefit from a reduction in salt. Drinking adequate water to help flush our system is of paramount importance, too.

Fighting the flab is equally critical; a healthy diet and plenty of exercise definitely go a long way in keeping us both well and fit. Recent studies conducted in the United States show obesity is once again on the rise.[32] Not smoking aids us enormously. For those who have heightened risk factors such as diabetes and high blood pressure, careful management of these conditions is vital to keeping them in check. None of these suggestions differs from what we are hearing from Health Canada. When I see my retired friends who are healthy, I notice the quality of their lives is absolutely beyond compare. Diets for people with kidney failure, however, do not follow the usual recommendations. We are asked to consume white bread, little fibre, limited types of vegetables and small amounts of fruit, in addition to having to drink less fluid. It is the antithesis of all that the general population is advised to do. If living a healthier life prevents us from developing kidney disease and becoming subject to its subsequent restrictive diet, then surely it is not asking too much.

Unknown causes

Now, try as we might to follow these strategies, sometimes there is nothing we can do to prevent us from succumbing to kidney disease or failure. In some cases, it is difficult to determine what causes kidney disease and kidney failure. Many of my fellow patients have revealed the cause of their kidney failure has never been determined. While applied mathematics, physics and chemistry are exact sciences, medicine is not.

One of my British consultants told me, "There was nothing you could do. You were a marked person." This was reiterated by one of the nephrologists I consulted. Why it happens remains a mystery. What causes some of us to develop a particular condition is sometimes a matter of speculation.

Treatment

Once a person is diagnosed with kidney failure, there are two forms of renal replacement therapy. One is dialysis and the other is a kidney transplant. For dialysis there are two options: peritoneal dialysis or hemodialysis. In peritoneal dialysis, a tube called a catheter is medically inserted into the abdomen. There are two types of peritoneal dialysis, one being continuous ambulatory peritoneal dialysis (CAPD), the form I used in my first kidney failure. It requires exchanging the dialysis solution every four to six hours during the daytime. It is less used today. The other is called continuous cycler peritoneal dialysis (CCPD). A machine is programmed to perform exchanges overnight during sleep. Exchanged solution is drained into washroom facilities. In the morning one exchange is performed that lasts all day.

There are a number of advantages to dialyzing using peritoneal dialysis. It can be performed at home and in a person's own time. It provides greater freedom of mobility and access to easier travel. People can more easily work while using this method. As well, individuals are able to eat a wider variety of foods containing higher amounts of potassium, while still being cautious of foods high in phosphate. A phosphate binder such as calcium needs to be taken prior to each meal, something that is necessary for all dialysis patients. Quantity of fluids is less restricted because solutions can be adapted to remove extra intake. In the early stages, training is provided and follow-up appointments are regular, but once a routine has been established and the system works well, it is only necessary to attend clinics every three months. Toxin clearance is very good because of the continuous dialyzing.

When my friend Allan Wheeler was diagnosed with kidney failure, he explained he was given three options: home hemodialysis, hospital hemodialysis and peritoneal dialysis. Peritoneal dialysis sounded revolting to him. Hospital dialysis was out of the question because he and his wife, still living in Whitehorse, had no access to a hospital offering hemodialysis. He opted for home hemodialysis but was told the waiting list just to take the course was about a year, and until then, he would need to be treated at a hospital. His only choice was to do peritoneal dialysis.

Once he had mastered the technique and found the discomfort to be minimal, apart from having a bit of a pot-belly, he felt fine. Allan worked as an electrician, while his wife taught in a college. Their home was a rustic cabin with no water or electricity. The sole source of heat was a wood stove. Living an informal lifestyle suited them. While using peritoneal dialysis, he and his wife were able to continue living in their cabin. Allan could eat and drink whatever he wanted, continue working and even travel. Storing the solution boxes was a bit of a problem because he was worried that the solution would freeze in cold weather. The hospital staff assured him that this would not be a problem since the solution could be thawed. His ability to manage his exchanges amazes me.

Allan said the most important and the trickiest part, "especially in a smoky, dog- and cat-filled cabin" was keeping the connection to his catheter hygienically immaculate. The nurses who monitored his care emphasized this over and over. An inserted catheter is an open door to peritonitis. That was his biggest risk. So positive was his overall experience with peritoneal dialysis, however, that Allan would have no hesitation in doing it again, should his transplanted kidney ever fail.

Doing peritoneal dialysis worked for Allan, but there is the need to have space in which to store the many boxes of solution and the supplies that are delivered either monthly or bimonthly. Scrupulous hygiene to avoid infections when cleaning the exit site and when attaching the solution bag to the catheter is vital. Peritoneal dialysis users are now advised, in addition to washing hands, to wear a mask when cleaning their site and attaching the solution tube to their catheter. However, neither Allan nor I were encouraged to wear masks when we prepared to dialyze in the 1990s.

While the advantages of using peritoneal dialysis are many, it is not always possible for an individual to dialyze using this method. Sometimes the drained-in solution, instead of being easily removed, remains in the abdomen and becomes absorbed rather than being removed when the solutions are exchanged. This happened to me in my second kidney failure. The absorbed solution stayed in place and added water retention, contributing to swelling in my body, hands and feet. I could not continue using this method. For some, dialysis at home simply isn't an option, whether due to lack of physical space, physical or cognitive capabilities or concerns with hygiene. They have no other choice but to do hemodialysis, the second form of dialysis treatment. Some people simply prefer to do hemodialysis.

In order to perform hemodialysis, vascular access that can be used to remove waste products from the blood and return cleaned blood to the body is required. A vascular surgeon creates an arteriovenous fistula in a vein, most commonly in the arm.[33] In some cases the fistula may be inserted in other parts of the body, depending on the most appropriate access point. Sometimes veins may not be appropriate because they are too narrow or may have already collapsed. As a result of the effects of scleroderma, the doctors felt my veins were unsuitable, so instead I had a catheter inserted into my neck vein, directly connected to my heart. A catheter may also be used in the early stages of hemodialysis when it is necessary to perform immediate dialysis.

One advantage of hemodialysis is that, with specific training, it is possible to do it at home. Unlike peritoneal dialysis, the machines are larger and the training longer and more complicated. It also requires access to both water and electricity and, in some cases, modifications to accommodate the machine. At home, individuals typically perform at least five to eight hours of dialysis four to five times a week. This means there is a possibility of greater toxin removal because the process is done more slowly over a longer period of time. It also frees up the day and is more amenable for those who are able to and wish to work. Some hospitals provide overnight dialysis. The outcome is similar to home hemodialysis.

Another advantage of hemodialysis is having access to a hospital or community clinic where nurses connect the individual to the hemodialysis machine and monitor the process throughout a session.

One of the disadvantages of having to perform hemodialysis in an external setting is the inflexible necessity of having to attend three times a week. The American postal service expression, "Neither snow nor rain nor heat nor gloom of night stays those couriers from their swift completion of their appointed task,"[34] is equally applicable to hemodialysis patients. Holidays and socializing have little relevance; there is no option but to attend the sessions. For most, a session is four hours in duration. I have met some people who attend three times a week but for up to six hours at a time in order to maximize clearance efficiency, and still others who attend four times a week for three hours because they cannot tolerate a longer time frame.

Diet and fluid restrictions are much greater. It is possible to adjust potassium levels using different levels of solution, and taking phosphate binders prior to eating can reduce phosphate levels, but there is nothing to replace fluid intake. It requires constant watchfulness. Fatigue factors into the mix, too. Following a session, an individual feels weary, tired and drained.

Both fistulas and catheters can be sources of infections. A fistula needs to be checked twice a day to ensure it is working effectively, and it needs to be washed prior to treatment. For anyone such as myself who has a catheter, it is essential that it remains intact and clean. I cannot have a proper shower and need to wash my hair in a sink to avoid water getting into my site. Because it is a direct conduit to my heart, any infections could be fatal. The advantage to having a catheter is that once the dialysis tubes are removed and my catheter tubes cleaned, I do not need to check blood leakage, because there is none. The downside of having a fistula is the potential for bleeding following dialysis. All dialysis patients need to hold their site for some time following needle removal. As one of my friends reported, this can take up to fifteen minutes, meaning a delay in getting home. As well, a person's arm can be quite sore following treatment.

Another challenge is that over time veins can narrow, leading to less blood flow. This can hamper the dialysis treatment and require a procedure called angioplasty to open up or dilate the narrowed area. A wire with a deflated balloon is inserted through a catheter at the fistula site over the narrowed area. Once inserted, the balloon is inflated, dilating the vein. I have been told this treatment can be very unpleasant, terribly painful and uncomfortable, and it can result in severe bruising. A fellow dialysis patient informed me recently that it is necessary for her to have this procedure every few weeks.

Fistulas may also need to be replaced, again an uncomfortable process.

Not all hemodialysis patients are well. Some are considerably ill and require greater care than others. In one of the rooms where I dialyze, there are a number of patients who come by hospital-transfer ambulance. One such patient is an older man who is accompanied by his wife. She is his constant companion, never leaving her husband's side for the entire dialysis session. She caresses his head and hands to comfort him, adjusts and fetches blankets if she feels he is cold and calls for aid as needed. The wife's dedication to her husband is without equal. It is an incredible experience to witness this depth of such open affection. Open affection is not often seen in a hospital ward, wards being public places, but they can also be an enormously private refuge for some.

As a renal patient, I have frequent blood tests to ensure my internal systems are in balance, and I have regular consultations with a dietician regarding my diet to make sure my potassium, phosphate and protein levels are good, as well as to help me work around the food restrictions. I also meet with a specialized pharmacist to keep abreast of medications I need. It is helpful for me to learn why I have been prescribed certain medications. All medications can have side effects; some may interact badly with others. What proved effective once may not continue to be effective. I am always a work in progress; nothing is static. I have access to a social worker, an important service because renal failure is stressful. Doctors provide medical coverage during the day and evening routine to check on my progress or medical needs.

The effectiveness of the hemodialysis treatment is closely monitored. My blood flow and clearance are checked periodically to ensure it is working well. Once a month this is checked by using a Transonic machine, explained in a previous chapter.

As I discussed in chapter 4, I have received pneumonia, hepatitis and TB vaccinations, and I have yearly flu shots as well as yearly bacteria checks to prevent further complications from occurring as well as to keep me safe while I am in a group environment. No matter how efficient the hygiene—the cleaning and changing of bed sheets, machines, equipment, even our TV remote controls—the danger of acquiring an illness is heightened when groups of people are brought together. Every three months I fill in a form to personally assess my own condition, effects and feelings; all this is part of the medical staff's vigilance in keeping me well and safe. I am appreciative of their continuous care and attention.

All dialysis nurses have specialized in hemodialysis as well as in peritoneal techniques. The technicians, who prime the hemodialysis machines, organize the dialysis solutions and attend to malfunctioning machines, are also specifically trained for this job. The technicians work the same hours as the nurses and are considered part of the team.

One particular evening, a call of nature required my nurse to perform an intervention on my behalf. Using the washroom facilities carries its own set of challenges. The nurses need to unhook us from the dialysis machines in order for us to be mobile. This requires clamping the tubes to prevent unwanted blood flow, returning some of our blood so that we don't experience dizziness or become too weak to move, and flushing our lines to ensure they are clear. On this singular occasion my nurse had not only just concluded her probationary period but was also working on her own for the first time. Because I was attached to the specialized hemodiafiltration machine, it was essential that my lines be clamped prior to their being removed; my newly trained nurse forgot to complete this part. She began to unhook me when an enormous geyser of blood spurted out, covering not only me, my bedsheets and the surrounding area, but also her. We were a drenched sight! My poor nurse, humbled beyond words and covered in both blood and embarrassment, stuttered her profuse apologies. No damage had occurred other than to her own feelings of discomfiture. When I returned, upon my refreshed bed was a huge bunch of flowers from my ashamed nurse. We often laughed about this occurrence afterwards. My nurse has since told me, "Never again have I done this. Lesson learned the hard way."

To have or not to have treatment remains the individual's choice. For some, the prospect of having to dialyze for years is not inviting. For others, a transplant may not even be a possibility. When I was first diagnosed with my second kidney failure and contemplating peritoneal dialysis, my peritoneal dialysis home nurse told me a patient had been on peritoneal dialysis for twenty years. A distant relative of mine had been on hemodialysis for forty years, discontinuing on his seventieth birthday. With a prospect of a long wait for a kidney transplant, and the possibility of further health risks accompanying kidney failure, it is easy to understand why some may prefer to forego treatment, trusting their lives to nature. The medical staff are entirely supportive of an individual's decision. Sadly, many people do die before they receive a transplant. This may very well happen to me. I have been on hemodialysis for almost three years; statistics show that over 50 percent of patients on hemodialysis do not live beyond their first five years of treatment.

The second form of treatment is a kidney transplant. While it is not a cure for kidney disease, it does provide an enormously improved standard of living. A spokesperson for BC Transplant told me their greatest wish would be to be able to offer transplants as a preventative measure even before a person needs dialysis, as soon as end-stage kidney disease has been diagnosed. That is not currently an option due to shortages of organ donors.

According to Kidney Research UK, the leading national research charity dedicated to kidney treatment and cures in the United Kingdom, a transplant functions exactly in the same way a normal kidney does. In two original, fully functioning kidneys, the estimated amount of blood filtered is approximately 180 litres per day. The number of times blood is filtered is approximately sixty times every twenty-four hours. This continuous filtering removes the body's waste products such as creatinine (a by-product of normal muscle function) and excess fluids, and they are eliminated in the urine. Fully functioning kidneys produce a natural hormone, erythropoietin, to prevent anemia and also convert vitamin D into an active compound that helps to keep bones healthy. They additionally work to excrete the effects of some drugs and help control blood pressure.

A normal kidney performs these functions continuously, day and night, year in, year out completely unnoticed. Healthy people are usually oblivious to the complexities of how a kidney carries out its work in maintaining their overall well-being.

Kidney Research UK further states, "It has been shown that kidney transplantation gives a better quality and quantity of life than dialysis treatment."[35] When kidneys fail, converting vitamin D no longer occurs, nor does the blood produce red cells. As previously described, EPO injections are given to us renal patients to simulate the production of these. Transplantation is the preferred course of treatment. Nephrologists, organizations and agencies in Canada, Britain and other countries agree on this.

All forms of dialysis are enormously expensive, the most expensive being hospital hemodialysis because of the equipment, solution, nurses, technicians and medical staff as well as the space required. In my unit, the ratio of patients is two to one nurse for those requiring extra care and attention, three patients to one nurse for more independent patients who are able to perform some of the many required tasks, and five patients to one nurse for those on nocturnal dialysis. Dialysis is also environmentally unfriendly, given the number of tubes, equipment, various needles and amount of solution and chemicals used, as well as the empty solution containers needing to be destroyed and the filtering of solution into main drains.

A report undertaken by the Canadian Institute of Health Information (CIHI) stated that over a five-year period, a kidney transplant patient's care can cost approximately $250,000 or less than an individual on dialysis.[36] Transplantation is the most economically feasible and healthiest form of treatment. It doubles the life expectancy of a dialysis patient. For me, it meant twenty-two years of additional life and income. Economically, countries gain. My healthcare costs dropped considerably. I was able to work during my first kidney failure because my health permitted it, and my time on dialysis was short in comparison to the norm, so I benefitted from having an income, which, being taxable, meant the governments in both the UK and Canada benefitted from collecting the extra revenue. Just imagine if all dialysis patients who are unable to work could return to work following a transplant: a country's gross national product would increase incrementally as would government revenue from the ability to collect taxes on the earned income. Healthcare costs saved could be invested in other areas of need.

> The Canadian Institute for Health Information (CIHI) is a non-profit organization whose responsibility is to report on health information data for Canada. Its mandate is "To lead the development and maintenance of comprehensive and integrated health information that enables sound policy and effective health system management that improve health and health care."

A further consequence for me was that my earning capacity enabled me to become self-sufficient, provide for my son, contribute to a pension fund and save for my eventual retirement. Having a salary likewise meant I had both buying and spending power, so could continue to help keep the economy flowing.

To date, the longest recorded kidney transplant in BC is forty years. This person is still going strong.[37] A woman in the UK received a kidney from her mother in 1973 and is still alive, forty-three years later. In reality, this kidney is over one hundred years old: the woman's mother was fifty-seven when she donated her kidney.[38] On average, the life span of a living donor kidney is twenty years. These two exceptions are astounding.

Conclusion

Our kidneys are one of the most important organs in our body and are of vital significance to our well-being. By replacing the word *person* for *patient,* then, truly their guardianship perfectly reflects that, *"For the secret of the care of the person is in caring for the person."* Our person, our own health and the treatment of it matter indeed. For those of us who enjoy the benefits of good health, it is we ourselves who must maintain our own vigilance. For those of us whose health has been compromised, we rely on the know-how, compassion and good judgement of our doctors, nurses and caregivers to keep watch over our welfare. To them we are indebted for their efforts in protecting us from further harm and helping us survive another day.

Chapter 7 | Among the Nocturnal Elite

Gently does it!

A friendship made then lost

We instinctively recognize from the moment of first encounter, words aside, the intangible understanding that we are in the company of one of those rare people who by their very being exude true kindness and genuine empathy for others. A person who not only instills in us a wish to be better ourselves but also leaves us in awe of their innate humaneness. Charity, her pseudonym, personifies such a being. She arrived one evening in the waiting room as a new hemodialysis patient. Immediately those of us present recognized her appeal. There was something entirely open and hugely friendly emanating from her personality. We easily fell into conversation with her.

Charity had had diabetes for thirty years and had been diagnosed with kidney disease in 2009. Blood tests following a knee replacement surgery revealed a very high level of creatinine and potassium. Charity was subsequently referred to a nephrologist who performed a myriad of tests and confirmed kidney disease. The disease eventually led to kidney failure in November 2015. When we met her, she was a new initiate into the world of hemodialysis. Charity's story is similar to many others whose kidney failure was caused by diabetes. Although she has managed to avoid some of the accompanying side effects of this disease, her eyesight has been affected. She is virtually blind in one eye and requires painful monthly injections in an attempt to save her good eye. She requires two injections of insulin a day and takes water pills and medication for high blood pressure.

At the time of our meeting, she was on six-month disability leave from her full-time work as a provincial civil servant. Too young to retire and not old enough to receive a pension, she had to keep working. Having kidney failure and the subsequent need for treatment had had significant consequences for her life. She was feeling physically exhausted the day after her dialysis sessions, too drained to do much socializing or any activity. Dialysis on Mondays, Wednesdays and Fridays made Sundays her only time for participating in social activities. Not easy for someone who was a people person. As well, the financial fallout of kidney failure had been extensive.

"Everything costs more, given that I don't have the energy I once had to do things for myself, so ordering in food, hiring someone to clean has become a priority for me. I also find using public transport a challenge sometimes and have had to rely on taxis. It all adds up," she said.

Emotionally, the toll had likewise been devastating. Charity felt fragile and discouraged by the limitations of kidney failure. "Travelling was the greatest pleasure in my life," she said. She was not complaining but found it hard to imagine her long-term future. Although she had been accepted as a potential kidney transplant recipient, her blood type and the lack of available kidneys could lead to a wait of eight years before a matching donor is found. Charity further confided, "I have suspended my dreams for now, based on the premise that I may only be disappointed if further challenges occur to thwart them." This feeling is not uncommon among kidney patients. We are not naturally pessimistic, but given the current climate, we are inclined to become more pragmatic in our expectations.

The doctors had told her that once on dialysis, she would feel better and would lead a more conventional life. This had not been the case. She said, "I am not feeling better," something that further corroborated her then-current attitude. She was learning to take one day at a time and in doing so advised: "Savour the good moments and accept the others." She was continuing to produce urine, thereby not needing to restrict her fluid intake. I drooled upon hearing her talk of having had a large bowl of soup. Something long forbidden me since my production is much less than hers. None of her worries or concerns affected her outgoing, warm and sympathetic nature.

Charity's time with us was brief. She was switching to the nocturnal dialysis program hoping that in so doing she would feel well enough to return to work full-time. She and I kept some contact by email. She would occasionally stop by my bed on her way to her nightly treatment. Then another blow: a diagnosis of possible breast cancer. Soon we lost contact; I doubted I would ever have the pleasure of her company again. I felt sad, left yet again with an unfinished story. How wrong I was. We met again when I transferred to nocturnal dialysis.

Nocturnal dialysis: What it is and how it works

Dr. Robert Uldall, working at Wellesley Hospital in Toronto 1993, developed the concept of nocturnal dialysis. The previous year, Dr. Charra, in Tassin, France, had pioneered an overnight dialysis program consisting of three lengthy nighttime sessions per week. Dr. Uldall in conjunction with another Toronto nephrologist, Dr. Andreas Pierratos, converted this program into an overnight, home-based hemodialysis treatment consisting of six sessions per week.[1] The premise was that a longer, gentler dialysis run would provide better toxin clearance, thereby reducing some of the existing side effects of dialysis and leading to an improvement in a patient's health. In 1994, the first patient was trained to perform dialysis at home. Unfortunately Dr. Uldall died in 1995 before further research proved his theory to be effective.

Dr. Pierratos, therefore, continued the research, publishing a paper in 1998 in which he laid out the benefits of nocturnal dialysis. It confirmed that the longer, slower, gentler form of dialysis not only removed more toxins and fluid but also led to improved blood results. Lower potassium and phosphate levels were achieved, reducing the need for rigid food restrictions. Also, patients no longer needed to take phosphate binders to control phosphate levels. They reported an improved appetite, leading to better health in general. Results included an increase in albumin, the most abundant blood plasma protein, and a decrease in urea, the major waste component of urine which gives urine the ammonia smell and, for dialysis patients, its taste in their mouth. Lower levels of urea are a major indicator of healthy kidney function. Its levels rise drastically with impaired kidney function.

Some patients experienced lower blood pressure levels, too, no longer requiring blood pressure medications. Additionally, an improvement in blood circulation was noticed. A further benefit was shown in 2012. Professor John Agar, at the Geelong Clinic in Australia, demonstrated that the thickness of the muscle wall of the left ventricle of the heart normalizes as the strain is lifted from the heart and calcium deposits in blood vessel walls diminish.[2]

Other benefits included a reduction in post-dialysis nausea, fatigue, headaches, weakness and vomiting. During dialysis, many patients experienced painful cramping: this, too, disappeared. Skin colour improved, and patients reported increased energy as a result of a better quality of sleep. Many patients could return to full-time work and lead more conventional lives. One of the most valued benefits was having greater daytime freedom and more time to pursue activities—a real bonus for dialysis patients. As one nurse told me prior to my embarking on my new journey, "Many patients who have had to stop nocturnal dialysis for a while can't wait to return. They find it a much more positive form of treatment." When I learned this information, it instantly made sense why the fellow whose wife I had briefly met earlier in my dialysis sessions explained that her husband was content to continue with his home dialysis treatment and did not necessarily want a transplant.

Today, it is accepted that the benefits of nocturnal dialysis outweigh the downsides that can include difficulty in disconnecting the blood access sites, whether via fistula or catheter. Disconnection problems can contribute to excess blood loss and site infections.

Becoming a nocturnal patient

Towards the beginning of my second year on dialysis, I started experiencing greater unpleasant side effects after my two evening and one afternoon hemodialysis sessions. Nightly sleep, a restorative balm, became harder to achieve. Fatigue, a by-product of dialysis and kidney failure, intensified. I felt perpetually weak, shuffling my way through the day. My constant neuropathic pain became excruciating to the point of being unbearable. I had been able to salvage some semblance of conventional life with the exceptional help of my pain doctor and my solid determination—on good days. I began, however, to return home from dialysis with my hands and fingers burning as though on fire, my elbows and feet in turmoil and my body grasping for any sort of relief. During the night, my pain was intolerable. No pain medication afforded me any respite; any that I did take ended up compromising my intestines so that I suffered for days after having taken a single dose.

During each dialysis session, I shivered profusely, regardless of how many layers of clothing I wore or the number of blankets I requested to cover me. I even resorted to covering my head with towels—what a picture I must have been. The dialysis machines' temperature is purposefully kept low to enable better blood flow. The low temperature was even more important for me, because I was using a hemodiafiltration machine, the aim of which is to increase the level of toxin removal to lessen side effects, in my case, severe restless leg syndrome. My Raynaud's disease worsened. My hands were virtually numb throughout my sessions and continued to be so even after I had been detached from the dialysis machine. Even though I wished to sit up during my sessions so that I could read rather than having to lie down watching television, my blood pressure frequently dropped so that I had to lie down. As soon as I lay down, I experienced torturous neck pain, something that occurred off dialysis, too, but with less frequency, another result of my spinal damage.

Entering the dialysis unit was similar to walking into a living nightmare. I dreaded my sessions and the agony I was to endure. The degree to which I could cope began to fade drastically. Any quality of life I did possess eroded. My already diminished social life was non-existent. I was simply existing rather than living. I wanted to find a solution to ease my suffering.

I knew my hospital offered nocturnal dialysis; I asked my doctors if I could switch to it. It would mean rescheduling my days, changing my patterns and no longer being able to meet with my new friends. This caused me some sorrow as I had formed some good bonds. But if such a switch proved successful, then perhaps my life would also improve. And who knew? I might rekindle my friendships in some other way. A few of my doctors were skeptical because not everyone can sleep during nocturnal dialysis. I, nevertheless, was willing to take my chances. I first needed to be assessed by one of the clinical nurses. This was my opportunity to plead my case.

Then I had to read and sign what seemed to be reams of paper work. In reality, there were only three different forms, each consisting of several pages outlining the prerequisites to which all potential nocturnal dialysis patients are required to conform. They include agreeing to be on time—an essential factor for overnight dialysis patients, because it requires adhering to a pre-determined eight-hour schedule—arriving sober and substance free, being quiet, respecting other patients' need for sleep and accepting feedback from medical staff if, in their view, treatment was not proving to be successful.

Papers read and duly signed, I received my pass—a programmed card to open the doors permitting entry into the hospital and ward after hours. I had been accepted! However, now I needed to wait until a bed was available. The clinical nurse in charge who had performed my assessment asked me if I would be willing to switch my days, in which case a bed was immediately available. Since I really desired to keep to my existing schedule, I was told that it might take a little while to arrange. I was prepared to wait. This would give me time to organize my overnight paraphernalia.

My good friend Elizabeth and I went shopping for a suitable carrying case, the first time I had really been in casual company with another person in some time, and good fun it was. We enjoyed a lovely lunch and fabulous catch-up conversations prior to our shopping foray. The venture was successful. We found a case I could use. I was ready. A little less than a week later, I learned I was to attend my first overnight session. The clinical nurse had worked hard to move patients around so my wish could be accommodated. I acknowledged the kindness of this act.My social worker organized a new schedule with HandyDART. This was a new adventure—not of the same order as a kidney transplant, but I was excited. Excited that another solution had been found that might just alleviate some of the problems I had been experiencing.

I couldn't wait to join my fellow nocturnal patients. While many patients perform nocturnal dialysis at home, a number of hospitals provide in-house treatment. My hospital created its own program in 2011. It began as a pilot project based on one undertaken at St. Michael's Hospital in Toronto and in response to a cry for help from a patient who had been experiencing severe post-dialysis effects. As the founding doctor explained in an interview at the time of its inception, "We already had a lot of the infrastructure in place at the hospital, so the pilot project has moved forward very smoothly. ... We've also been fortunate to have a group of dedicated and skilled nurses who have been integral to the program."[3] The pilot project was offered six days a week and followed the usual three-treatment sessions. Today, in my hospital, there are fifteen patients for each of the two three-times-a-week sessions—only thirty patients in all. I think of us as the elite. The turnover is often more frequent than in the day sessions, because some patients prefer daytime sessions while others are waiting for their living donors to be cleared before receiving a transplant.

A new connection

A few weeks before I began nocturnal dialysis, I met a twenty-three-year-old woman whom I had noticed during my evening dialysis sessions. She seemed to be well known and fondly greeted by the nurses, who often hugged her whenever she entered the unit, something not commonly seen. She and I happened to be together one day in the waiting room. We began talking, something most dialysis patients do with others. We are both curious and supportive of our fellow patients. She was known as Princess Marie, a name she had acquired sometime during her life. I found her to be a gregarious, energetic and amiable companion, another real people person. We had an enjoyable time together. I learned she had had congenital kidney disease and had recently succumbed to kidney failure.

Since beginning dialysis she has had innumerable complications from her fistula site. Princess Marie told me, "I tried nocturnal dialysis but my blood pressure would seriously drop resulting in my spending my remaining time in the ER. I now require dialysis treatment four times a week in order to clear my toxins effectively. Furthermore, my fistula has caused problems with my blood flow. I have had it changed several times. As a result of my veins seizing during dialysis, my hands and arm are numb."

She showed me that she could neither easily open nor close her hand.

"I have carpal tunnel syndrome and have to have surgery to repair it," she added.

The doctors had finally decided to exchange the fistula for a catheter that also seemed to be still causing her problems. Because of her constant need to spend time in hospital, not only being a frequent visitor to ER, but also as an in-patient, she confessed to me, "I have little social life."

In spite of her confession, and after hearing more of her story, I discovered Princess Marie lives her life to the full. She has a full-time job, is attending college and is engaged in many extracurricular activities. Her educational goal is to study social work so she can practice in this field. She told me, "I want to help people."

As a child and young teen, Princess Marie spent a good proportion of her youth attending medical clinics, seeing doctors and therefore missing a lot of school. The happy, carefree, fun-laden days of her peers were forbidden her. She had found the transition from childhood care into adult care a horrific experience, often filled with medical misconceptions and a lack of understanding by her new care providers, and she wished to rectify this situation. She said, "I do not want other young people to experience what I did when I was transitioned into adult care."

Princess Marie put all her energies into creating a volunteer position for herself with a local children's hospital, helping to prepare the children who were to move into adult care for what lay ahead. Her initial focus was kidney driven. The result of her enterprising efforts has been the creation of a new position as a transitional worker at the local children's hospital. She works full-time in this position now, concentrating on all children as well as visiting those attending clinics in our hospital.

Princess Marie has been an active participant in hospital life, as well. She has designed a special T-shirt for dialysis patients and staff to wear marking Dialysis Month and other occasions. The T-shirt is now sold in the dialysis unit and worn frequently by many in the dialysis unit. Since my joining the nocturnal elite, Princess Marie finds the time to visit both Charity and me. She is always upbeat and never downtrodden, a truly incredible young woman whose schedule makes me breathless just listening to her recounting her day's activities.

Reconnecting with a friend and being a nocturnal dialysis patient

My day arrived. It felt peculiar because it happened to coincide with my daytime dialysis session. Although normally I would have been picked up by HandyDART midmorning on this day, I was not collected until after 8:00 in the evening. I passed the day in suspended anticipation, not really settled, accomplishing very little, willing the hours to pass. I was like a child waiting for the great treat, which explains a lot about my reduced currency—that this change in routine bore the weight it did. I packed and repacked my suitcase to ensure I would have the necessary bed comforts—pillow, warm blanket and suitable night attire that would help me nestle in my new surroundings. Information I received suggested we bring headphones, a snack if required, a mask and earplugs if we were light sleepers. All these items I packed in my new suitcase. Together with my other accessories—glasses, toothbrush and extra meds, as well as a book that I stowed in one of Roland's old backpacks—I was beyond ready. I did not know what to expect.

Who were my pajama mates to be? The unknown seemed thrilling. Of one thing I was sure: I would once again see Charity. What a pleasure it would be to reconnect.

The hour arrived for my first night. I was the only passenger on Handy-DART and told my driver I felt as though I were going on a camping trip as, cane in one hand, suitcase in the other and knapsack on my back, I made my way to my seat. The driver kindly towed my case to the hospital door and helped me use my new privileged card to enter the hospital. I made my way to the dialysis unit where I once again needed to key in my entry and was enthusiastically welcomed with a lovely smile and friendly greeting by a nurse whom I knew from my day sessions. The casualness and calmness of the unit—a far cry from the hustle and bustle of the day ward—struck me.

"Would you like to meet your mates?" the nurse asked.

"Love to," I replied.

I was introduced to three men whose beds were on the same side of the room as mine. We exchanged a few pleasantries. One had been dialyzing for ten years and for the last three years at night.

"You'll feel much better following nocturnal dialysis," he assured me.

The other two had been on dialysis for only a year and a bit. Other patients, behind closed curtains, had already been settled for the night. I was the lone woman in the company of nine men—three of whom I had just met.

Having quickly deposited my case and backpack, I couldn't wait to meet Charity who was in another ward across the hall. She had yet to arrive, so I returned to my ward and made my bed for the night. Still excited to see my lost friend, back to the room I went, calling her name. There she was, in full view! We hugged each other and I asked how she had been faring. Her breast cancer diagnosis had been a tempest in a teacup. All was well. She had developed a peculiar cyst just behind her nipple. She had not gone back to full-time work but was doing well, finding it easier to sleep, if only for about four hours at a time, and getting out more on her days off, living an improved quality of life. She told me she was a bit weary following her sessions and slept for a further three to four hours, after which she felt well and energetic. She remains the genial and optimistic personification of her namesake.

Charity has had some problems with her fistula and has needed to have an angioplasty several times during the past year. It appears her veins open for a while and then narrow, preventing blood from flowing easily to and from her body. It is a painful and unpleasant experience for her but a necessity if she is to maintain a good dialysis. She was due to have another one the following week.

After our quick catch up, Charity introduced me to one of her roommates, a woman she called Queenie because of her regal demeanour. A fitting description, since she is indeed elegant and graceful. There are three women and two men in this ward. Charity has never met the men, because they are already behind closed curtains when she arrives and leave in the morning before she is up. The other woman, who had yet to arrive, was an older woman. Her daughter brings her, picks her up early in the morning, drives her home and then goes to work. Another very caring family.

Queenie had been dialyzing for twelve years. She had already suffered kidney failure, the cause of which had never been diagnosed. She had received a transplant that lasted fifteen years. In 2012 Queenie decided to try nocturnal dialysis because she felt it would help her more.

"Has it?" I asked.

"It took me a long time to adjust, and just as I thought I would give up, I was able to sleep. I can now eat mangoes!" she said.

She drives herself to and from the hospital. She lives on her own but has a grown-up son. Until her transplant failed, Queenie held a job and wanted to continue working while on dialysis but her union put a nix to that, illustrating some of the lack of accommodation for those who suffer from ailments. It is a sad reflection of what we call a modern, equal-opportunities society. As a result Queenie has suffered financially. Her greatest wish is to have a transplant and return to work.

A complication for her is a high degree of antibodies in her system that makes matching difficult. Apart from having a terrible experience with undetected narrowing veins, which caused her to have heart problems that were finally resolved by an angioplasty, she has no other health issues. However, during the procedure, the balloon used to widen the veins burst, requiring surgery to repair the damage.

After I had taken my weight, temperature and blood pressure standing up and sitting—which I was accustomed to doing during my day runs—the nurse calculated the amount of fluid to remove and began the process of preparing me for my hookup to the machine. One change I immediately noticed was the pump speed. On nocturnal dialysis the pump speed is reduced to 250 ml per minute, a much slower rate because of the longer time spent dialyzing. During the first week of nocturnal dialysis, our blood pressure is taken once an hour, the second week every two hours, and the third week every four hours. Thereafter, it is taken twice: once when we are first connected and again at the end of our session in the morning.

Patient hookup times are staggered between 8:00 and 10:00 pm to enable the three nurses time to tend to all of us. The last hookup time is at 10:00 pm, necessary if we are to be finished by 6:15 am so that the beds and machines can be ready for the morning group who arrive at 7:00 am. When our runs are completed, the machines peel out a sound similar to the one heard in casinos following a win. I call it winning the lottery. Prior to starting my new sessions, I knew we were expected to sleep earlier so we could accommodate the eight-hour time period.

At home, my bedtime had been between 2:00 and 3:00 am because of my difficulty sleeping. In the days leading up to my nocturnal, I had tried to adapt the new routine so that I would be better prepared for the earlier sleep time. That first night I was already connected shortly after 9:30 pm, far too early for me to even begin to think about sleeping. With the slower machine speed, I was able to sit and read without the worry of my blood pressure dropping or the machine beeping at every little movement I made. This was already turning out to be an improvement for me. Except when I tried to sleep at midnight—to no avail.

Other new friends

That first morning, HandyDART was picking me up between 6:00 and 6:30 am. Weary from lack of sleep, I dragged my suitcase to the exit door where I was greeted cordially by Al, my bedside mate. Kindly, true to his nature as I learned, he opened the locked door, holding it for me while I walked through. On my own I doubt I would have had the strength to push it open. Al appeared to me as a very pleasant individual and we had a brief chat, during which he told me he had been on dialysis for a year and was on the transplant list but was not too worried about the wait. "I have had a good life, and it doesn't matter to me if I have to wait for a long time," he told me. We parted company. My ride came quickly and I arrived home a little after 6:30, whereupon I donned my pajamas once again and slept the sleep of the dead, not waking until midday. I felt a little grogginess for a good part of the day, gradually being replaced by an enormous sense of well-being. I had no horrible neuropathic pain, no semblance of Raynaud's frozen fingers. Instead I was experiencing an improved feeling of wellness. That night I enjoyed a full night's sleep, the first one in a long, long time. The next day I could not believe how energetic and well I felt! Even after one night of nocturnal dialysis, I was already reaping the benefits.

When I arrived for my second night, I noticed Al collecting his supplies. I knew we were expected to gather our own supplies, record our stats and eventually calibrate the machine ourselves so that the nurses could tend to other patients. Some patients even perform their own connection to the machine. I wasn't sure I could do that due to the limited flexibility in my hands, but the other three tasks I certainly could handle. Normally the nurses teach us how to gather our supplies, but seeing no reason for not taking the initiative myself, and Al being a genial fellow, I felt I could ask him to help me collect mine. "Absolutely," he said and immediately began to point out the things I needed. With my supplies in hand, I couldn't resist adding a note to my Dialysis Record Sheet, writing, "Good girl, collected my own supplies with help from a roommate."

In good spirits, the nurse wrote, "Well done."

I thoroughly enjoy the freedom of being in control of my preparation. Being on dialysis is a form of institutionalization, because of both the routine we need to follow and the limited diet to which we need to adhere. Travelling by HandyDART adds a further sense of institutionalization. Thus, the more we do ourselves, the greater our sense of independence and self-worth. A few months later I was taught how to calibrate my machine and to calculate the amount of fluid to remove. My poor arithmetic skills, which I thought would be truly tested, have not been. Whew! Fortunately, I do not need to prepare my catheter site and perform my own connection. One extra task I do is to prepare my morning supplies and get the nurses' sterile gloves. I tell them it is part of my job. They laugh.

Al and I have become good buddies. He is terribly modest for someone so kind. He has turned out to be my guardian angel. He arrives before I do and always has extra blankets, a pillow and table and chair waiting for me. He is an incredibly helpful soul and willingly offers to do whatever he can to assist me. Following our first brief discourse I asked him more about how he came to be on dialysis. He told me, "I am new to all of this. I have only been on dialysis for a year and a bit. I don't have much to tell other than I fell down a few times and went to my doctor who told me I had kidney failure." I have since learned Al has diabetes, a common cause of kidney failure.

Al lives with his sister, his mother, his long-haired Chihuahua and his sister's two Shih Tzus, whom Al told me all get along together. He came to be on nocturnal dialysis because, when he started dialysis, his scheduled sessions were erratic.

"I wanted to have a regular session, so I opted for nocturnal dialysis," he said.

"Are you able to sleep?" I asked.

"Oh, I sleep like a log," he said.

He generally feels fine following his dialysis sessions. As far as the needles used to connect his fistula to the lines are concerned, he tells the nurses, "I can't stand the sight of them. I turn my head away. I also feel a searing pain in my arm as they are being inserted."

We have lovely short conversations when I first arrive because, soon after, he is connected for the night, and I need to perform my own preparations, making my nest, taking my stats and recording them. Al, our sweet guard ian angel, ever cheerful and upbeat, continues to ensure all our beds are made properly. He is a genuinely kind and considerate person, never complaining or expecting a return for his generosity.

Jeffery, a youthful twenty-eight-year-old, is another patient who impresses me. His kidneys had failed one-and-a-half years ago because of a suspected, undetermined autoimmune condition. He had tried peritoneal dialysis with limited success. He has a thin peritoneal membrane that hindered his ability to drain the solution. He did not like having to store the solution boxes or walking around all day feeling bloated from the extra fluid in his abdomen. He chose nocturnal dialysis due to his work schedule as a computer programmer.

Jeffery performs all the tasks associated with connecting himself to the dialysis machine. In one conversation, he told me, "I sleep fairly well depending on whether or not I have calculated the correct amount of fluid that I need to have removed. When my calculations are inaccurate, my blood pressure drops, and I wake up. Mostly I calculate correctly but I usually feel 'shitty' following my dialysis, but soon regain my energy so I can work productively."

Jeffery sleeps for a few hours after arriving home before heading off to work in the mid-afternoon. He also said, because his is a desk job, he is not required to move around much which helps him retain his energy. He is the youngest member of our nocturnal group. Well, it should be said, at least to me, who once remembered having been sixty-five! Jeffery has a living donor lined up who is having the last set of tests to assess eligibility. Because of his youth, Jeffery certainly merits having a transplant so he can resume living a better quality of life.

The results and further friendship

After I had been on nocturnal dialysis for three weeks, I had the so-called monthly blood work, which in reality is drawn at six-week intervals, to ascertain if any difference had occurred since starting nocturnal dialysis. Yes, there had been a difference! My creatinine had dropped from 600 to 493 micromoles per litre (μmol/L). My potassium was well within the normal range, and my phosphate level had dropped quite a bit. The protein levels in my blood had increased, as well. I was really pleased. These were incredible results.

One result that was not as good, though, was my hemoglobin. My hemoglobin had dropped from the high 90s to 88 grams per litre (g/L). Hemoglobin is basically a protein of red blood cells that contains iron and carries oxygen from the lungs to the tissues and carbon dioxide from the tissues to the lungs. Normal hemoglobin levels vary between women and men. For women, a marker ranges from 120 to 160 g/L; for men, it ranges from 140 to 160 g/L. While on dialysis our levels are lower, mostly in the range of 95 to 115. This, I am told, is better for our overall health. My drop, then, was quite significant. To counteract my hemoglobin drop I was administered doses of iron intravenously for eight days. On the third day, my hemoglobin had risen to 90, and on the sixth day, to 97. A drop in hemoglobin is not uncommon for dialysis patients, since our kidneys are no longer able to create red blood cells without intervention such as EPO injections or iron infusions, usually given on a monthly basis, depending upon the individual patient's needs. Charity, for example, has bi-weekly iron infusions.

A week later I was due to meet my pain doctor before attending a clinic appointment. My pain doctor had agreed to meet in the cafeteria, a halfway point between his office and the clinic. I didn't think I would be able to go to his office lugging my suitcase and bearing my backpack, because I then had to go back to the clinic. Since our meeting was scheduled for 8:00 am, it would give me time to have something to eat first. I was sitting deliberating about whether or not it was safe to leave my belongings while I grabbed some porridge. Hospitals are, sadly, notorious places for theft. I spotted another fellow whom I had seen on my ward but had been unable to have a conversation with because he could not speak. As he came towards me carrying a cup of coffee, I asked his advice. "Should I leave my things while I get some porridge?"

"No problem." He gestured he would get me my porridge. I tried to give him money for it. He waved it aside and bought me my breakfast. This was a most charitable act and one that I felt I needed to repay.

My pain doctor arrived on cue. We had a good session, during which I told him my latest results. He was delighted and said, "I hope you are going to include this in your book because these are definitely measurable improvements." I assured him this was a given. We also talked about a rather bad dream I had had. He told me that 98 percent of dreams are more negative than positive. It is a way for our brains to process our thoughts and sort out our daily lives. An interesting fact, and something I had not known. Our session over, I needed to move on to my next appointment, so I did not have time to find out the price of my porridge. I would need to ask others.

I reported to the receptionist who right away greeted me by my name. I am well known in this part of the hospital, having attended the transplant clinic for almost twenty-two years. I was immediately seen by a doctor, who, when learning how much I liked the nocturnal session, told me she was very pleased to hear this since the hospital was trying to encourage more patients to do home dialysis. She would use my positive feedback as further proof of the benefits of nocturnal dialysis. It would add more power to her recommendations. "Of course," she said, "home dialysis would be difficult for you to do." Later I met with the pharmacist, who decided to keep me on my current medication, and the dietician, who explained to me that after my next blood work results I would probably be able to stop taking my phosphate binders. She further said that I didn't need to take any extra, should I wish to have a snack between meals, and that I could extend my range of diet to include more potassium-rich foods. A wonderful bit of news for me.

Before I was due to leave the clinic, one of my regular nephrologists popped in to see me. I again explained how well I was doing, except for the sleeping bit. I still could not sleep well. Her response was that it takes a long time to adapt, and to wait until I felt really settled. One of the things potential nocturnal patients need to agree to is to give this change at least a month before deciding if we wish to continue or not, due to the time it takes to feel comfortable. The doctor agreed to my continuing. My second clinic appointment was to be in three months.

Not forgetting my fellow patient's good deed, I asked the nurse at my next session if she knew the cost of a bowl of porridge. No, she didn't but would make enquiries. Since I would not see her for another week, I wanted to find out sooner.

I knew Charity frequented the cafeteria. The following morning, while we were waiting together for HandyDART, I asked her if she knew the cost of a bowl of porridge. Yes, she did, at least a ballpark figure. The following dialysis session I placed an appropriate amount of money in an envelope, writing my gratitude on the outside, suggesting that it might be used to purchase a lottery ticket. I placed the envelope on the table beside the fellow's bed. In no time, it seemed, he came to my bed with the envelope in hand, having written, "Not necessary. I shall invest the money in a lottery ticket for both of us. I would, however, love to be mentioned in your book." I said I would be absolutely delighted to include his story in my book. Thus began our friendship, and his story.

Arjay, a replica of his initials, was diagnosed with glomerulonephritis, an acute inflammation of the tiny filters in the kidney, over thirty years ago. His first visit to his doctors landed him in hospital for a month. He was put on four hours of hemodialysis, three times a week. A year and a half later, he received a transplant that lasted for twenty-one years. During this time, he worked around the world installing the radar and computer systems that air traffic controllers use to keep aircraft from bumping into each other. Many of his jobs included working on military bases for foreign governments. His friends and family considered him a spy in disguise and therefore nick-named him "Spy." Arjay is an avid James Bond fan, thoroughly enjoying the movies, so "Spy" stuck.

Following this work, he taught computer science in a local college before moving to the Interior of British Columbia, where he taught in a university for five years. Because he loved working there, he and his wife, Tessa, pur-chased a little cabin on a lake nearby, where he stayed while Tessa continued to work in Vancouver. They saw each other at weekends and planned to retire in the Interior. However, when his health took a turn for the worse, they rather sadly sold their cabin and returned to Vancouver permanently, to be close to a major health centre.

Arjay's reason for moving to Vancouver: he had been diagnosed with throat cancer. He knew something was wrong when it took him three at-tempts to swallow a McDonald's French fry. Chemotherapy and radiation had little impact on his cancer. A year and a half ago, he had a total laryn-gectomy that later led to him losing his voice. This was followed by more bad news: he was diagnosed with lung cancer.

Having been raised in a Christian home, Arjay retained his faith, al-though he did not attend church as regularly once he lived on his own. Now, though, despondent about this latest bit of bad news, he sought solace in prayer, asking to be rid of his lung cancer. A month or so later, he had an MRI of his throat and chest. That same day his wife received a call from the oncologist: "We cannot explain it, but Arjay shows absolutely no indication of cancer anywhere."

Whether or not it was a miracle, further exams show he remains cancer-free. As can be imagined, he is happy with his current status. His kidney transplant failed twelve years ago, and while he would love to have another transplant and has two sisters who are both perfect matches and willing to donate a kidney, the doctors have said no. A compromised im-mune system could trigger a return of the cancer. A transplant could actu-ally prove fatal for him. Still a relatively young man, he will spend the rest of his life on dialysis. Arjay's story is an excellent example of the far-reaching impact the effects of kidney failure have on our livelihood and well-being. Additional health issues create more complications for us than they do for some other illnesses, often making it more difficult to receive transplants.

Nocturnal dialysis has worked well for Arjay. He has better blood work results; he is able to eat anything he wants and to drink freely. The one downside for him is that it has disrupted his sleep patterns. Like many of us, after dialysis he goes home and sleeps until noon. He does not wish to perform home hemodialysis since he feels he would forever be reminded of his kidney failure.

True to his word, Arjay purchased a lottery ticket. We did not win anything, but it was the beginning of a new enterprise. We are pooling our money to continue to purchase more tickets. Arjay proposed we call ourselves "the renal gamblers." Who knows? We may win "the big one" yet.

Sleep continues to elude me, although my Zorro-like mask does shield me from the pervasive hospital light. I often drift off towards the end of my run. My dreams are incredibly vivid and busy, replete with all sorts of unusual people coming and going. The sights and sounds of the morning preparations must be foremost in my mind; I am always amused to find upon waking that all was illusionary and I am still ensconced behind my curtains. I am, however, determined to stay on nocturnal dialysis because of the benefits such as improved blood results, increased warmth (I am able to increase the temperature on the machine), reduced neuropathic pain, more energy and better health overall. As well, lying down at the same time as most people provides me with the freedom of having more days to socialize and complete tasks.

Unfortunately, my neck pain has not been alleviated and can be agonizing as I lie awake suffering its relentless throbbing. However, as expected, my latest hemoglobin blood test showed it had risen to 100. My iron had also risen. I currently receive iron infusions monthly. I have told my nurses I do not want to return to the "frozen north," my euphemism for the day sessions.

Recently I had a phone call from Candy Man inquiring as to how I was doing. It was wonderful to pick up the threads again. We agreed to stay in touch. I have, after all, managed to retain a vestige of contact with my former pals.

While Charity and I wait for our rides in the morning, we pass the time discussing a wide range of topics and subjects, sometimes trying to solve the world's problems, but invariably our conversation returns to talking about our mutual kidney failure. Not surprisingly, our lives are engulfed by our condition. Charity has been experiencing some further problems with her fistula, necessitating her to have angioplasty procedures approximately every two weeks. Her last procedure was exceptionally painful and unpleasant, reducing her to tears. She has requested that the procedures be performed only by the main doctors and not resident doctors.

Since I have been on nocturnal dialysis, Charity has also had her first adventure in a long time, and one that she had never contemplated happening in the early days of her dialysis therapy. It was a three-day trip to San Diego, where she stayed in Little Italy, near the water, close to downtown. While there, she dined in her favourite Italian restaurant, eating 1950s-style Italian cuisine. She felt healthy, almost normal. She has done more on her days off, enjoying meals out with friends, even travelling to a casino near Seattle. While there, not a gambler, she feasted on the grand buffet. I think it is plain to see from her comments about food that she is a foodie. It is wonderful to see her in such good spirits. As she sees things, she said, "I have survived two years of dialysis. Six more to go before I could receive a transplant, unless some kind soul donates one in the meantime." We are now in the same room.

Charity, who enters the ward like a beacon in the night, bringing with her lightness, laughter and warmth, arrived not too long after one of her ventures to the States in a more sombre, heavier mood. Her light and airy presence had been replaced by a darker shadow. I asked her if something was bothering her. She replied, "I don't think my friends really understand just how ill I am."

I replied, "I understand. Others have expressed the same feelings."

Charity continued, "I am able to work, albeit only part time, but I do as much as my colleagues and am able to socialize far more than I could before switching to nocturnal dialysis. I look fine, but the reality is that I am alive only because I am on dialysis. Following dialysis I don't feel well. I need to recover. If I didn't have dialysis, statistics tell me I could be dead within two weeks."

I agreed with her. Having vented her moment of despair, she once again returned to her customary sociable self. Her words were the stark reality of kidney failure. We live a see-saw life, never knowing how our condition could change.

Despite living with these uncertainties, I am incredibly glad I have transferred to the "gently does it" method for a number of reasons. I feel better, I have more energy and I have been able to rekindle a friendship and meet new friends such as my gambling pal Arjay, among others. Over the months, Charity and I have had lunch together before exploring a shop she wanted to go to. Al has switched to the other nocturnal schedule. Some of our fellow bedmates have had transplants so we have welcomed new members to our "Nocturnal Elite." Transplants remain the number one dream for many dialysis patients and are an important area to discuss.

Chapter 8 | Receiving a Transplant

For it won't be long
Till I'm gonna need
Somebody to lean on
—Bill Withers, *Lean on Me*

Some stories

"I got up, went to the bathroom and was getting dressed for work when I got the phone call to come," said the young man to the nurse as she was inserting an intravenous needle into his arm on the Friday of a hot August long weekend during my hospital in-stay. The young man had come in street clothing and was lying in the bed next to mine. He had had a call from the Transplant Department requesting he come immediately.

The nurse explained, "Yes," a kidney was waiting for him, but the doctors needed to retrieve it sometime later that day. When, though, was the unknown factor.

Shortly after this, the young man was moved to another room. I next saw him a few days later lying in his bed with an array of tubes trailing from various parts of his anatomy. He had had his transplant. The doctors were waiting for his new kidney to start working effectively.

Three other transplants were performed that weekend. Not a record, but more than usual. Three were from deceased donors and one from a living donor. The recipients were three men and one woman. The woman's kidney had been donated by a friend of hers who had offered to do so because they shared a less common blood type.

Transplant patients who are waiting for a kidney from a deceased or even anonymous living donor experience a pattern. They never know when a kidney might be available. The waiting time can vary from months to years—mostly years because of the scarcity of available donors. There are no forewarnings; the long-awaited call could come while on dialysis, perhaps in the middle of the night, during a leisure activity or simply when at home or work. These potential recipients are on hold, hoping tomorrow might be the day. For recipients receiving living donor kidneys, the time frame can be different and more predictable. Depending on locale, procedures may take less time to complete.

Art, whose story I recounted earlier, had this experience with his transplant. One day, Art's wife answered the phone. Because confidentiality when dealing with kidney transplants is extremely important, the caller, who asked to speak personally to Art, did not reveal their identity. His wife explained that he was having his dialysis treatment. The caller said, "Thank you," and hung up.

Subsequently Art received a call at his dialysis unit; it was the hospital letting him know he was to receive a transplant. He was so excited that he said, "I'll come at once, now."

The caller replied, "No, complete your dialysis first so you are as toxin-clear as you can be. It is better for the transplant surgery and your recovery afterwards."

Once home, Art could hardly pack his bags quickly enough. So uncontainable was his excitement that he arrived at the hospital sooner than expected. He had a long wait. Two kidney transplants from one deceased donor were scheduled for that day. His was the second one. The first one took longer than anticipated. Concern grew among the doctors. It was imperative that both surgeries be completed within an allocated time period. Otherwise the kidneys were no longer viable. Finally, Art had his operation late into the night, a success that provided him with a renewed lease on life.

Allan Wheeler, my twin, whose story I also related earlier, received his call while visiting his sister in Victoria. The doctor, having first called his home in Whitehorse to learn from his wife, Annie, of his whereabouts, woke Allan's sister at home at about 2:30 in the morning. Alarmed by being wakened so early, she was about to hang up, thinking it was a prank call, when the doctor reassured her it was real. Could Allan go immediately to the hospital in Victoria where a helicopter was waiting to fly him to Vancouver for his kidney transplant?

"Most certainly," was his response. Groggily, Allan grabbed his bags and rushed to the hospital. Sure enough, a helicopter, engines prepped, was waiting. He was flown to Vancouver, received his transplant and as he said, "Began the unimagined rest of my life."

"How did you feel?" I asked.

He replied, "Odd, not only to have received the call when I did, but also to have been personally transported to Vancouver. Amazing experience."

Things might not have gone so quickly now, since transplant patients are asked to move closer to their transplant centre. Allan's transplant was in 1991.

One summer, Henry Upton, whose story of faith and hope continues to impress me, was listening attentively to a band at a local music festival. The band stopped abruptly. Silence fell. Audience participants turned to each other perplexed. A man appeared on the stage and said two words: "Henry Upton." Stunned at first, Henry "stood his ground." The man repeated his name with greater urgency and instructed him to go to the back of the stage. This time Henry complied. There he saw two policemen standing by a squad car. Henry assumed that an emergency of some sorts had occurred. It had: they were taking him to the hospital for a kidney transplant. "Sitting in the back of the police car, with siren blaring, hurtling between traffic while being rushed to my transformation was a most incredible experience for me," he said later.

At the hospital, Henry was "pumped full of immunosuppressants," as he said, and wheeled into the OR. Recovering from surgery, pain searing through his body and in a "haze of drugs," he, like me, felt a sudden sense of wellness as his kidney, functioning properly, began removing built-up toxins. Henry vowed, upon returning home, to lose weight, join a gym and begin cycling again. He no longer required blood transfusions, nor was he to suffer from lack of energy due to low hemoglobin. His transplanted kidney re-energized him. He could do anything he wanted.

Henry described one particularly outstanding moment in his journal: "*It was a warm spring day, and I was riding my bike. I noticed all the plants and flowers that were coming to life. The birds were singing, I felt connected to it all. It was a picture perfect scene, my mind, body and soul were together in complete union.*"

He couldn't have been happier. His rent in social housing was inexpensive, and he had enough left over to cover his bills. Needles, meds, dialysis and endless rounds of hospital visits were no longer required.

For two years Henry lived fully until he once more succumbed to kidney failure. The following year, his sister donated her kidney, affording him a further ten years of priceless living and, with that, an immense gratitude to her. Not all kidney transplants will fail. Some transplants are hard to sustain because of rejection, the effects of medication or other ailments, while others have fewer challenges. We transplant recipients are incredibly grateful to our donors for their charitable gift, enabling us to enjoy an improved quality of life irrespective of the length of time our kidneys continue to perform well.

Haida recently asked me to ensure that readers were aware of her appreciation for her transplant and for the twenty wonderful years it gave her. All of us recipients know we are the caretakers of something precious, a privileged gift. And for those who have received one from a deceased donor there is an underlying sadness that someone had to die in order for them to benefit.

> When I received my transplant in 1991, because of confidentiality all I knew was that it had come from a young man who had died in a road accident. One of the first things I did was to write a thank you letter to the donor's family, sending it in care of the British Transplant Society who would pass it on to the family. It is common practice for transplant recipients to do this in acknowledgement of their gratitude.

Joan, in her early twenties—happy, fun-loving—is enjoying her university studies, unencumbered by health concerns. This was not always the case. Joan was born with childhood congenital kidney abnormalities and spent most of her childhood undergoing medical care. She began peritoneal dialysis while still a young child. At night, her tubes would frequently entangle, causing the nocturnal peritoneal machine to beep, interrupting her sleep and making her fatigued for school the next day.

Early in her teens, one of her parents donated a kidney, but it soon failed to function properly. Once again Joan required dialysis. A few years later an abdominal infection meant she could no longer continue with peritoneal dialysis; she needed to switch to hemodialysis, leaving her even more drained and tired as she worked to complete her high school studies.

In her late teens, while at home, the call came: a kidney was available for her. Still, a positive outcome seemed beyond belief, but her fears were unfounded. As with Henry, and me, after surgery Joan immediately experienced her new kidney's recuperative affects. Even her looks changed. Kidney failure, coupled with dialysis, often changes a person's appearance. Skin can yellow and become sallow, and eyes can be dulled. The first time Joan looked at herself in a mirror, she was stunned to see a vibrant face with glowing skin and bright, lustrous eyes staring back. "Miraculous," thought Joan, feeling grateful for her kidney and even more appreciative since it had come from an anonymous living donor.

Determining eligibility for a transplant

Receiving a kidney transplant is a long process. The assessment itself is lengthy, convoluted and not necessarily linear, often taking months to complete. First we candidates need to complete a preliminary questionnaire regarding our existing lifestyle, concerns, hopes and dreams before being interviewed by a team of nephrologists, surgeons, a nurse coordinator and a social worker. The social worker is an integral part of the process, offering advice on how to deal with the transition from dialysis patient to transplant patient, how to handle the ensuing emotional upheaval and how to cope with the new medical regime required by having to take immunosuppressant medication. At the interview we need to demonstrate that we will be compliant with medical requirements and are not clinically too ill to receive a transplant.

Following the initial interview, we candidates need to have a series of blood tests to determine blood type, antibodies, immunities to infections, potential risks for further infections, HIV status and any other issues—up to twenty-seven blood tests in total are drawn. Since I was in the system, my nephrologist told me I did not have to complete the questionnaire, but I needed to be assessed to find out if I qualified to be on the waiting list. Our medical conditions can change both from kidney failure and new ailments. I was required to have my blood type retested and other blood tests conducted, my records having long been lost since my transplant in England. When I recall having the blood tests, the number and array of different coloured vials astounded me. It felt as though I were to be held captive with a needle jutting out of my arm for hours. In actuality, the tests took moments to complete.

Blood types were first discovered by Dr. Karl Landsteiner, an Austrian biologist, physician and immunologist, in 1900. He categorized them into three types (A, B, O). A year later, two other doctors, Adrian Sturli and Alfred von Decastello, working under Landsteiner, discovered a fourth blood type, AB.

Establishing blood type is of primary importance for a kidney transplant because not all types are compatible. The types are known as O, A, B and AB. Transplant recipients with type O can receive a kidney from type O only, type A can receive from types A and O, type B can receive from types A and O, and type AB can receive from types A, B, AB and O. AB is the universal recipient type: recipients with AB blood are compatible with any other blood.

Likewise, people with blood type O are universal donors: their blood can be matched with types O, A, B and AB. Type O blood is the most common. Type A can be matched with types A and AB. Type B can be matched with types B and AB. Last, type AB, the least common blood type, can be matched only with type AB.[1] Individuals vary so it is important that each case is assessed separately.

Equally important is discovering the kind and number of antibodies an individual has. We all have antibodies. They are large, Y-shaped proteins whose purpose is to fight foreign substances such as bacteria or viruses and protect our immune system. The challenge lies in identifying the antibodies and whether or not they are compatible with another kidney. A greater number of antibodies present in our blood creates increased difficulty in finding a suitable kidney match. Tissue matching is carried out through blood tests similar to tests for blood types. Both donor and recipient undergo a series of blood tests to determine kidney compatibility and blood group.

During my second kidney transplant assessment, I had fitness tests and heart tests including an electrocardiogram (ECG), an echocardiogram and nuclear heart examinations, the latter called by its abbreviated name MIBI. This test took place over several hours and was divided into two sections. Following the first exam, I was asked to have a drink and told to wait a period of time before being tested again to ensure my health condition was stable and I would not be at risk during surgery. The doctor suggested I choose green tea for my liquid intake.

I also had a FIT test, a Pap test and a mammogram to search for signs of cancer. Many of these tests are carried out depending on the age of the candidate. Men, I believe, are given prostate examinations. My rheumatologist was asked whether I was a suitable candidate for a kidney transplant. I was further tested to ensure I could physically withstand the surgery itself. All these tests were completed over many months.

> A fecal immunochemical test (FIT) is a noninvasive stool test for low-risk individuals.

Once I had been thoroughly assessed—"been through the mill" as it were—I met with the team. The doctors decided that my placement on the transplant list should be deferred because I had a number of issues that required attention: I was far too thin, so needed to gain weight, and I needed to have my nephrectomy and throat cyst surgery. Happily, follow-up appointments since then have determined I am now a suitable candidate for the transplant list. Even though it has been several years since my kidney failed, I will not lose my original place on the transplant list.

One of the nephrologists told me that, in many instances, the doctors prefer to accept someone rather than reject them. They would, at the very least, rather err on the side of favouring a transplant, thereby affording an opportunity for a better quality of life than denying someone that potential.

There is no age barrier for organ transplants in Canada. A person's existing health condition, risks from having surgery and availability of organs are the main deterrents for a person of any age. Recently, a seventy-nine-year-old woman and an eighty-two-year-old man received kidney transplants in my local hospital. In most cases, donor organs and recipients are age-matched as much as possible. With regards to the eighty-two-year-old man, however, his donor was considerably younger than him.

Complicating factors in receiving a transplant

Candidates waiting for a transplant, whether from a deceased or living donor, may encounter a variety of circumstances delaying their receiving one. Conditions ranging from rare blood groups, socio-economic circumstances, increased number of antibodies and health issues can add additional complications to the waiting time.

Janet, the woman I met in hospital and mentioned earlier in the chapter, received a transplant even though she had a rare blood type. The doctors had informed her that she could be on the waiting list for a very long time.

She had been extremely fortunate because a friend who, surprisingly, shared the same blood group said she would be more than willing to donate one of her kidneys. My new acquaintance accepted this as an absolute blessing.

Because Janet lived out of town, the waiting had become expensive for her. With the combination of tests required and the need for frequent visits to Vancouver, the bill had been mounting. For renal patients living outside a hospital's area, the waiting process is expensive because accommodation, travelling and living costs are not considered medical expenses. By the time of her surgery, my friend had spent thousands and thousands of dollars. She still needed to plan a further two months' accommodation following her transplant in order to ensure her surgery had been successful and to complete bi-weekly clinic appointments. She may be blessed again because in some regions the Kidney Foundation of Canada has furnished suites that can be rented for little or no cost for up to eight weeks.

Socio-economic circumstances play an important part as well. We are fortunate in that our Canadian health system does not distinguish between those who have and those who do not. The playing field is level as far as treatment is concerned, but life is not. Circumstances differ. The same applies for renal patients. Not all patients have supportive families or are surrounded by a caring community. Statistics show that the more favourable a person's environment, the greater their likelihood of enjoying a healthy life and the more chances of receiving better care. There is frequently a correlation between health and education. Many of my fellow renal patients are not financially well off, are often hampered by additional health issues and do not enjoy the backing of either family or community.

I am reminded of my friend Mischievous Marty and his wife whose lives have been anything but an easy ride. They have to deal with considerable financial constraints, coupled with serious health issues. They fight for survival alone, unaided by either family or community support. They are but one couple of many patients I have met. Without family support or community protection, someone like Mischievous Marty is less likely to have a person who could donate a kidney as a living donor or could act as an advocate, providing the extra help required to promote his case.

Furthermore, with his health already compromised, Mischievous Marty did not have sufficient energy or the resources to verbalize his need for help.

Kidney failure has been draining on his ability to self-advocate. His road could be long and isolated. His only recourse is to wait years in the hopes he will receive a deceased donor's kidney or one from an anonymous living donor. As one of my fellow patients, who has been dialyzing for eleven years and is now at the top of the list, quipped, "It is like spending time in prison and I already did that years ago, so this is like a double sentence."

The level of antibodies in an individual's blood can increase the length of time a potential transplant recipient remains on the waiting list. Someone who has a greater number of antibodies in their blood is more likely to find a compatible match harder to obtain. Antibodies can occur as a result of pregnancy in women or of blood transfusions and kidney transplants themselves, because they are a foreign body. I recently met a tremendously energetic and positive woman who explained to me she has been on the waiting list for ten years due to an extremely high level of antibodies in her blood. In every other way she is healthy and has no additional complications. I learned from Renee that she had been diagnosed with high blood pressure leading to kidney failure and had fortunately received a transplant that had lasted for five years but then failed because of high blood pressure. Renee did tell me, rather wryly, she had been working during this time, looking after her family and, for some reason, not taking blood pressure medicine, alas causing her transplant to fail. She had developed a large number of antibodies in her system for various reasons that meant it created difficulties in finding an appropriate match. She has tried peritoneal dialysis, evening hemodialysis and nocturnal dialysis over the course of her ten years on dialysis. A nurse who happened to be near us, hearing our conversation, ventured the following comment, "If anyone has a story to tell, it is Renee. You can learn a great deal about her challenges. She has experienced it all."

My new friend is currently attending the afternoon session. Renee told me she feels it is important to stay positive, not dwell on things that might have been and keep her sense of humour. She also said that it is really important for her not to think of herself as a victim, but rather as someone who can overcome obstacles. Renee further told me, "I make sure on my days off from dialysis I go out, even if it is nothing more than to window shop. And in the summer I take my dog for long walks when the weather is better." I have been enormously impressed by my new friend's verve and positive outlook.

To reduce the challenges of blood incompatibility and tissue matching, especially in the case of high levels of antibodies, the US Food and Drug Administration in 2004 approved high-dose intravenous immunoglobulin (IVIG) therapy at the Cedars-Sinai Medical Center in Los Angeles. It reduces the need for the living donor to be a compatible blood type or even a tissue match. IVIG is derived from the pooled blood of hundreds of donors. The therapy reduces the incidence of rejection in highly sensitized patients. So far, Cedars-Sinai has performed more than 200 kidney transplants after desensitizing the recipient with IVIG therapy.[2]

The Johns Hopkins Hospital and Mayo Clinics rely on plasmapheresis, a blood cleaning process that can eliminate the dangerous antibodies, generally followed by low doses of IVIG. Plasmapheresis is used only in cases in which the patients have a living donor. Cedars-Sinai accepts patients without a living donor to prepare them with IVIG for a transplant from a deceased donor. IVIG therapy is an expensive treatment and costs in the region of $20,000. In a report published by Cedars-Sinai, it was suggested that between 25 and 30 percent of patients on the American National Transplant Registry could benefit from this therapy.[3] During my dialysis sessions I have observed transplant recipient patients who have begun to show signs of rejection having this treatment. The purpose is to alter their blood to prevent further kidney rejection. The machine used has a number of extra revolving wheels and many bags attached to it containing various solutions.

While this treatment has been used with some recipients attending my hospital who have a living donor, it is not commonly used in Canada, because the success of the Kidney Paired Donor Program (KPD) or Living Donor Paired Exchange (LDPE) has meant better compatibility of matched donors. The KPD Program, an interprovincial program, is run in collaboration between Canadian Blood Services and Canada's LDPE and transplant programs. It is one of three central registries run by Canadian Blood Services and called the Canadian Transplant Registry. This registry differs from the organ donation registers organized by the provinces and territories. The provincial registers record individuals' requests to become intended donors following death. Canadian Blood Services' three registries have three separate responsibilities and concern immediate organ availability.

The first registry, the National Organ Waitlist (NOW), is responsible for monitoring all urgent organ transplant cases across Canada, such as individuals whose lives depend on immediately receiving a transplant, and procuring an organ for them. This covers all organs.

The second registry, the KPD Program, is primarily concerned with co-ordinating paired kidney exchanges. For example, if a donor in BC is not compatible with the intended recipient, this registry will find a matching donor in its national registry from anywhere in Canada. Therefore, the BC donor could be paired with a compatible recipient in Nova Scotia, and the recipient in BC could be paired with another compatible donor from Manitoba. The purpose of this registry is to extend the horizon of pairing opportunities for donors and recipients as well as enabling anonymous (altruistic) donors to participate in the donation process. According to a BC Transplant Society spokesperson, even one altruistic or anonymous donor helps speed up the waitlist. This registry was created in 2008 and is one of the reasons why the number of living donors in Canada outperforms the number in some other countries such as Spain. Canadian Blood Services estimates that by 2018, ten years after its inception, because of the success of this registry, they will have recouped both the costs of setting up the registry and the expenditures required to maintain it.

The Highly Sensitized Patient (HSP) Program is the newest of the three registries, having been established in 2014 and implemented in 2016. Its purpose is to match hard-to-match recipients with compatible kidneys. Hard-to-match recipients are those whose levels of antibodies have been increased through pregnancies, blood transfusions or past transplants and whose compatibility for receiving a kidney through normal processes is significantly reduced, making it more likely they would reject a kidney. Access through deceased donor pools will increase the likelihood for an individual to receive a compatible match. This program will take time to be fully operational and will require candidates to be reassessed. My friends Renee and Queenie could be beneficiaries of this program. But being a new registry, it will take some time for results to be recorded.

Co-morbid issues, meaning a combination of health issues, as discussed in chapter 2, often create difficulties for renal patients waiting for a transplant. Although they may have been cleared for a transplant, their wait time can be affected by other issues. Kidney failure also contributes to a number of other health problems for dialysis patients. A patient told me he had experienced a heart-related challenge that meant further exploration was needed. He had been put "on hold" while tests were being conducted and his situation monitored. Just when he had begun to feel his chances for being a recipient had been increased, the rug was pulled out from under him. He will eventually resume his original place on the list, but the delay takes its toll both emotionally and physically. This is problematic because research has indicated the longer a person waits for a transplant, the greater the recovery time and the lower the chance of a successful outcome.

About deceased donors

There are two distinct waitlists for potential transplant recipients: one with deceased donors, and the other with living donors. Transplant candidates can only be on one or the other. A deceased donor is someone who has healthy organs and is on life-support in a hospital intensive care unit, having suffered irreversible brain damage from conditions such as a stroke, aneurysm or trauma or died from cardiac arrest. Generally, cardiac arrest is the most frequent cause of death, but if organ donation is to be undertaken, then it is necessary to respond promptly because organs deteriorate quickly after cardiac arrest due to loss of blood flow. Why this is so relates to the body temperature. In the case of a person suffering irreversible brain damage, the body remains warm. With cardiac arrest, the body cools rapidly. Deceased donors can also be those whose hearts have stopped beating, but the retrieval and survival time for organs to be donated is much shorter.

> The most common category of deceased donor is donor after brain death. According to Dr. Squifflet, brain death was described by Coulon and Mollaret, who were French critical care specialists, as being *le coma dépassé*, or beyond coma. It means that while the brain is not functioning, the body is warm, the heart beating and the individual breathing, all maintained by a ventilator. Once a diagnosis of brain death has been given, it provides physicians with time to speak with family members about their wishes to donate their loved one's organs, procure organs and then allocate them according to need.

Deceased donors are critical sources of organs because each donor can provide up to eight organs, and more if tissue is taken into consideration for transplantation. The eight organs are two kidneys, two lungs, heart, liver, pancreas and intestines. In 2014 hands and faces were included on the US list. It is essential that an organ be fully functioning upon its retrieval;

in other words, blood flow has been maintained. It seems, though, according to a recent report from the Canadian Institute for Health Information (CIHI), that many potential donors are not being realized. Potential donors are missed because they either have not been ventilated soon enough or are unidentified. The barriers seem to arise from few resources being available and insufficient numbers of trained medical staff to respond to the problem. According to the CIHI report, there is a need to address the shortcomings.

On a more positive note, the report states that, fortunately, medical advancements in the donor process, and in response to the growing demand for organs, the criteria to determine who is medically suited for organ donation is evolving and expanding globally.[4]

Canadian regulations detail a long list of contraindications to organ donations. These include malignancies, infections and neurological disorders. Exceptions can be made on a case-by-case basis by local medical teams. Many countries have shortened their lists of contraindications significantly in order to encourage as many people as possible to register as a potential organ donor.

Age, another criterion, has undergone a shift in status as far as organ donation is concerned. While no described age restrictions apply in Canada, only a decade ago, donors older than seventy-five were never even thought of. With increasing demand on waiting lists and an aging population (statistics indicate a greater number of people over the age of sixty-five are being diagnosed with kidney failure), today older patients are increasingly being accepted as potential organ donors. Doctors are now considering older donors who have died of stroke or other underlying conditions that would have previously disqualified them. In the UK, the cut-off age for potential donors has been extended from seventy-five to eighty years.[5]

In Europe, a non-profit European consortium called Eurotransplant was created in 1967 by a group of medical students who decided a cooperative approach in the area of deceased organ donation and transplantation would improve patient outcomes. The concept is based on one of cooperation and trust. Cooperation means that all countries will work together matching donors to recipients and trust that if one country donates an organ to another, the receiving country will reciprocate. The recipients are prioritized; those in urgent need in any of the participating countries are matched first. Participating countries either follow the opt-out method of donation or adhere to the consent structure in which it is presumed citizens are willing to donate [continued] their organs. The international framework includes all transplant centres, tissue-typing laboratories and hospitals where organ donation takes place. Its headquarters are based in Leiden, Netherlands. Currently, eight countries are working together: Austria, Belgium, Croatia, Germany, Hungary, The Netherlands, Luxembourg and Slovenia, which have a total population of 135 million inhabitants. Statistics show that, in 2016, there were 14,560 patients on the active waiting list, an increase from 10,808 in 2015. In 2016, there were 7,145 patients who received organ transplants. October 2017 celebrated the fiftieth anniversary of Eurotransplant's inception.

In an effort to address growing concerns over deceased organ shortages and the aging population, Eurotransplant has developed:

- a senior program where deceased donors are sixty-five or older, and recipients are also sixty-five or older
- the use of non-heart-beating donors
- the use of deceased after cardiac death donors[6]

Canada does not have a national organization responsible for monitoring or registering potential transplants. This domain falls within provincial health authorities that provide their own rules governing the transplant process. This often leads to differing numbers of transplants performed across Canada and a lack of overview, creating difficulties in answering the question of how to increase the number of potential donors generally.

Becoming a deceased donor is much more involved than simply registering an Intent to Donate consent form. Several procedures need to be followed: The first step is to identify the individual as a suitable candidate for organ donation. Then, for someone who has previously signed an organ donor consent form, the hospital needs to refer the family to the organ donation organization to consider the deceased person's request so organs can be used as soon as possible. This is the stage where there is the most potential for increasing the number of donors. In reality, only about one percent of deceased organs are used. In many cases, individuals do not die in a hospital setting, so eligibility to be a donor cannot be determined. In others, suitable donors are not identified quickly enough. And in others, there are no trained specialists on hand.

If an Intent to Donate form has not been signed, doctors are required to ask families the heart-wrenching question: Do you wish your loved one's organs or tissues to be donated? Families have the right to agree or decline. In Canada, families are always involved in the decision process, as I believe is the case in many other countries, hence the importance of having a conversation with families early and while a potential donor is in good health.

A private member's bill was introduced in the House of Commons on June 13, 2016, proposing the creation of a National Organ Donor Registry. Two days later it was defeated on its second reading based on the sitting government's statement that since 2008 more than $64 million had been spent by the previous government to develop a Canadian transplant registry. The Minister of Health's press secretary said that, "While the government supports the objectives of the bill, its passage would infringe on national, provincial and territorial responsibilities and create judicial issues." The Minister's press secretary said, "It would also duplicate an existing initiative managed by the Canadian Blood Services and Héma-Québec that is focused on kidney transplants." The Minister instead urged all Canadians to consider becoming organ donors themselves.[7]

Gerri, a friend who had been an instructor in a food science program and whose story I related earlier, is a recipient of a deceased donor kidney. His recovery was a bumpy road but now he is doing well and living life to the full. He told me what he most appreciated about his new, unrestricted diet; water and Coca-Cola were at the top of his list.

He said: "I had become very disciplined in the amount of water I took in when I was on dialysis. I generally allowed myself about one litre a day and developed all kinds of tactics to keep my intake down, including drinking from a shot glass. This kept me from having to remove excess amounts during dialysis and reduced the strain of the treatment. Now I can drink limitless amounts of water. I enjoy drinking large glasses of ice-cold water from my fridge supply. The downside is that now I get up frequently during the night to pee it out, but this is a small complaint compared to not needing to get up during the night to pee it out because I didn't have anything to get rid of."

Upon hearing this, while sucking on an ice cube, my current method of quenching thirst, I salivated as visions of fully charged glasses of ice-cold water on open tap sparkled before my eyes.

Gerri continued to explain about the pleasure that had been restored by his transplant. "I love Coca-Cola! I always have. On dialysis I had to give it up because of the phosphates it contained, and, of course, much of your activity on dialysis is restricting. Food containing high levels of phosphates are not absorbed effectively. Too-high levels rob your body of calcium. Since I received the transplant, phosphates have been transformed from a 'bad thing' to a 'nutrient' and I am expected to eat foods that contain them. So, of course, I drink Coke!

"Now, I know you will tell me that Coke is bad for me, but this is really not true. It has essentially the same nutrient profile as all common fruit juices (which nutritionists tell me I have to drink) in terms of sugar content, etc. except that it is missing some vitamin C that we get lots of with normal eating. The societal problem is that we consume too many soft drinks and get too much sugar overall. It is not the fault of the drink, but the lack of discipline by the consumers that leads to problems. And drinking fruit juice is no solution. It is a control issue.

"A side benefit of drinking Coke is that I get to tell the nutritionists I'm doing it during the clinic sessions and then get to watch their reactions! Bless their hearts, they struggle with the desire to tell me to drink fruit juice instead of Coke but can't really come up with a good argument for doing so. I sit quietly after enthusiastically proclaiming my new-found introduction to Coca-Cola and enjoy their reactions. Good times."

Registering to be a potential donor

Every province has its own governing rules for managing transplants, waiting lists and donor programs. However, not every province has a provincial registry. BC Transplant is the only provincial organ donor organization in Canada interested not only in knowing who would be willing to be a deceased donor but likewise, who would not. All information is confidentially recorded on a registry, as indeed is the information on all provincial registries. A BC Transplant spokesperson explained to me, "It is a help to us to know so that, if a situation arises and we have a registered person on our files, we can then inform their family member of the person's request to become a donor or not. It streamlines the process much more effectively, especially during an emotional and critical time."

There is no official registry for living donors. In BC someone wishing to become a living donor can do so through the Kidney Paired Donor or

Living Donor Paired Exchange programs.

Too few people signing up

Why so few people sign up to be potential organ donors is something that plagues health providers throughout the world. There is a worldwide shortage of donors, according to a recent Canadian Institute for Health Information (CIHI) report. Kidney donation either from deceased donors or living donors does not provide sufficient kidneys needed for the number of people on waiting lists. Canada in particular lags behind other countries in the world for deceased organ donation. Countries such as Spain, Australia, the UK and the US all lead Canada. Some of the reasons relate to better-informed public and professionals, meaning more financial investments have been provided to educate citizens, more professionals trained, greater numbers of hospitals/practitioners able to retrieve and perform organ transplantation and greater utilization of deceased organs. While living donors in Canada remain high in comparison with other countries, there does seem to have been a slight drop in the number of living donors coming forward in recent years. There are, according to BC Transplant, about five hundred people waiting for a kidney transplant in BC at any given moment. CIHI statistics for 2014 reveal there were 3,473 people throughout Canada waiting for a kidney transplant. In the same year, sixty-seven Canadians died while waiting for a transplant.[8] The numbers are significantly higher when factoring in other patients waiting for heart, liver, lungs and pancreas organs.

Improved road safety features have resulted in fewer accidents contributing to fewer casualties and decreasing the number of available deceased donor organs. Improved medical treatment for those suffering from severe head injuries are resulting in fewer deaths. Also, the authors of a 2012 CIHI report wrote, "Unfortunately, very few prior consenting patients' organs are suitable for recovery. Sadly only a small number of people who die are clinically suitable candidates for organ donation in Canada. In many cases their deaths may be attributed to other diseases or conditions rendering them unsuitable to be donors."[9] The challenge lies not only in encouraging individuals to sign their intention to be an organ donor but also in deciding to be a donor in the first place.

While there are advertisements encouraging people to register as potential organ donors, as well as a week in Canada—National Organ Donor and Tissue Awareness Week—the number signing up to become potential donors or offering to become a living donor, while increasing, remains low. Recent polls show that, when asked, 81 percent of Canadians are willing to donate their organs and tissues, but only 20 percent have made their intentions clear either through registration or by informing their family.[10]

The barriers we face

Understanding that barriers to donating organs existed, I decided to explore what they might be by asking my doctors, fellow patients, family, friends and agencies. The responses I received covered an array of opinions. I offer them in no particular order.

A recurring theme seemed to be fear: fear regarding the prospects of surgery itself and fear of the unknown. One person put it this way: "I am simply too chicken to even consider going down this road." Others worry that, should they be hospitalized, the doctors would not work in their favour to save their lives but let them die so they could use their organs for transplantation. This is a myth and does not happen. Doctors are committed to saving lives, not to ending them.

Although donating a living kidney requires surgery, which does carry inherent risks for the donor's health including post-surgery complications, kidney surgery is performed using laparoscopic or minimally invasive methods. For my own nephrectomy the surgeon made four small incisions about one inch in length, one on my side and three others in my back near my kidney. He then pumped air into my abdomen making it easier to remove my kidney. After having severed the kidney from the arteries and ureter, the surgeon increased one of my incisions by about four inches and removed my kidney. My surgery lasted about three hours. I was required to stay in hospital for four days to ensure all was well. The surgeon told me not to drive for two weeks and not to lift heavy objects for ten weeks. Had I been working, I could have returned to my job two weeks following surgery. Had I been a living donor, I would only have routine monitoring to ensure my health remained in good condition.

In January 2009, the first all-robotic kidney transplant was performed at Saint Barnabas Medical Center through a two-inch incision. In the following six months, the same team performed eight more robotic-assisted transplants.[11]

A further barrier to donation is geographical distance. This can be difficult in Canada, considering its rural areas, as well as internationally. A lack of understanding as to the important role transplants play in providing a better quality of life for recipients adds another dimension. I was directly impacted by these two things. A friend of mine who resides in the UK, a director of a significant charity, had offered to donate a kidney. While some of the tests could have been carried out in England, according to one of my nephrologists, and her expenses here would have been covered, the chair of her board of directors said that, while they were sympathetic to my friend's wish to help me, a six-week absence from her work could not be accommodated. Others with whom I have spoken have encountered similar situations. Some changes in policies have been implemented in BC so that any citizen who becomes a living donor is not financially impacted. They receive compensation for time lost from work, and expenses incurred through having surgery and for recuperation are covered. This is not the case everywhere. A need exists for more employers to be willing to grant their employees time off work without being penalized, should they wish to become living donors.

Cultural and religious views regarding the human body, which some see as sacred and therefore not to be tampered with, can also create barriers to transplantations. In reality, nearly all religious groups support organ and tissue donation as long as it does not impede the life or hasten the death of the donor.

Surprisingly, even among the culture of the medical world, there can be blind spots. A friend who works closely with a group of doctors has observed a lack of understanding among doctors about the need for donated kidneys. While they recognize the need for dialysis treatment, not all are even familiar with the different types of therapy. Most assume hemodialysis is the main method of dialysis. This lack of awareness was confirmed by one of my nephrologists.

Misconceptions create another stumbling block for many in the general population. Many are ignorant of the fact that an individual can live perfectly well with one kidney. Recently a close relative of mine, someone who would consider herself to be well informed and who knew that I had lived with one kidney from a deceased donor, surprised me. When I asked her if she had ever considered what she would like to do if her kidneys failed her, she said, "Well, I just hope I could have one from a deceased donor."

"Would she ever consider having one from a living donor?" I asked.

"Oh, no!" she said. "Why, that would be absolutely jeopardizing another person's health and life."

I agreed that while some risks were attached to the living donor, for the most part living donors fare well, living an unimpeded life with only one kidney. That's why nephrologists and kidney organizations are able to advocate for living donors.

Many people overestimate the risks for donors. One person during Organ Awareness Week told me, "I am hearing advertisements urging us to become donors, but they say if we were to suffer kidney failure ourselves the consolation would be that we would be placed high on the waiting list. That doesn't sound like much of an incentive to me."

I agreed that, yes, some risk is involved. There is a possibility of acquiring an infection, experiencing an allergic reaction to general anaesthesia, contracting pneumonia or developing a blood clot. However, the likelihood of this happening is minimized through rigorous tests to determine an individual's eligibility. Only the healthiest individuals are considered acceptable as donors, and their health is then monitored throughout their lives.

Some with whom I talked have also expressed concern about being too old to donate. While age is important, the health of the individual and kidney is the most important criterion. The oldest known living donor is ninety years old,[12] and an eighty-three-year-old UK resident donated a kidney to a forty-two-year-old man. To date, the eighty-three-year-old continues to live a healthy life.[13]

Another deterrent can be the challenge of accessing and filling in the donor form. It can seem very complicated. Donor organizations are investing considerable resources into raising public awareness and making the forms easily accessible for everyone. However, I fear more needs to be done to encourage people to become donors and to ensure the forms are promoted and obviously available.

The greatest barrier, though, is the general unawareness of kidney disease and what it means to have kidney failure. Some diseases have a very high profile; kidney disease is not one of them, although that is changing slowly. A number of people with whom I have spoken and who know I have kidney failure have confided they know absolutely nothing about it. Indeed, had it not been for my own situation, talk about kidney failure would have been only words on a page or screen, mumbo-jumbo to my eyes and buzzing in my ears. My friends seem to skirt around the issue. They might ask me how I am doing or even if I am still needing to dialyze, but that is the extent of our conversations. The topic becomes the elephant in the room.

Even mentioning the subject of organ donation seems to be another huge barrier. I have no idea what my friends' thoughts are regarding kidney disease and organ donation. I am reticent to bring it up. I fear a lot of stuttering, shifting in seats and eyes turned in the other direction, wary I might ask them to be a donor. Many of my fellow patients have experienced similar reactions.

May I encourage any readers who personally know people in need of organ transplant: please talk to them. They will not wilt, nor be maudlin in response. Judging from the other patients with whom I share my dialysis life, they are the least complaining and most open-minded and level-headed of people. Questions asked will be answered without fanfare or fuss. Greater public and professional awareness, as well as a cultural shift, are necessary to help remove some of the barriers preventing people from becoming donors. Unless citizens and governments are willing to engage in more conversations about organ donation, no one will be any the wiser, and organ shortages will prevail. It is well worthwhile contacting a living donor program to learn more about what being a donor entails. The Resources listed at the back of this book include websites and phone numbers of organizations across Canada.

Why some register their intent to become deceased donors

Since my research revealed the low number of people registering their intent to become potential donors, I was interested in looking at the other side to find out why people would ever wish to be a donor. What I learned amazed me. The reasons were not what I had anticipated. What had I anticipated

I would learn? I have no answer to give to that.

One person I asked told me, "We are always being solicited for money or financial contributions of one sort or another. While I am happy to do what I can, I do not have an endless source of money. Becoming a donor costs me nothing, but it could help many others. I am told as a deceased donor I could help up to eight people and even more if I were to donate my tissue. How good is that! I may be able to do more with my body parts than I could with my money."

Another explained, "Well, I look at it this way. If my kidneys or other organs were to fail and I wanted to have a transplant, then I feel it is only right that I become a donor. You know, what goes around comes around. I can't expect someone else to give me an organ if I am not prepared to do the same for another. Simple fact."

A further respondent said, "You know we are all going to die eventually. Why not do something with my organs? They are no use to me six feet down, but may be a lot of good six feet up."

One of my nurses told me a funny story. Working with kidney patients has made her more conscious of the struggles we kidney patients endure, the toll dialysis takes on our bodies, the endless hours of brutal treatment and the years of waiting patiently for a transplant. This awareness consolidated in her mind the reasons for becoming a donor. She and her husband had many discussions about her wanting to become a donor, and while she had not yet done so, she decided to keep it forefront in her thoughts and posted a note on her fridge. The note stayed in place unattended to, until one day she felt it was time to act. My nurse proceeded to enter her application online only to receive an instant message in response. The message: "You are already registered." The date given: many years earlier! How quickly we forget our actions, but what it did show was that the registry is alive and active. Anyone who registers is never forgotten. A great benefit of the computer age.

Someone else gave me a compelling reason to register as a donor. The person told me, "None of us wants to die. We all want to leave a legacy behind us. We would like to be immortal, but we cannot be. This is one way in which we can do both. We may not have amassed fortunes, become famous or solved the world's problems, but perhaps we can enable someone else to do any or all of these. What better way to end our lives? Can you imagine how we can shape the world of tomorrow by one simple gesture and a signature on a piece of paper?"

About living donors

When I received my first kidney transplant, deceased donors were mainly used. Historically, living donors were used in early transplants, but they were mostly monozygotic twins whose successful matching was more guaranteed or those who were related to the recipient through birth. But as shortages of deceased donors became more evident, the trend to use living donors increased, and the living donor pool extended to include relatives such as uncles, aunts and so on, then to friends and gradually to strangers. I recall that, while I attended a seminar in the mid-1990s, a discussion concerning how to best assess the suitability of living donors arose. Now some twenty years later, we candidates who are eligible to receive a transplant are advised to consider advocating for a living donor ourselves.

There are many reasons why living donors are important sources for those of us on the waiting list. Firstly, as previously discussed, there is a shortage of deceased donors; therefore, the wait time for a deceased donor can be lengthy. Secondly, a living donor can be tested in more ways than a deceased donor for obvious reasons: they are living and their medical history is easier to access and assess. Testing can be more thorough and complete. Thirdly, recipients have a better chance of receiving a kidney sooner if they can find a living donor.

The ratio of kidney transplants from living donors as opposed to deceased donors is better. In 2013 in Canada, living donors exceeded deceased donors. There were 588 living donors versus 553 deceased donors.[14]

However, advocating for a living donor is not always an easy task, especially if family members are unable to provide a kidney. It can be riddled with complications. There are the ethical concerns regarding whether or not another person's life is being jeopardized. Risks, while minimized through rigorous tests, are still possible. Whom to ask? How to do this knowing the many obstacles? It can be a sensitive issue, particularly if friends or acquaintances do not offer to become donors. Not everyone is willing to donate a kidney. A transplant candidate's social worker can provide advice and support with the quest. It still remains a challenge because candidates are often not well enough or do not have the energy required to do this. Many use social media to advertise their need to greater or lesser degrees of success. Friends and family can also help spread the word if they feel they can help.

Being a living donor

When someone decides to become a living donor, regardless of whether they are related to or familiar with the recipient or they are an altruistic donor, it is necessary for them to be thoroughly and meticulously assessed for suitability. One nurse told me, "Tell anyone who might wish to become a living donor that they will receive the best treatment and most up-to-date assessment of their health status that anyone could imagine. It is an excellent opportunity for an absolute, complete physical examination. A win-win for all. No other examination equals it. And it is free!"

I happened to talk to Sue, who had donated a kidney to her brother. She explained the process to me. She said, "First I was required to fill in a lengthy and detailed questionnaire concerning my medical history and related questions, as well as how I spent my leisure time. Once I had filled it in and it had been reviewed by the transplant team, I was interviewed. One of the questions the medical team asked me was, 'Why do you want to be a donor?' At first, I was put off by this question and inwardly thought, 'Well, I'm here, aren't I? Why are you asking me this?' The team must have thought me rude or not interested while I paused to answer. Instead I asked them why they were asking me this question. I was told that this was important since they needed to know how I felt my contribution could benefit my brother, and to make sure that it really had been my decision and that I had not been coerced or offered payment to donate. That made instant sense.

"Once the team felt confident with my reasons, the next step was for me to be medically assessed to rule out the possibility of future kidney or other diseases occurring. This, I was assured, was required to be done, since the nephrologists needed to be absolutely certain I was a 100 percent fit, well and healthy, and would not succumb to kidney failure. They wanted to be sure I would survive the surgery and was not susceptible to other serious conditions. I had a full physical examination to determine my overall health and physical condition, as well as tests for infectious diseases and blood disorders, in fact anything that might compromise the quality of my life.

"Additionally, I had tests checking the health of my blood vessels, organs—kidney, heart, lung and liver function—as well as blood type. I was required to have an echocardiogram and ECG, stress tests, as well as a mammogram, Pap test and a FIT test. I think men have other tests. Because my tests showed I was physically healthy, I then had my tissue tested to see if it matched my brother's. I had no idea I would have as many tests as I did (over 68 blood tests alone), nor the process be as time-absorbing as it was, or the length of time it took before I was cleared to become a donor. In fact, at one time, because everything seemed to be taking so long, my brother confessed to me he had tried to find out how my testing was progressing. He was told because I was the donor, my information was strictly confidential and even though he was my sibling, it made no difference. Confidentiality was just that! The waiting was well worth it to be able to help my brother. I don't regret my decision for one moment.

"I was also asked if my tissue or blood type turned out not to be a suitable match for my brother, would I be willing to donate to another person through the Kidney Paired Donation Program. Again, it caused me to think it over. Not a question I had expected. I agreed. I knew about kidney shortages. The doctors explained in that case they would need to find a match donor for my brother and a recipient match for me before the surgeries could proceed."

My friend Rebecca, whom we met in an earlier chapter, had been a participant in the Kidney Paired Donation Program. She was able to find a woman who was not a match for her but willingly volunteered to become her pair. Both were tested for compatibility with other donors and were elated to learn in the early summer of 2016 they were cleared, in Rebecca's pair's case to donate to a suitable recipient and in her case to receive from a suitable donor.

Rebecca's living donor underwent a nephrectomy. She texted Rebecca almost immediately following her surgery to let her know: "Everything went very well; in fact, better than expected!" The donor's recovery was incredibly rapid and she was discharged two days later. Again she texted Rebecca to tell her, "I have just gone for a long walk today after being discharged from hospital."

Rebecca received her own donor's transplant a few days later. Her surgery was likewise successful. She called me to tell me her doctors were thrilled with her results, as indeed was she. Rebecca was expected to leave hospital about five days later and begin her new dialysis-free life. Rebecca said she could hardly contain her excitement when she informed Baxter, the company responsible for delivering dialysis supplies, that she would no longer require their services.

When a number of donors are involved it is commonly called a "chain." Multiple chains occur when a number of incompatible matches are paired with other incompatible matches. The concept of open-ended chains was developed by Dr. Michael Rees at the University of Toledo, Ohio, in 2007.[15]

The advantages of kidney chains means there is a greater likelihood of a greater number of people receiving kidneys. Anonymous altruistic donors play a significant role in reducing the number of patients waiting for transplants. A spokesperson from BC Transplant explained to me that altruistic donors are an incredibly important source of organ donation and that, by their charitable act, not only do they help one patient but they ultimately help everyone on the waiting list. In July 2008, an altruistic donor kidney was shipped via commercial airline from Cornell in New York to UCLA in California, thus triggering a chain of transplants. The shipment of living donor kidneys, computer-matching software algorithms, and cooperation between transplant centers has enabled long, elaborate chains to be formed.[16]

A similar situation happened for a number of living donors. Sandra's boyfriend needed a kidney and had been on dialysis for a while. Sandra was willing to donate one of hers and was duly tested for suitability, only to find hers was not a good match. She was asked if she would be willing to donate hers to someone else, which she readily agreed to. She said, "I wanted to help my boyfriend in any way I could."

The hospital contacted the local renal agency that replied that Sandra's kidney would be a perfect match for a recipient living in another area, and asked if Sandra would be willing to travel there. Again Sandra agreed. The slated second recipient had a donor who likewise was not a match; that donor was asked the same question as Sandra. Would they be willing to donate to another recipient? Yes, was the response. What ensued was a wonderful flow of events as a number of donors exchanged kidneys. Through several people's generous consent, more recipients were given new lives.

In the end, Sue, in her quest to help her brother, said, "I was relieved to learn that my own social, financial and physical well-being were important considerations." All surgery and changes in lifestyle have ramifications for an individual. The upheaval caused to donors during the tests, the surgery itself and the following recovery period does impact their lives. In BC the Kidney Foundation of Canada administers what is called the Living Organ Donor Expense Reimbursement Program (LODERP). The purpose of this program is to reimburse the living donor for expenses, including travel, accommodations, parking and meals, and for residents of BC, any loss of income related to assessment tests and donation of, in this case, a kidney.

Following Sue's tests for compatibility, she did discover she was a match. "I was so glad to find out I was a suitable donor for my brother. It just made everything easier, and our surgeries were successful too. Such a relief to have been able to help him when he needed my help. Although, now knowing more about the KPD Program, I would have gladly done what was best to assist my brother."

As a result of my research, I learned that living donors invariably have a higher quality and more fulfilled life following donation. Several schools of thought suggest this is so because family members who have donated to their relatives can see how their help has enabled their recipient to live a healthier life, too. Others believe that many donors, particularly altruistic donors, feel good about having helped another and by doing so have enriched another person's life. They are regarded as modern-day heroes. So positive is the outcome for the donors that a nephrologist told me this is something we tell potential donors. We tell them that, "We can guarantee you will reap enormous benefits from having been a donor." It is one of the most selfless acts an individual can do for another.

Who are living donors?

Those heroes who have become living donors intrigued me. What prompts someone to do this was something I wished to explore, so despite the barriers, I began to ask donors, where possible and confidentiality permitted, what convinced them to become donors.

In the first place, it does seem to hold true that families are the number one source of living donors. Families not only include parents and siblings but also other relatives such as aunts, uncles and cousins, to name but a few. In fact one older hemodialysis patient told me she was waiting for a transplant offered to her by her grandson who lives outside Canada. He had been tested and cleared. His reason for wanting to donate one of his kidneys was because he wanted his grandmother to have a better quality of life than she was presently experiencing. It is understandable why families would be the first port of call, because they are more likely to share similar blood groups, provide better tissue matching and reap the benefit of seeing a loved one's life improve close at hand.

The Kidney Foundation of Canada in its *Facing the Facts* bulletin for 2016 stated that 51 percent of kidney transplants are made possible by living donors, and that 37 percent were unrelated donors, including spouses who are not considered related.[17] Interestingly, wives are more likely to donate to their spouses than the other way round. A nephrologist confirmed this fact, and in so doing said, "You can quote me on this."

A father's story

Several months ago my fellow dialysis patients and I were waiting in the lobby for HandyDART when a man, rather wearily pushing an intravenous infusion machine, passed our way, presumably walking towards the exit door for a breath of fresh air. For some reason, he stopped and talked to us. When he learned we were dialysis patients, he told us, "I have just given my son a kidney. He is my son and it is the least I could do for him." Although weak from the after-effects of his recent surgery, he was extremely proud of what he had just accomplished and further added, "By the way, he is doing really well," then carried on his way.

A brother's story

Nick is a fairly new dialysis patient who had received a kidney transplant five years ago. It failed, not from being a bad match, but for other reasons. He told me he had received his transplant from his sister. Nick, who is Greek, had lived in Vancouver for a long time but he decided to return to Greece where he worked for a number of years. When he wished to return to Vancouver, because he was diabetic, he thought it prudent to have a medical checkup. The checkup showed he was beginning to manifest the signs of kidney failure. Nick immediately contacted his three siblings. Each one of them automatically offered to donate a kidney to help him. They were duly tested and the doctors suggested his brother would be the best match.

One of his sisters who lived in Greece would have none of that and said she would become a donor. She travelled to Vancouver and persuaded the doctors to use her kidney. The doctors obliged and, because of her persistence, they told her she was a real fighter. Although she stayed with Nick, her fare and subsequent medical costs were covered by Nick's own public health number (PHN). Nick told me he was really fortunate because everything happened so quickly he bypassed the need for dialysis. But, he ruefully added, had he had to wait he might have appreciated his kidney more now knowing what it is like to have dialysis.

Today, Nick's other siblings are prepared, tested and waiting for the all clear to become further donors. Nick explained that he was fortunate in having a supportive family willing to help him. He recounted something that happened following his transplant surgery. Apparently he and his sister were in gurneys side by side. His sister wailed to him as she was wheeled by, "They never told me the surgery would be so painful!" It is not uncommon for a nephrectomy patient to experience pain following surgery. It is related to how the kidney is extracted. In order to expedite the laparoscopic removal, air is pumped into the interior region and it causes discomfort before gradually dissipating. Following my nephrectomy, I too experienced considerable pain. But once it had been cleared, I cannot recall experiencing further pain.

George's story

"Are you a visitor or are you here for dialysis?" asked one of my waiting room mates following the arrival of a robust-looking young man who had joined our group.

The young man replied, "I am here for dialysis. I am here because I am going to have a transplant in two days."

George, it turned out, had come to Vancouver from out of town so he could prepare for his imminent surgery. He related his story. About eleven years ago, while still attending university, he had been diagnosed with chronic kidney disease resulting from a protein leak in his kidneys. He knew his kidneys would eventually fail but continued with his post-secondary education, met his girlfriend and future wife, and began a career in business.

George said that by July 2015, "My kidney function had dropped to about 18 percent. Dialysis was on the horizon. I had been trying to avoid dialysis before having a transplant but it was not to be. I started hemodialysis in March 2016."

He continued, "When my mother-in-law discovered that it was time for a transplant, I believe her first words were, 'Well, how do I get tested?' Truly a remarkable person! I guess mother-in-law jokes are now outlawed for me."

George's mother-in-law was duly tested and proved to be a perfect match. His blood type was A, and his mother-in-law's O.

He said, "The crossover was easy."

George's story continues. The transplant surgery was performed as planned. At first the results were good, but within the first week, George experienced a rejection episode. He was given a biopsy that confirmed rejection was occurring and to counteract the effects, he was given three days of intensive, high doses of IV prednisone. The therapy proved successful.

George said, "My creatinine has continued to drop so the prognosis is good. Around 10 percent of transplant recipients go through something like this. It is not the end of the world. I will continue to be monitored closely for signs of further rejection and will need to be kept on low doses of prednisone for the rest of my life."

Meanwhile George's mother-in-law continues to recover well from her own surgery and is delighted to have been able to see her son-in-law resume a healthier existence. It is a wonderful story of generosity and devotion.

A spouse's story

Recently, while attending a non-renal social function, I happened to meet a fellow who told me he had donated a kidney to his wife. It had been some years ago. Although the transplant had been a success, his wife later succumbed to a lung infection. Jack informed me that his wife had been diagnosed with focal segmental glomerulosclerosis (FSGS)[18] in the early

1990s. That led to her having kidney failure. Jack added that, while he and his wife were conversant with kidney disease and understood a transplant would provide her with an improved lifestyle, they were unaware that they shared the same blood type as well as other factors contributing to a suitable match. It was a tremendous surprise for both him and his wife when Jack's tests revealed how well his blood type and tissue matched those of his wife, a miracle that enabled him to become his wife's donor. It so happened that when Jack had his nephrectomy, the laparoscopic machine had just been introduced. He said he is probably one of the first people to have had surgery performed using this method. He only has what resembles a small C-section scar. Current methods are even less invasive.

Jack told me, "By giving my wife my kidney, I was able to afford her eight more years of dialysis-free life. I learned very rapidly the reason why donating kidneys is so important to the well-being of others."

A woman overhearing our conversation asked Jack, "But how is your health now? Do you not suffer from the effects of only having one kidney? Are you able to live a healthy life?"

Jack replied, "Apart from recovering from the surgery itself, I am perfectly healthy. I can participate in any activity I wish. I have absolutely no adverse side effects."

The woman was amazed by what she had heard. "I had no idea," she said and shook her head in astonishment.

Perhaps with this new knowledge she may now sign up her intention to become a deceased donor or even become a living altruistic one.

A friend's story

Friends are another source of donors. Being a donor or even the notion of being a donor had never crossed Ruth's mind. The concept didn't even exist for her. As with many others, not only did she not know anyone with kidney failure, she knew even less about it. But when a friend had kidney failure and she realized how much it had affected her ability to socialize, travel and lead a life as Ruth could, she said, "I knew I needed to do something. I believe friends are there to help friends. It is what we do. I could not stand by and watch as the disease changed her life. My friend was suffering. I debated with myself what I should do. It was not an easy decision to make.

Of course, I was worried about the tests, surgery and after-effects. But when I applied and met with the doctors, they seemed to put me at ease: I was to be applauded for my actions. The procedure took a long time but in the end it was worth it to see my friend regain some of her old energy and vitality. I feel that I did something good for someone else."

A stranger's story

Mere acquaintances and strangers form a third source of donors. Peter worked in a large firm. There were many employees, some he knew, others not. A workplace environment can be—well, to put it mildly—like a telegraph pole; news spreads quickly. Somehow, he learned from one source of the telegraph pole or another that a colleague required a kidney transplant. Peter had never met the person. But, as he said, something triggered his brain. He said he does not know what it was. He did not know the person in question, had no relationship with him and most likely never would. Whatever it was that set his thoughts in motion is hard to explain, he said. All he knew was that he needed to help.

He was healthy and it came to him in a flash: perhaps he could donate a kidney. Why? To this day he cannot explain it. Peter began the process of applying to his local hospital and found himself, many questions and endless tests later, lying in the pre-op waiting to have a nephrectomy. All was successful. His colleague survived and continued working, a much-reinvigorated person. Peter likewise survived the surgery and its aftermath. He told me, "I cannot feel more satisfied than I do now. I have no regrets, only pleasure that I responded as I did. I am no hero, just an ordinary guy, but I know I helped another person. That is enough for me."

Anonymity is usually fiercely maintained, as is confidentiality regarding known living donors. Sometimes, however, a shared experience brings people together and friendships develop. Where an acquaintance has helped another, a bond had been formed and new relationships evolve. Again, a win-win for each person.

Anonymous or altruistic donors

Anonymous or altruistic donors are another source. But because they are anonymous, they are harder to track down in person. For these I needed to talk with doctors and agency representatives, who told me that many become donors either because they have experienced some major trauma in their own lives or because they understand what it is like to have suffered and feel they want to repay the support they received. Others are more likely to feel a spiritual connection and view this as contributing to the broader universe. Still others may have no family, be single and see this as their way of ensuring they leave a legacy of some kind. Some are simply generally benevolent and become donors for no other reason than wanting to share an act of kindness. An act of unsolicited selflessness can never be trivialized. "Kindness can become its own motive. We are made kind by being kind."[19]

Donors save lives and costs

The Kidney Foundation of Canada bulletin, Facing the Facts, in 2016 reported that one-third of the people who died waiting for an organ were waiting for a kidney. In that year, there were eighty-eight deaths recorded.[20] The report contained a detailed account of the healthcare cost of a kidney transplant, including donor costs. It is approximately $100,000 for the first year following a transplant, reducing to $20,000 in the second year. Each year the transplant survives, the healthcare costs lower so that over a five-year period, in addition to the improved quality of life afforded the transplant recipient, the healthcare system recovers over $250,000 in dialysis costs. However, in reality, as soon as one recipient is removed from the waiting list, another takes the removed recipient's place so the savings are transferred to the new wait-list person. Real cost savings would be most notable were there fewer people on the waiting list and a greater number becoming recipients.[21] It is true to say that the saving grace for kidney patients is that the ability to dialyze preserves life; a similar treatment is not available for people requiring a heart, lung, pancreas or liver. For this reason, all organ donations are valuable and equally required.

Regardless of any of the reasons supplied by the donors I spoke with, I am left with a feeling of tremendous humility and thankfulness for their generosity in considering others before themselves. We can only be a richer world when people are willing to support those in need. We are all eventually *"gonna need somebody to lean on."*

Chapter 9 | Some Solutions to Transplant Challenges

Houston, we have a problem.

Elementary, my dear Watson.

Finding a way to preserve kidneys

Following my first failed transplant surgery, I was informed that two kidneys had been harvested—the old terminology used in the 1990s—that day from the South of England; mine was sent to London and the other to the North of England. Being new to the world of kidney transplants, I had never considered how they had been transported. My curiosity was piqued. The story behind their preservation has now been clarified.

Researching not only appropriate solutions in which to store the retrieved kidneys, but also the length of time kidneys could be preserved before losing their viability for being transplanted, took several decades and many attempts before the problem was resolved. Preserving a kidney is of extreme importance if it is to be transplanted effectively. The process is much more involved than the following indicates and has been simplified for the non-medical reader.

Today, a donor's retrieved kidney is first cooled prior to removal. Unlike many hibernatory mammals whose bodies can adapt to rapid changes in temperature, human bodies are not so conditioned. The term used is static cold storage. An ice-cold preservative solution is flushed into the organ. This begins the process of preserving the donated organ. The body cavity is also filled with sterile ice to aid cooling. Following removal the kidney is placed in fresh sterile solutions and double-bagged. To cool the preserved kidney further, the sterile containers are surrounded with an icy slush mixture. It is important to keep the kidney cool but not frozen. A mixture of chemical solutions is used to counteract the effects of the cooling process.

For a non heart-beating donor, a different method is used. This is carried out using a hypothermic machine perfusion. Machine perfusion systems continuously pump cold preservation solution through the kidney. A kidney can be kept anywhere from one to twenty-four hours before it loses its ability to be transplanted. These preservation methods allow kidneys to be transported to other areas. This has afforded greater opportunities to locate a suitable recipient.[1,2]

The hunt for appropriate supportive medications

Gerri, whom we met earlier, after having been on dialysis for almost five years, received a telephone call from the Transplant Department. He was to receive a transplant—his second one—that evening. He went out for lunch and then, with packed bag in hand, headed to the hospital where he was immediately prepped for the surgery. Early the following morning, he had his surgery. Upon waking, he told his wife his new kidney would be named "Bob."

"Don't ask me why," he said. "It just seemed appropriate."

Gerri's road to recovery was long and arduous and is an excellent example of the types of modern medications used to prevent rejection. To prevent further potential kidney failure, he was given what he termed "a strong drug treatment with initially high levels of anti-rejection drugs called Cell-Cept, tacrolimus and prednisone." The plan was to start with high doses and gradually reduce them as his body adjusted to the new regimen. He didn't tolerate them well and had to deal with side effects such as dizziness and intestinal disturbance. As well, his low hemoglobin level of 78 grams per litre (g/L) led to a lack of energy and stamina. He was also required to take insulin for a type of diabetes that Gerri calls "Type 3," caused by the prednisone and tacrolimus.

Additionally, his urine output was minimal. Lack of urine output over a number of years can cause the ureter to shrink and become blocked. This was Gerri's case. He required an operation called a transurethral resection of the prostate, or TURP. A laser probe was used to open up his ureter and remove a significant portion of his prostate. He was prescribed alpha-blockers that enabled him to urinate reasonably well, but he had brutal side effects. He said, "I was delighted to get off these drugs. The TURP was no fun at all but about two weeks after it, I began urinating vigorously. I delightedly told my wife I was now capable of putting out the campfire without reaching for a bucket!" Gerri gave "Bob" the kidney a proper name following this: "Bob Tupper."

"For future reference," he added.

Gerri was not done quite yet. He experienced heart issues primarily related to a reduction in tacrolimus in order to correct overly high blood pressure. Pulse rates of around 130 beats per minute (bpm) and heart flutter resulted in Gerri being taken to the emergency department where a cardioversion was eventually performed to snap his heart back into rhythm. Removing the alpha-blockers created a further ordeal for Gerri, including a heart rate of 130 bpm for thirty hours. Then it dropped back to the more normal level of 80. For four months Gerri lived with a see-sawing of health issues.

Then, he said, "One day, I woke up full of energy and raring to go. I haven't looked back since. My hemoglobin level recovered to 125 [g/L]. I regained energy and the ability to walk and explore." He and his wife are in a new phase of life. They have planned trips to Hawaii and Europe. They moved to a seafront condo and got their bikes out to pedal around Vancouver's seawall as frequently as possible. Gerri said, "I am actively reducing my drug levels to a maintenance level and can feel the improvement in well-being and normalcy that comes with living like a regular person."

Finding appropriate medicines, namely immunosuppressants to stave off rejection, took many years. First uses included corticosteroids in the early 1960s, followed by prednisone in the later 1960s. In 1962 azathioprine (Imuran) was used. Each successive medication increased patient survival rate, but they had been given separately, not together. In 1963 a new discovery was made when Dr. Thomas Starzl (1926–2017), Associate Professor at the University of Colorado, used both prednisone and azathioprine together from the start of the transplant process with success. This ushered in the start of dual drug therapy and led to the largest number of kidney transplant undertakings at that time throughout the world.

In 1972 a Swiss doctor, Jean-François Borel, and his team at Sandoz in Switzerland discovered cyclosporine A in Norwegian soil samples that had been sent to a laboratory for routine testing for new antibiotics. Cambridge Professor Sir Roy Calne (1930–present) experimented with cyclosporine first in skin grafts on animal models and then he began using it in humans. It was discovered that large doses of cyclosporine were toxic for kidney survival. Adjusting and monitoring the doses increased the patients' survival rates from 50 to 80 percent over a one-year period. The introduction of cyclosporine transformed the perception of organ transplantation from a hazardous exercise to a clinically feasible procedure.

Dr. Starzl introduced cyclosporine in the United States in the early 1980s while combining it with steroids. Dr. Squifflet told me that during this time, while he was a transplant fellow at the University of Minneapolis, he and his colleagues performed a number of animal experiments in combining cyclo-sporine with azathioprine. He said that this was the basis for the triple-drug immunosuppressive regimen in transplantation. When I had my transplant in 1991, cyclosporine, azathioprine and prednisone were my prescribed im-munosuppressants.

In 1987, Dr. Starzl, then working at the University of Pittsburgh Medical School, introduced a new drug, tacrolimus that was initially used for liver transplants. In 1994 it was used for kidney transplants and proved to be even more effective than cyclosporine. Currently there are a number of im-munosuppressant medications in use.[3] Today CellCept is one of the latest anti-rejection medications used.

Solving the mystery of tissue matching

One patient I met during my daytime sessions told me, "My mother wanted to donate her kidney to me but she proved to be a wrong match. I am now waiting to see if I can find a donor who will be a better fit." The match may have proved difficult due to incompatible tissues.

A friend, when told I was writing a book, said to me, "What I am really interested in finding out is who discovered tissue matching." I hope the fol-lowing provides her answers.

Tissue matching proved necessary in order to provide compatible kidney pairing. Two early physicians noticed problems using different tissue types, but it was centuries before the solution was discovered. First, Dr. Gaspare Tagliacozzi, a 16th-century physician who had performed skin grafts on patients, prophesized that different types of tissues were incompatible.

Second, Dr. John Hunter, a Scottish physician and surgeon in the 18th century, having successively transplanted the spur of a young chicken from its leg to its comb, attempted to graft a spur from a young cock onto the leg of a chicken. That was not successful. Hunter concluded their failure happened because they were two distinct animals with two different tissues. He had concluded different types of tissue would not necessarily provide a compatible match.

According to Dr. Squifflet, there are several fathers of "tissue matching" discoveries in modern times. For example, in 1963 in France, Professor Jean-Baptiste-Gabriel-Joachim Dausset (1916–2009), who became head of immunology at the Hôpital Saint-Louis, together with Felix Rapaport (1929–2001) discovered the human leukocyte antigen (HLA) system by performing skin transplants on volunteers. They showed that success depended on what is termed histocompatibility or tissue compatibility. Similar tissues are better matched. HLA is a protein found in most body cells. Dausset received the Nobel Prize for Medicine or Physiology in 1980. He also founded France Transplant and Greffe de Moelle, the latter an organization that matches recipients with donor organs and bone marrow transplants.

Further research was carried out in the Netherlands by Professor Jon Van Rood (1926–2017) and by George D. Snell (1903–1996) who discovered additional HLA antigens leading to better tissue matching. Dr. Paul Ishiro Terasaki (1929–2016), who as a child had spent three years in a Japanese-American internment camp during World War II, later studied at UCLA in California and became professor emeritus of surgery at the David Geffen School of Medicine. Dr. Terasaki developed an even better method for cross matching tissue. As a result of his experimental research work, the method he discovered has become the standard practice for matching all organ donors and recipients, as well as making matches for bone marrow transplantation. Dr. Terasaki also created the UCLA Kidney Transplant Registry, the largest in the world.

HLA tissue matching gained prominence when Dr. Starzl contributed to improving the importance of the ABO blood group in transplantation.[4] Tissue matching is carried out through blood tests similar to blood type groups. Both donor and recipient undergo a series of blood tests to determine kidney compatibility and blood group.

Dr. Starzl retired from clinical practice in 1991. A research building on the University of Pittsburgh campus is named the Thomas E. Starzl Transplantation Institute in his honour. His numerous distinctions include the Medawar Prize (1992) and the Lasker Award for Clinical Science (2012). Dr. Starzl passed away at age 91 in March 2017.

Today improvements in medical technique, knowledge, immunosuppressant medication and follow-up care for kidney transplant recipients are considered the norm for people with kidney disease. An individual receiving a transplant has a better survival rate than an individual on dialysis. Figures suggest that even someone seventy-five years of age who receives a transplant will live four years longer than someone who does not.

Resolving further challenges

Doctors and researchers are continuing to seek ways to solve the challenges of insufficient deceased donor kidneys, heal ailments causing kidney failure, increase transplant survival rates for recipients and improve methods of patient management.

Chapter 10 | Some Research Projects

We keep moving forward, opening new doors, and doing new things, because we're curious and curiosity keeps leading us down new paths.

—Walt Disney

My own involvement in research projects

"How would you like to participate in a study project? It won't necessarily help you but may well be of value to later kidney recipients whose kidney transplant has failed?" The nephrologist had sought me out while I was waiting to be called in for my dialysis session. I was intrigued.

"What is the purpose of this research project?" I asked.

"It's a five-year national project in seventeen study centres across Canada involving nine-hundred-and-eighty participants whose first transplant has failed. We want to find out if continuing with immunosuppressant medication is important in preventing the transplanted kidney from being rejected and therefore creates additional complications, or whether or not we should remove the kidney itself." He went on to explain, "Fifty percent of all deceased donor kidney transplants stop working within ten-and-a-half years. Transplant failure is now the fifth leading cause of dialysis initiation in Canada."

The study would not include patients whose second kidney transplant had failed or who had had double kidney–pancreas transplants. The study proposed two questions. The first: Is it better to remove the non-functioning kidney after it has failed or should it be left? The concern was that it could contribute to further severe health complications. The second: Should immunosuppressant medication be continued or stopped after the failure of a transplanted kidney? The concern was that discontinuing immunosuppressant medication could contribute to an increase in antibodies, making it difficult to find suitable matches for a further transplant. Many people are waiting years to receive a second kidney transplant because of accumulated antibodies. Queenie and Renee are two examples of those who are affected by an accumulation of antibodies.

If we agreed to participate, which I did most willingly, we would have our blood tested periodically for several years. Our general health would also be regularly monitored throughout. Risks would be minimal to us, other than the discomfort from blood being drawn if we were not on hemodialysis. For hemodialysis patients, blood can be drawn from their fistula or catheter sites. The drawn blood would be kept on a confidential file for fifteen years. Only the nephrologist would have access to this information. This was my introduction to the world of kidney research. Unfortunately, half way into my second year, the study terminated. The reasons why were never explained to me because I rarely saw the nephrologists who were leading the project in my hospital.[1]

Since then, I have participated in other studies. One related to a research registry examining ways to create treatment that might reduce cardiovascular morbidity and mortality rates. Heart attacks are common in end-stage renal patients. Patients who consented and continued to consent were to be asked a series of questions: Would you be willing to participate in a trial evaluating a new drug like a heart pill? Do you have a history of diseases such as diabetes or heart disease? Those of us who had given our consent were given contact information relating to research studies. The registry is a continuous registry open to all renal patients. Its funding body is the Canadian Institutes of Health Research (CIHR), and the sponsoring agency is Population Health Research Institute, Hamilton Health Sciences. It is led by one principal investigator and three co-investigators.[2]

Another study, "Inter-rater reliability of exit site monitoring tool for hemodialysis catheters," sponsored by my own hospital, was created to validate an existing monitoring tool to assess potential infections in catheters. Since no similar system had been reported in medical literature, my hospital wished to determine if their tool could be used in other centres in my province, and possibly elsewhere. To do this, they needed to ascertain if the tool they were using conformed to their desired standard.

It was a short study, involving only a couple of dialysis sessions. Two nurses assessed our catheter sites, each marking a score independent of the other. Once the first nurse completed the assessment, the data results were recorded. Fifteen minutes later one of the co-investigators then found a second available nurse to complete the same assessment on me. Both nurses were unaware of the other's score. If the scores did not tally, then the higher score was used in which case the catheter site was swabbed again. My scores must have tallied because I never received further swabbing.[3] A report about the study has been recently published in a nursing journal, much to the delight of its researchers.

I also participated in a PhD candidate's thesis, entitled "A qualitative study of patient/family experience of health care quality improvement and safety initiatives from an ethical lens." The principal investigator was a Research Associate with Ethics Services, Providence Health Care, and also an Associate Professor of the School of Nursing at the University of British Columbia. The study was primarily concerned with finding ways to encourage patients and families to use alcohol-based hand rubs and wipes and to remind their healthcare providers to wash their hands. The researcher felt it was important to know how these kinds of projects helped to reduce infections, as well as what patients and families thought about these initiatives.

Part of the study involved the researcher observing everyday activities, focusing on interactions between health providers, patients and families related to hand washing. The study interviewed twenty-five patients and family members, of whom I was one. The aim of the project was to improve future patient care. After I agreed to participate, I was asked a series of questions pertaining not only to my knowledge of hygiene practices, but also about information provided to me by the hospital about hygienic discipline, about the hygiene used by practitioners and about the training I myself had received. At the time of writing this, the results have yet to be published. The study was carried out in various units of my hospital.[4]

BC Renal Agency conducted a postal survey involving all kidney patients in BC. The agency wanted to determine if renal patients' healthcare needs were being met effectively. The survey asked us what BC Renal was doing well and what required improvement. The results remained confidential but would be provided to health authority programs to help them improve their overall service delivery.[5]

Research involving fellow patients

Other patients have been involved in research studies or have tested new anti-rejection medications. Allan Wheeler deliberately asked his transplant nephrologist what new drugs were being used. He had been living successfully with a transplant for several years and was interested in knowing about current research. His nephrologist explained there was a new drug currently being tested. Would he be interested in trying it? There were no guaranteed effective results. Yes, Allan was willing. He was first required to have a kidney biopsy and some other tests to verify his kidney was functioning well. Everything was fine. Allan received his new drug and was monitored closely. Nothing adverse happened.

Allan believes the continued success of his kidney transplant may be attributed to this change in medication. "I am so glad I switched medicines. I do feel it has had a positive effect on my kidney's survival," he said. Another patient, Zoe, was not so lucky. When she recently tried a new anti-rejection medication, her results were less successful. The medication caused problems for her kidney and it subsequently failed.

Kidney disease research covers an array of projects, studying not only patient care but also the methods used for dialysis procedures. Jools, a patient in my ward, was one of the first to have a magnetic fistula inserted into his arm. The conventional AV fistula is created through a surgical incision that exposes the artery and vein, which are then cut and stitched together. The vein grows bigger and stronger over six to twelve weeks. This procedure requires anaesthesia and time for the wound to heal before dialysis can be started.

A magnetic fistula insertion, however, requires no anaesthesia, involves only a small incision and can be used soon after installation. Two flexible magnetic catheters connect the artery and vein. A small burst of radiofrequency energy, given through the catheters, is then used to create a connection between the artery and vein, creating the AV fistula. The catheters, having done their job, are removed, leaving no scars. The insertion is minimally invasive and does not lead to other challenges encountered with common fistulas. Jools is very glad to have had his fistula created in this manner. It works well for him.

Two other patients, Mischievous Marty and Deborah, were given the opportunity to test a new type of dialysis solution. Each was given the solution for a period of six months. Mischievous Marty found he could increase the speed of his machine, thus achieving better clearance, contributing to him feeling better following his dialysis treatment. He enjoyed having the opportunity to try the solution and was sorry when his test time ended. He did not know if others are now using this solution. Deborah never commented to me as to whether or not she found the solution worked well for her. Others have been able to try different styles of chairs for comfort and flexibility.

We are told we will soon be getting new hemodialysis machines. Machines are continually being refined for performance and speed.

International and national research projects and programs

UK project focusing on the use of iron infusions with dialysis patients

All hemodialysis patients develop anemia. It is a common occurrence and leaves us patients feeling exhausted, affecting our quality of life. Intravenous iron infusions are regularly administered to treat the condition. Some patients, like Charity, require bi-weekly intravenous iron infusions. She always tells the nurses, "It is my new favourite cocktail." I receive monthly infusions. So far, no study has been conducted into the amounts of iron administered, so patients receive an arbitrary amount.

To rectify this, in 2013, a groundbreaking clinical trial, the largest ever undertaken in the UK, was introduced. Designed to last four years, it is known as PIVOTAL—Proactive IV irOn Therapy in hemodialysis patients. It involves more than 2,000 first-year dialysis patients, as well as clinicians and research nurses in fifty renal units across the UK.

The purpose of this trial was to test two different approaches to administering iron fusions. Some patients received high, but not unsafe, doses of iron to increase their levels of iron, while others received lower doses. Those receiving lower doses had them either when their iron levels were beginning to decrease or when symptoms of anemia appeared. Having reached the target number of patients by 2016, the patients were treated for at least two years. It is hoped that results will affect the way in which iron is administered by the National Health Service in Britain and will be of value globally, too.[6]

> Patient involvement is crucial to the trial and a patient support group has been established to provide patient input and awareness about the ongoing trial throughout every stage of the trial including profiling, evaluation and analysis. An Advisory and Dissemination board, led by Kidney Research UK, the charity representing a range of stakeholders, will monitor proceedings.

Drug trials to control or prevent kidney failure

Other recent research studies undertaken in by Kidney Research UK, as well as in the United States and Canada, have concentrated on finding ways to control or prevent kidney failure from conditions such as polycystic kidney disease (PKD), focal segmental glomerulosclerosis (FSGS), and diabetes. In the UK, with a 173,000-pound grant from Kidney Research UK, Dr. Jill Norman and a team at the UCL Medical School, University College London, are studying the cells in the kidney that cause scar tissue to form in patients with PKD. These cells, called fibroblasts, are found throughout our body. They aid the healing process. Dr. Norman has been able to identify an enzyme that seems to encourage the fibroblasts to produce scar tissue in kidneys.

She and her team are trying to discover if, by using cultured kidney cells in a laboratory setting, they can explore the enzyme further to see if it does lead to kidney scarring. If this is the case, they are hoping they can find ways to inhibit the enzyme, creating a new treatment that could effectively maintain the life of the kidney. Her hope is that she and her team may find a new form of treatment for people with PKD that could slow the formation of scar tissue and possibly not only extend their lives but also delay the need for dialysis.[7]

In 2013 a report in the *Harvard Gazette* detailed a discovery made by a Dr. Peter Mundel, in the Division of Nephrology at the Harvard-affiliated Massachusetts General Hospital, regarding the treatment of FSGS. He had used a drug called abatacept (Orencia), normally prescribed for treating arthritis, with some considerable success with five test patients. The report was issued online in the *New England Journal of Medicine*.[8]

All five patients showed signs of remission of their FSGS, which causes proteinuria (proteins leaking into the urine). Two of those with recurrent disease have remained in remission for three and four years, respectively, after a single dose of abatacept. The other two required a second dose when proteinuria reappeared a few weeks later and have been in remission for ten and twelve months, respectively. The fifth patient—one who had not responded well to previous treatments and was at risk of developing kidney failure—went into remission for the first time in more than a year and, continuing to be in remission a year later, has resumed a normal lifestyle.

While the woman still receives monthly doses of abatacept, she no longer needs the high-dose steroids and immunosuppressive drugs that she had depended upon, some of which actually increase the risk for kidney failure.

Dr. Mundel explained that a larger trial needed to be conducted, and if it proved equally successful, then there may well be good reason for using abatacept for treating FSGS and even for diabetic kidney disease.

Cell transplants

In Canada, in 2015, Dr. James Shapiro, Director of the Clinical Islet Transplant Program at the University of Alberta, published a study in *Nature Biotechnology* in which he described an innovative way of transplanting islet cells underneath a patient's skin from a donor's pancreas. Dr. Shapiro, one of the world's leading insulin experts had previously, in the 1990s, co-developed the Edmonton Protocol to treat diabetes through transplantation of islet cells into a patient's liver. While this technique offered hope, Dr. Shapiro soon realized the liver wasn't the ideal site for transplantation as most of the cells were rapidly destroyed.

In his recent report, Dr. Shapiro said that until his present test, it had been impossible for transplanted cells to reliably function when placed beneath the skin. He further suggested his studies have harnessed the body's natural ability to respond to a foreign body by growing new enriching blood vessels. He feels that by controlling this reaction he and his team have successfully and reliably reversed diabetes in their preclinical models. Dr. Shapiro feels the new approach marks an evolution of the protocol and could soon become a new standard of treatment, not only for diabetes but also for other diseases.[9]

Stem cell implants

Stem cell implants have also been used to grow kidneys. A number of researchers have attempted to achieve success. One Japanese nephrologist, Dr. Takashi Yokoo, and colleagues at the Jikei University School of Medicine in Tokyo, had tried to use a stem cell method to grow kidneys. They were unsuccessful since urine drainage caused the kidneys to balloon under pressure. To counter the negative outcomes, they grew a drainage tube for the kidney in conjunction with a bladder to collect and store the urine.

Laboratory rats were used as incubators for the growing embryonic tissue. They found the system worked when they connected their new system of plumbing to the rats' existing bladders.

The transplanted kidney continued to work well when they checked their experiment eight weeks later. The doctors repeated the procedure on a much larger animal, a pig, and much to their satisfaction achieved the same results. Pigs' organs are more comparable to human organs than rodents' organs. Comments from other stem cell experts noted that the research was interesting and that while the science had produced good data in animals, it was impossible to know whether or not it would work in humans and would take years to achieve such a positive outcome. It was felt that the experiment did, however, move doctors closer to understanding how plumbing might work. The Japanese doctors continue to refine their experimental trials.[10]

Chimera projects

In the United States, doctors at the Salk Institute in California are attempting to grow human organs also in pigs. This is known as a chimera project.[11] It is based on a Greek mythological beast, Chimera, who had the body and head of a lion, the tail of a snake, and a fire-breathing goat head coming from its back. The Greeks believed in the notion that blending two different components created a new being. The modern use of the word chimera or chimeric properties was introduced in the 1940s.

An American geneticist, Dr. Ray Owen at the University of Wisconsin-Madison, was the first to describe chimerism in what are known as Freemartin cattle. Freemartin cattle are fraternal twins. Each twin had some of its own and some of its twin blood cells. A British immunologist, Sir Peter Medawar, a Nobel Prize winner, noted that a skin graft from Freemartin twins were permanently accepted and never rejected. He continued to notice the same thing in mice. This has led to the injection of human cells into animals.[12]

Human stem cells have been injected into pig embryos to produce more compatible organs for human use. The doctors say they should look like and behave like normal pigs except that their organs will be composed of human cells. The human–pig chimeric embryos are being designed to develop in sows for twenty-eight days since that is the normal gestation time for pigs. After twenty-eight days, the pregnancies are terminated and the tissue removed and analyzed. It is a controversial program and funded by private resources, the National Institutes of Health Informatics having disapproved the use of animals in experiments in 2016. Currently the researchers are waiting to find out if the regulations will change.

This experiment has evolved after many years of research on stem cell engineering. Stem cells have two main characteristics: one, they create more of themselves, and two, they can become any type of cell in the body. The term used to describe this is pluripotent. Embryonic stem cells are those that are most often surrounded by controversy, and are the ones used for the chimera project.

Blastocysts that form the basis of cells are formed in the early development of mammals. In the middle is what is known as the inner cell mass, which ultimately becomes the entire organism. In its early stages the cells are undifferentiated, that is they have no determined cell fit. When they receive messages from surrounding cells and their environment, they begin to change or differentiate into specific types of cells such as brain, heart, kidney, skin and pancreas, for example.

After following a certain path, the stem cell cannot become a stem cell again. Researchers at Japan's University of Kyoto in 2006, however, identified a way of reprogramming these cells so they resembled the original cell. These cells are called induced pluripotent stem cells (iPSCs). The advantage of these cells is that differentiated cells such as skin cells can be isolated from patients, transferred into iPSCs and then used to model diseases. Since these cells come from patients, the hope is that they will not be rejected by the patient.

The Salk researchers first tested their theory on rats as models and then decided to expand their test using pigs. Human iPSCs were injected into pig blastocysts. The first results were exciting as they saw the cells could be incorporated with the inner cell mass in blastocysts. Next they injected the newly introduced iPSCs into female pigs. The results were not necessarily as they hoped them to be. The embryos were sickly and small. The experiment, although opening doors, shows there is still a long way to go before successes may be obtained. Controversy also continues with worries that the pigs could be affected in other ways, such as having human brain cells. To offset these concerns further experimentation is proceeding with considerable caution.[13,14]

Less controversial and one that has proven effective has been the use of bone marrow tissue for a number of cancer treatments. The literature discusses using bone marrow tissue as an augmentation to organ transplantation since the 1950s when Dr. Peter Medawar also used the term *chimera* in relation to monozygotic twins. Since then further studies and research using bone marrow tissue for patients with multiple myeloma kidney transplants have shown good results.

Immunosuppression research

Lifelong immunosuppression carries with it problems for a transplant recipient, and can in itself lead to further health issues as well as kidney failure. The ability of the recipient's body to maintain the transplant without having to use immunosuppressant (anti-rejection) medication on a daily basis has been termed in the literature as The Holy Grail of transplantation. Some cases use animal models and a few reports of patients being taken off immunosuppressant medication have shown some success.

Those that have shown the greatest success are the cases where infusions of the donor's bone marrow have been used during the transplant. The donor's bone marrow becomes blended with the recipient, and the new bone marrow cells re-educate the recipient to accept the new organ, thereby eliminating the need to take anti-rejection medication. Considerable work still needs to be done in this area, but scientists and researchers are working on ways to avoid having to use lifelong immunosuppression. The Canadian National Transplant Research Program (CNTRP) is the first program to bring together and integrate solid organ transplant, bone marrow transplant, and donation and critical care research communities nationally.

The Canadian National Transplant Research Program (CNTRP), established in 2013, is a national research network designed to increase organ and tissue donation in Canada and to enhance the survival and quality of life for Canadians who receive transplants. The CNTRP's purpose is to develop new knowledge [continued]

The way in which immunosuppression medication is administered may have an adverse effect on the longevity of transplants, a recent study has discovered. What had not been known or ever really investigated was whether or not the role of the recipient's gender played any part in a kidney transplant's longevity. A recent study documented on the CNTRP's website described a project undertaken by Dr. Beth Foster, Lead CNTRP Investigator and Associate Professor of Pediatrics at McGill University Health Centre, and several other investigators at the Centre de recherche du Centre hospitalier de l'Université de Montréal (CRCHUM). Their work showed that young women had poorer transplant outcomes compared to young men, whereas women of post-menopausal age had similar or slightly better outcomes than men of the same age.

This was the first time a study of this kind had been conducted. Most studies had been conducted using adult models, whereas this study concentrated on younger ages. It showed that young women between the ages of fifteen and twenty-four have a 30–40 percent higher risk of transplant failure than young men of the same age range. Interestingly, it also revealed that women having a transplant over the age of forty-five fared slightly better than men similar in age. What had been known from studies unconnected with kidney transplants was that the female sex hormone estrogen is inclined to activate the immune system, while the male testosterone tends to suppress it. Young women's estrogen levels are at their peak, while women over forty-five have declining estrogen levels.

Dr. Foster feels this study leads to questions regarding how sex hormones can influence the effectiveness of anti-rejection in recipients of all ages and gender. She also believes this observational study reveals how little is known about the role of sex, gender and age on the immune system, transplantation and medical care in general. Presently male and female patients are treated similarly, but with improved understanding, potential kidney transplant longevity could be improved through the development of age- and sex-specific immunosuppression strategies.

Dr. Foster suggests another possible explanation for the sex differences observed in this study is that sex hormones may influence the function of anti-rejection medications, making them less effective in females than males. Outcomes open the door to a new approach for organ transplantation that could lead to personalized immunosuppression strategies based on age and sex. It is an entirely new area of research and has significant ramifications for future recipients.[17]

Cross-Canada studies

The CNTRP is involved in numerous cross-Canada collaborative studies focusing on six projects and four supporting core platforms. The six projects include *ex vivo* (out of body) organ transplant and repair; increasing solid organ and hematopoietic (pertaining to the formation of blood or blood cells such as bone marrow) cell donation; understanding, predicting and preventing early graft (transplant) rejection and graft-versus-host disease (GVHD); strategies for immunomodulation (adjustment to immune response) and transplant rejection; predicting and controlling viral complications in transplantation; and improving pediatric transplantation outcomes.

The CNTRP has several core platforms that support its research. One of the platforms is called the ethical, economic, legal and social platform, and within this area falls Canada's new law regarding medical aid in dying (MAID), which received royal assent in June 2016. Issues that have arisen from this new law, and ones that have confronted other countries that have similar laws, are whether or not a person who has requested help with dying may be eligible to donate their organs if so requested. A number of cases have existed in Canada where this has been possible.

Because the MAID law is new, it will be surrounded by controversies for some time to come. To explain how the new law works so far in Canada, the CNTRP has created a fact sheet in which it details what the law has decreed and how it works regarding organ donation.[18] There are three categories in which the law applies: voluntary euthanasia, assisted suicide and medical assistance in dying. Voluntary euthanasia happens when an individual, at their own request, is administered a substance resulting in their own death. Donating organs following voluntary euthanasia is legally permitted.

Assisted suicide occurs when an individual requires a prescription to hasten their death in their own time. Organ donation is not allowed in this case. This is because death is not predicted for a specific time and organs may not be suitable for retrieval. Medically assisted dying covers both euthanasia and assisted suicide. One or both of these methods may be available within certain jurisdictions. The Netherlands has also developed specific policy regarding the three types. In Belgium organ donation following authorized death has recently been permitted.

Innovative procedures in transplantation

An example of an *ex vivo* procedure used in a lung transplant was reported by Alberta's Transplant Institute. A young mother of two children who had suffered from cystic fibrosis all her life required an immediate lung transplant. The young mother was offered a "reconditioned" set of lungs, which would otherwise have been useless because of massive blood clots. Through a clinical trial of *ex vivo* perfusion technology, the first of its kind done in Canada, the clots were treated outside the body to make the lungs safe for transplant. The process involved a three-to-four hour period during which the donated lungs were placed inside a sterile plastic dome attached to a ventilator, pump and filters. The lungs were maintained at normal body temperature and treated with a bloodless solution containing nutrients, proteins and oxygen. Once assessed to be suitable, the lungs could be transplanted into the waiting recipient. This is an innovative measure.[19]

Other trials have been conducted in which organs from deceased donors have been reconstructed for use. For example, at the Texas Heart Institute, researchers are working with deceased organs, which they prepare by "washing" them of their living cells, similar to ex vivo perfusion. According to Dr. Steven Paraskevas, the past president of the Ottawa-based Canadian Society of Transplantation, what is left are "ghosts." These ghosts are the remaining connective tissue and form a scaffold that can be seeded with stem cells. Dr. Doris Taylor, in Alberta, who appeared in the CBC's *Nature of Things*, aired November 16, 2016, added that the stem cells seem to take cues and know where to go and what kinds of cells to become. This process has been used to bioengineer heart, liver and kidney tissue. The approach holds great promise for using scaffolding from human tissue discarded during surgery and combining it with a patient's own cells to make customized organs that would not be rejected by the immune system.[20,21]

> The first successful kidney transplant using the *ex vivo* organ preservation method was performed in Toronto in November 2017. Patient and kidney are doing well.[22]

The Kidney Project

Since 2015, Dr. William Fissell of the University of California San Francisco and Dr. Roy from Vanderbilt University have received funding to pursue what is known as The Kidney Project. The aim of their project has been to create an artificial, implantable kidney in patients with end-stage kidney failure, in an attempt to address the shortage of available organs.

The problem has been to re-create an organ that matches the recipient's tissue, filters blood and waste material effectively, and does not require anti-rejection medication. To solve their challenge, the pair have been designing a prototype that resembles a coffee cup and uses a combination of silicon nanotechnology and living kidney cells to filter blood. A series of fifteen microchips serves as scaffolding for the living cells to grow on and around, creating a bio-hybrid device. Apparently kidney cells grow well in laboratory dishes and can then be grown in a bioreactor of living cells. Dr. Fissell has referred to the device in a recent article as a "Santa Claus system" because it can reliably distinguish between the "naughty" waste chemicals and the "nice" nutrients a body should reabsorb.

According to Dr. Fissell, the device is powered naturally by the recipient's own blood flow. He and his colleagues are working hard to ensure that blood can flow through the device without clotting or causing further damage. The device would be inserted into the recipient close to their natural non-functioning kidneys and attached to their bladder tube. A Vanderbilt biomedical engineer, Amanda Buck, is studying the device's fluid dynamics and further refining the channels for maximum blood flow efficiency. Currently the bioreactor can survive sixty days without intervention. In February 2017, the team announced they could soon be performing human trials using the device. Should their work prove effective, another solution to the organ shortage may have been realized.[23]

Transplant candidates becoming advocates

Modern technology has paved the way for considerable transplant experimentation. It has also created a social network for people seeking transplants to advocate for themselves. Some recipients have been successful in trolling for their organs, but it does have its drawbacks. Doctors have become worried that not everyone who needs a transplant can be successful. They feel touching stories or those with access to social media may have an unfair advantage over those who need transplants but do not have similar access. At a CNTRP conference in July 2016, a number of doctors suggested the need to create appropriate guidelines so that the playing field becomes equal. Other doctors have written similar suggestions in a number of medical journals. This situation is similar to that when kidney transplants were in their formative stages.

The Canadian Society of Transplantation in conjunction with the CNTRP and Canadian Blood Services are taking the lead in developing practices in the use of social media for soliciting anonymous living donors. A committee consisting of transplant physicians, ethicists, legal scholars and two patients presented a position paper in which they recognized the issue of the lack of available deceased donor organs, the numbers of patients waiting for a transplant and the number of public appeals in recent years. The paper acknowledged that acquiring anonymous living donors via social media raises ethical questions such as fairness and equity, donor and recipient autonomy, and anonymity, among other considerations. In conclusion the committee felt that it could be acceptable for transplant centres to consider solicited living donors on the proviso that they did not contravene Canadian law and did not involve monetary exchange in the process. In their statement the committee provided guidelines to transplant centres relating to informed consent processes and necessary evaluations of those who have come forward through social media.[24]

Improving patient care

While new methods made available by our latest innovative technology are in the works, patient care itself remains forefront in researching improved ways of treatment. A groundbreaking $47-million research project funded by the Canadian Institutes of Health Research, the Kidney Foundation of Canada and a variety of donations, including one for $500,000 from St. Paul's Foundation, into chronic kidney disease (CKD) was announced in 2017. It is being led by Dr. Adeera Levin, Head of the UBC Division of Nephrology and world-renowned researcher. The project, termed Canadians Seeking Solutions and Innovations to Overcome Chronic Kidney Disease (Can-SOLVE CKD), is a unique and innovative partnership of patients, researchers, healthcare providers, policy makers, industry and renal agencies. Its aim is to establish a patient-oriented research network to transform the care of people affected by kidney disease. Its targets are ambitious, according to Dr. Levin, who hopes that in ten years, every Canadian with or at risk for CKD will be screened and able to access the best possible treatment. She is also hoping the treatment will mean that new dialysis centres will no longer be necessary, because the researchers will have found a way to delay disease progression.

Currently, not everyone attending kidney care treatment centres is part of an ongoing research program, something that is a natural part of cancer or cardiology care. This project hopes to change the existing landscape and involve all patients in its research. All patients, whether they live in urban or rural settings and regardless of ethnicity, gender or age, will be included. What Dr. Levin is aiming to do is to look at the ways current patients with chronic kidney disease are treated. Some of the research will include trying to find new methods for catching kidney problems early in spite of additional complications such as diabetes, trying stem cell therapies, and testing established drugs proven to show promise in helping kidney patients.

Dr. Levin has said, "Everyone desires to remain alive forever, their wish strengthened when their quality of life is not in jeopardy. For those carrying the extra burden of kidney disease, longevity does not hold great appeal. Should this research lead to patients not only living longer but better lives then its success will be a proven reality."[25]

There is no doubt each generation benefits from the previous generation's unstinting toiling to improve methods, techniques and survival rates for transplant recipients. The irony of this was brought home to me recently when I asked a scleroderma research doctor about current research regarding scleroderma and kidney disease. His reply: "In short: there is none. When new medications such as ACE inhibitors, channel blockers and ARBs were found to be effective deterrents in 1998, the risk of kidney failure was considerably reduced."

I replied, "If I had been diagnosed with scleroderma in 1998, I may have never had kidney failure?"

"That is so," he said, reminding me that timing in medicine is everything.

The search is never ending and will be so until doctors have been able to satisfy their insatiable curiosity, and we humans reap the benefits of their hard work. Much of the current trials will take a long time to come to fruition. In the meantime, the need for donated organs remains absolutely imperative if our fellow human beings are to survive and live improved lives now.

Epilogue

To dream the impossible dream
—Joe Darion, *Man of La Mancha*

The mountains proudly statuesque under a cloudless blue sky created an exquisite backdrop to the scene before us. The early autumn sun, still radiating heat from long summer days, cast strong rays on the water. Everywhere blinked little sparkles of diamonds as the sunbeams tickled the sea. A soothing, swooshing sound emanated from the gentle incoming tide as it brushed the beach's edge. A perfect setting for our visit. Roland and I had once again sought comfort from the peacefulness this view provided. It was a repetition of our visit two years previously when I had been diagnosed with the kidney cancer that had turned out not to be.

This time was different. Christopher had recently been diagnosed with pancreatic cancer. He would not recover. Roland had returned to Vancouver to be with his father and had taken a short break from his caregiving to be with me. Roland's stay with us was short as work demanded his return to Belgium, but he was able to spend quality time with his father before the cancer had ravaged his body and stolen his ability to think and speak. In this cathedral of ocean and sky, we found renewed energy, solace and sanctuary from our worries and concerns.

Christopher had borne his illness with incredible fortitude, courage, verve, zest and good humour. To a friend's telephone question of "How are you?" Christopher replied briefly: "Terminal." Forever an optimist, despite the horrible side effects of chemotherapy and his slowly deteriorating state, he attended social events, entertained friends and sang in two local choirs. He had been well supported by three of his siblings and a multitude of friends, but in his final days had been admitted to a palliative care facility. Withered by his spreading cancer, he accepted the end with little regret.

In a journal, he wrote that he was looking forward to spending his remaining days in a place of care surrounded by goodness and kindness. The excitement of future endeavours, and those seemingly pressing concerns of the healthy, held little importance for him. What had been in his past and what might have been in the future bore little meaning now that his end was certain. Whatever thoughts he had remained his private territory. All we know is that he felt at peace. After nine months of suffering, Christopher succumbed to the effects of cancer with Roland and Christopher's sister by his side.

Christopher has left a lasting impression through his eccentric lifestyle and noteworthy paintings. When clearing out his things, we discovered he had over four tie racks filled with hundreds of ties, and many carefully selected clothes. Among these were five different Scottish kilts representing his provincial, military and Scottish dancing associations. He could appear impeccably dressed one day only to be shabbily dressed the next. His "joyful, pleasant and fun-loving disposition," fondly described by many from abroad as well as locally, even touched the heart of the province's lieutenant governor, whom he had known for years through his various connections with Government House. Roland, Christopher's family and his friends will miss him.

We would all like to perceive our life ending peacefully at home in our beds as we sleep, having accomplished our goals. The reality, however, is often different. Many people spend their latter years, months and days unable to enjoy themselves or their surroundings, betrayed and incapacitated by their disease or illness, in pain, and brain befuddled by medication. This is not the imagined Hollywood ending. Such was the situation for Christopher. It was gut-wrenching to watch helplessly as his body shrivelled under the burden of illness, his mind fogged, his once dynamic personality and robust physical appearance atrophied. Death was heartless and soulless.

'Tis truly a world without end. Two-and-a-half weeks following Christopher's passing, Roland and his partner, Veerle, welcomed a healthy nine-pound baby boy, Arvid Christopher Paul. Roland, having swapped his computer keyboard for a pastry brush three years ago, has become a chocolatier. His artistic skills incline perfectly to this profession. Following a year in intensive study, learning both the theory and practice of making chocolate and confectionary delights, he served a practicum with a small, award-winning, well-established, family-run boutique chocolate and confectionary company. Today he is one of their main chocolatiers, producing delectable chocolates and fancy pastry goods. The first thing he is asked whenever he visits is, "Have you brought chocolates with you?" Woe betide him should he arrive empty-handed.

• • •

What of me, and my other friends, since I began tapping the keyboard almost two years ago? Writing, surprisingly, has afforded me some respite from my own trials. The act of writing and telling others' stories has been elevating. I found myself entering an entirely different sphere, a world both distracting and stimulating, greater than myself, only to return to reality either when I woke in the morning feeling the effects of my spinal cord injury or when I entered the dialysis unit.

I had envisaged completing my manuscript in a few months. "Four months," I boldly declared. I have learned that the truth is far different. Writing is a lengthy procedure, solitary and all-engaging. It requires both enormous discipline to stay the course and lengthy time to collect thoughts, research information, have chapters scrutinized for correct medical information and gather other patients' stories, a most important component of this book. It can be frustrating when fatigue or pain creates problems for typing and joyful when a day's work has been completed effectively.

• • •

I continue with nocturnal dialysis, sleep drifting slowly over me, and then recuperate from the effects of dialysis the following day. Both Charity and Arjay sleep for several hours following their arrival home but find by evening they have recovered sufficiently. As indeed do I. Charity is planning for her retirement at the end of September and a three-day trip to Las Vegas. She retains her good-hearted benevolence, bestowing her kindness and "charity" to all and sundry. Arjay and I, "the renal gamblers," cling to the hope of winning big one day. So far, the most we have won is $20. My kind guardian angel, Al, has moved to the other nocturnal schedule. Jeffery, who had been booked for his kidney transplant for last July and had it indefinitely postponed, his donor having unexpectedly encountered some medical problems, suddenly received the call from the Transplant Department. He would receive a transplant after all. To date he is doing well. Queenie has returned to the evening dialysis session, a preferred option for her.

The benefits of nocturnal dialysis for me continue to outweigh the downsides of attending a day session. I have better toxin removal, improved blood results and can enjoy the longer days. It is nearing three years since my transplant kidney failed. As with many other patients, the longer I remain on dialysis, the greater the fallout. The effects of my scleroderma and Raynaud's condition have worsened. My mobility, in spite of continuous stationary cycling, has deteriorated, and my neuropathic pain relentlessly perseveres. Medication, meditation practices, acupuncture, physiotherapy, massage therapy and other distracting occupations are of little avail.

With my blood pressure beginning to elevate and causing my anxieties to increase, I have decided to try a different strategy to deal with the incessant pain. I have two options: one, to live in misery, and the other, to live in happiness. I have decided the latter is the preferable choice. Based on the adage "if you can't beat them, join them," I am learning to live in the present, accepting my bodily condition. At its worst I try to feel only positive and loving thoughts towards my enemy within. Whatever stoutheartedness and strength I have to follow this path have come from other people, whether they have been in my pain management course, those affected by spinal cord injuries, my Scleroderma Association of BC friends or people I have met in the surgical ward, the kidney ward or the dialysis unit. I have been impressed by their resilience and fortitude. It is as though a stamp has been impressed on my heart, helping me to remember them and to strive to emulate their courage. We live with the knowledge that, while we may be experiencing trying times, we are not alone. We share a common bond. Their fighting spirit is my sword and shield.

My pain doctor, however, believes a transplant would alleviate many of my symptoms. If I am to receive one, though, I have recently learned it would have to come from a living donor. The older the patient, the less well they respond to a deceased donor's kidney. It is apparently a shock to their system, adding complications, even leading to death.

My enthusiasm for going to a dialysis session somewhat wanes on cold, snowy, wintery evenings when most creatures wish to be curled snugly in their own nests. Likewise, it is a struggle for me on balmy, summery evenings when the sound of laughter, the enticing merriment from worry-free, fun-loving people bursts through my open windows, or when I have to excuse myself from participating in exciting special events or social occasions. Holidays are particularly difficult to miss.

I am not alone in my feelings. None of us patients really desires to go, but we must if we are to feel some respite from the effects of kidney failure. To counteract our rumblings, many patients have told me they consider attending a dialysis session akin to going to a job, one in which the pay is excellent camaraderie with the medical staff and the vacation is two days off. There is no fixed retirement date and the benefit package is superb care.

. . .

A recent incident illustrates my concerns to be prompt for my evening HandyDART pickup. HandyDART drivers wait only so long for stragglers before continuing on their journey. I usually wear contact lenses but for my nocturnal sessions I replace them with glasses. Having received my Handy-DART pickup call one evening, I grabbed my coat, bus tickets, overnight bag and cane. I locked my door and walked to the elevator as quickly as my stumbling gait allowed, overnight bag in tow. Almost to my destination, I felt something seemed slightly askew, my eyesight not as clear as usual. I had left my glasses on the kitchen counter. Immediate anxiety engulfed me. I would be late for my ride and miss being driven to the hospital. I absolutely needed to get my glasses. I returned, almost falling, post haste to my door, leaving my bag in the middle of the hallway. Finding my door, cane in one hand, I clumsily fumbled with numb fingers to retrieve my keys from my coat pocket. Having finally wrested them out, I furiously tried to unlock my door, but without success.

Ever more desperate, I bent closer to the lock, foggily trying several times to unlock my door. The key would not work. So intent was I on my mission that I failed to hear a quiet voice behind me. The voice became louder, startling me, and finally registering. I turned around to see my neighbour and her daughter who had evidently come home.

"This is 205. Wrong door," she said. No wonder my key didn't work. Laughing from the humour of my situation, I limped quickly towards my own door, where my key immediately struck gold. I grabbed my glasses and was able to say to my neighbours who had remained *in situ* keeping a vigilant eye on my bag, "You'll have a good laugh about this tonight." I hurried to reclaim my bag and then caught the elevator and was just in time for my ride.

...

Since beginning hemodialysis, I have witnessed some innovative practices designed to support us through our journey with kidney failure and hemodialysis. Two artists volunteered their time twice a week for almost a year to provide art classes for those patients who wished to create artwork during their session. The artists supplied the materials, expertise and support to the patients. They organized an evening exhibition and reception of the patients' work on a dialysis-free evening. Participants, family, friends and others were invited to join them. The completed works were absolutely delightful, proving that one doesn't have to be a gifted artist to produce masterpieces, and lying in bed or sitting in a chair with one arm attached to a machine doesn't prevent someone from completing a creative piece of work.

Current scientific literature highlights the important role exercise plays in maintaining and increasing physical strength. Intending to prolong dialysis patients' well-being and general health, one of our dieticians has introduced the concept of a walking exercise called "Walk and Roll." It is based on her recent MSc thesis entitled, "Is there an association between dietary protein intake, Nordic walking exercise, and sarcopenia risk factors?"[1] She received a grant to purchase Nordic walking sticks and funding to train volunteers. Sarcopenia, the loss of muscle tissue and strength, occurs during the natural aging process. It contributes to shaky hands, broken bones and other ailments. Hemodialysis patients are prone to early aging because we lose protein through dialysis, follow a strict diet and spend at least four hours sitting or lying down three times a week. Lower levels of protein contribute to loss of collagen and muscle bulk. Thighs lose muscle more easily than other parts of the body. However, Nordic walking, a gentle form of exercise that incorporates using arm and leg muscles, enables patients to exercise at our own pace to improve circulation and promote strong muscles. Those who choose to exercise with the Nordic walking sticks receive initial training provided by a specially trained volunteer.

One of the hemodialysis social workers and the clinical nurse have created a mentoring program for patients. It is called the buddy project. Its purpose is to pair more experienced hemodialysis patients with less experienced ones in order to provide support. The pairs are carefully chosen and meet whenever they can and share their experiences. It is a new program and has so far recruited about three pairs. Mentor patients need to attend a training session. I have volunteered to be a mentor but have yet to receive my orientation. Princess Marie, who has been mentoring another patient, has recently received her training certificate verifying she is a fully trained mentor.

Another support group that was established three years ago by a social worker and a few patients has recently re-formed under the name The Kidney Krew. The aim of this group is to provide support to us patients through social activities, such as a summer BBQ and other events, and to act as an advocate for us. They wish to be financially self-sufficient; therefore, they undertake raffles. They meet once a month. One of its main innovators and leaders is our charismatic Princess Marie.

· · ·

It is a Friday in June, during an early part of my nocturnal dialysis session. A nurse is with me, preparing my catheter site for attachment to the dialysis tubes. Our curtains have already been closed to shade us from the dimmed lights so we can sleep better. Charity, likewise ensconced behind a curtain, is in a bed perpendicular to mine. There is a slight rustle in my curtains and a beaming face appears. It is Princess Marie. She says, "I have something important to tell you guys," ensuring Charity is privy to what she is going to say. "I have just been given the all-clear for a kidney transplant." That is wonderful news to our ears. We clap loudly.

Princess Marie continues, "Yes, because I have been having so many problems with my lines and dialysis sessions I have become top priority. The doctors have told me I should have the transplant within three to six months. I have lived with kidney disease all my life. It will be good to feel better finally." We cheer her news even more loudly. Princess Marie then rather wryly says, "Just when I have been accepted into my college program, am about to move and continue with my work. So now everything is on hold."

We say, "Ain't that the way, but it will all work out in the end." After her departure, we share our pleasure for her. All transplant recipients are a small victory for us, too, enkindling a renewed hope for us. Princess Marie is a most deserving person, and a real example of the goodness in others.

As far as my other fellow patients are concerned, Allan Wheeler has just celebrated his twenty-fifth transplant anniversary and continues to enjoy excellent blood results. His creatinine remains within the normal range. Allan's only challenges lie with the long-term effects of immunosuppressant usage. He is much more susceptible to low-level infections that heal slowly, and doctors are wary of carrying out a knee operation in case it might impact his kidney's performance. Allan remains healthy in all other respects and enjoys travels to local and distant climes.

Since my last discussions with Doctor X, he has again visited Ottawa, California and India. His spirited outlook remains positive. He has continued to benefit from good health in spite of his dialysis treatment and looks forward to living a healthy existence for a further few years. The Candy Man who has had an ear cancer treated, maintains his usual humour-laced, kindly, candy-distributing self. Bob had had a number of falls and suffered a heart attack. I saw him briefly before I began nocturnal dialysis. He had been switched to the morning session where the doctors feel they can monitor him more closely.

Mrs. Serena has had some ups and downs associated with her dialysis treatment and is growing weaker as a result, but she carries on with the devoted support of her family. Sasha, her daughter, frequently accompanies her, and in Sasha's absence, Mrs. Serena's granddaughter or brother fill in. It has been a long and remorseless journey for the family but they do not stint in their selflessness to provide the support she requires. Dan continues with his treatment, the result of his multiple myeloma, with the faithful support of his wife, Leah. Their journey has been long, too, and a reminder of the downsides of bearing the weight of an incurable illness.

Sain survives the side effects of his diabetes, but he is pain ridden and unable to walk, attending his dialysis sessions with the help of his family. He remains the pleasant, kind and warm individual I first encountered several years ago. Renaissance Man had been troubled by severe blood accumulation. The doctors told him he could be suffocated by his own blood were it not removed effectively. The culprit turned out to be a tumour in one of his kidneys. Following considerable discussion, the doctors decided to perform a nephrectomy. He has had the surgery and is doing much better.

Mischievous Marty moved to another province. I have lost touch with him. Wendy and Haida have moved to a community facility. Haida has had her transplant kidney removed because it had become infected and troublesome.

Will, who had switched to peritoneal dialysis, was doing well when we last had contact. Although he found the bloating in his stomach a nuisance, he was determined to persevere, having vowed to live to a grand old age. He has moved in with his daughter who lives outside Vancouver. I am no longer in touch with him, either.

I have been heartened to learn of friends who have received transplants. Among them is Rebecca, who, having had her transplant, is indeed proving herself to be a "mover and a shaker." Along with some employment prospects in the recycling industry, she has become a volunteer member of a BC Transplant committee and will be working with the Canadian Transplant Games this coming summer, organizing the recycling program. Additionally, she has been invited to be a guest on the Kidney Foundation of Canada–BC branch's TV show called *Plugged In* to share her story and promote the Kidney Paired Donor Program. She is also teaming up with a well-known beverage company that will be promoting a naturally sweetened product in sponsorship of a campaign to "Save a Life. Register to Become a Donor." Rebecca's work with them will involve helping with product designs, including for T-shirts.

David received his transplant in March of last year. He is doing well, enjoying his new life and visiting his beloved grandchildren more frequently, thanks to his new kidney. Gerri continues to enjoy his new transplant, "Bob Tupper."

Nick had his transplant in early spring. He was off work for three months and is doing very well. He told me he had had too many antibodies, preventing his second sister from donating her kidney to him. His story is a good example of how the Kidney Paired Donor Program works. His sister was matched to a recipient, whose daughter was matched to Nick. He shared his observations of what it is like to be a transplant recipient as opposed to being a dialysis patient. The transplant clinic, according to him, is a buzzing, joyful place where newly transplanted patients are happily discussing their future intentions, including taking long holidays, undertaking house renovations put on hold for many years, and dining out, no longer being restricted to the rigorous diet.

Not having heard from George, I can only presume all is going well for him. Matthew has now had his transplant for three years, is working six days a week, loving his new life and looking forward to his son's ninth birthday. His wife has been able to resume her college studies.

. . .

Not all has been joyful, though. In 2015 alone, we dialysis patients lost fifty-seven of our fellows. Some died from heart attacks, others from the endless wait for a transplant and others simply from the wear and tear of dialysis, their bodies worn out from its effects. Among the first was one of the young men who had impressed me so much with his need to work long, hard hours just to put food on the table and pay his rent, jeopardizing his health in the process. A donor might have saved his life. Mrs. Tims also passed away. Her husband told me, "I think she had just had enough." Mr. Tims continued to visit the unit once a week for many months to catch up on news from friends he had met while attending his wife's dialysis sessions for so many years. We are a closely knit family.

More recently further deaths have occurred. Nine of the patients were well known to me, either from my time in the dialysis unit or during my travels on HandyDART. One was Deborah, who, like Mrs. Tims, had had enough of the long-term effects of diabetes. Her death caused much sorrow for those of us who knew her. Charity found it particularly difficult. She said, "I was so warmly received by Deborah when I first started dialysis that I cannot forget her kindness." Similarly, Chatty Matty has been deeply affected, and told me, "I cannot get over losing Deborah. She has been my close friend for many years." Chatty Matty has been affected by further health problems, was hospitalized for over a month and is now hoping to move into an assisted living accommodation.

All deaths impact us. We patients live with this in mind. It is never far from our own world. There has been a great increase in areas of research, some that may in the future have significant effects in reducing the need for dialysis, others that may create newer and better kidney function following kidney failure, and still others that may provide artificial kidneys to perform natural kidney functions for the receiver, thus reducing the need for donors. Research is long and complicated. It does not happen overnight. We kidney patients will continue to rely on the kindness of our friends, family and strangers. Recent publicity has highlighted a renewed call for living donors. It is considered the best way of enabling patients to receive transplants.

We are indebted to those who have unselfishly donated a kidney. The Peters of this world, George's mother-in-law and Ruth's anonymous donor are among the heroes who have so kindly stepped forward to help us. We won't forget others who have themselves performed kind deeds for others.

We are equally obliged to the animals that have been part of scientific and medical research with the ultimate goal of our well-being. We must acknowledge their sacrifices if we consider ourselves to be caring individuals. It is important to think about our own role in helping others.

When I *"dream the impossible dream,"* I dream that one person reading this book will decide to become a donor, either by choosing to be a living donor or by registering their consent to be a potential donor. Of those who are able to become donors, who will be the next hero? Will it be you?

Appendix 1 | Transplantation: From Root to Route, a Layperson's Overview

The road is long
With many a winding turn
That leads us to who knows where
Who knows where
—Bobby Scott and Bob Russell, *He Ain't Heavy, He's My Brother*

Introduction

My evening dialysis session began exactly as others had: weighing in, taking my temperature and blood pressure and then the preparation of my catheter site for hook-up to the dialysis machine. All was quiet once everyone had been duly connected to the machines; the nurses were busy with their tasks.

Well into my scheduled four hours, two enthusiastic young women made their way to the empty bed beside mine. Why had they come so much later? I wondered. Why so enthusiastic? My curiosity was soon satisfied. One was to receive a kidney transplant from a living donor the following day. She had come in for a two-hour top-up dialysis session, leaving her better prepared for surgery. Both women were absorbed in a lively interchange, unusual for the dialysis unit. Even the nurses enjoyed the joyous spirits emanating from the pair and sent them off with good wishes upon their departure. I was glad to have witnessed the excitement, the hope of a transformed life and to have been reminded that a transplant is never routine for the recipient. Kidney transplant surgery, while still surgery, has been performed so frequently and the technique become so advanced that it falls within the category of routine mainstream surgery. This has not always been the case.

From the root

From a medical point of view, transplanting kidneys is a relatively new phenomenon. It has been slightly over sixty years since the first actual kidney grafting surgeries were performed. The concept of transplantation is older than Methuselah, who was said to have lived for almost 1,000 years.[1] According to Dr. David Hamilton, in his seminal work *A History of Organ Transplantation: Ancient Legends to Modern Practice*,[2] tissue replacement, both in theory and in practice, captured man's attention from antiquity—

across continents, nations and cultures. It is a history replete with myths, miracles, powerful gods, supernatural creatures, saintly cures, wondrous accomplishments and transformations. Mostly apocryphal.

Humans have always yearned to reverse and heal their own and others' afflictions, to replace limbs and body parts lost to war, disease, misfortune or punishment. There are recorded reports of missing hands, arms and legs having being replaced with new appendages. Many decapitated warriors had their heads replaced with new ones; sometimes leaving them looking backwards instead of forwards. One example, Nuada, a legendary Irish hero and warrior king, had his long-buried, severed hand replaced by Micah, a renowned physician.[3,4] Hamilton cites two Chinese classical tales. In one, a Chinese doctor exchanged two men's hearts in order to create better energy and treated them with potent herbs to maintain their success. Was this a possible precursor to modern anti-rejection drugs? In the other, a judge provided an illiterate man with a new heart carefully selected from thousands of human hearts in the netherworld.

To carry out the cures and restorations, practitioners used local help and shamans within their own communities, but they also sought guidance from supernatural realms. They believed that divine powers could re-create injured body parts, thereby restoring an individual to full capacity. Moreover, they believed that someone who died with fully functioning body parts could more easily be resurrected than someone who died in a mutilated state. This still holds sway in many cultures even today and has a bearing on organ donation.

Traditionally, the restoration of disfigured body parts, failing organs and lost eyesight was performed on those deserving help because their situations had arisen through no fault of their own. The stories had a positive moral outcome and were used as lessons in character building. Much discussion ensued regarding who was the most worthy of receiving cures. Similar arguments occurred during the early years of modern transplantation. One of my doctors told me that when he was a young medical resident in England during the 1970s and early 1980s, specialist doctors would meet to discuss a list of patients waiting to receive transplants. The decisions were arbitrary, not solely based on pertinent medical facts, since guidelines had yet to be established. Today it is no longer the case, guidelines having been firmly established.

Tissue fusion was expanded to bridge the gap between humans and nature, specifically animals, to create superhuman beings like Marvel Comics characters today. Wherever animals roam, man is surely not far behind. Humanity seems to have a perverse relationship with its fellow creatures. Bewitched by their grandeur, while at the same time bewildered by their brawn, their seeming freedom, their rugged independence and their omnipotence, people desire to harness their energy and tame them for personal uses. Through history, animals have become devotionals, treasures, pampered and protected, often decorated and adorned on one hand while being happily sacrificed or slaughtered, tortured and maimed on the other, in the pursuit of divine salvation, pleasure, greed or recuperation.

This desire to re-create human lives as part animal is witnessed in many ancient myths. People believed that the amalgamation of humans and animals would result in the creation of qualities hitherto unavailable. Hybridization, the creation of a new being by combining human and animal parts, and xenotransplantation, the transplantation of organs or tissues between two separate species, were viewed as pathways for creating new, improved beings.[5] Gods naturally possessed the ability to fuse supernatural animals and man, thus creating even more spectacular hybrid beings. The 12th century BCE story of the Hindu god Ganesh is one such example. A goddess, Parvati, created a son, Ganesh, from her womb to protect her during her bathing rituals.[6] Ganesh was wrongly beheaded by Parvati's husband, a belligerent warrior named Lord Shiva, who didn't recognize Ganesh after having returned home from a series of wars. In an act of deep repentance, he replaced Ganesh's head with one of an elephant. The newly restored son became known as Lord Ganesh and provides one of the first examples of tissue fusion.

Greek and Roman myths also feature accounts of transplants performed by gods. Chimera, described by Homer in the Iliad, was a fearsome creature with the body and head of a lion, a snake for a tail and a fire-breathing goat head coming from its back. The mere sight of Chimera was a bad omen.

There are many descriptions of Chimera. According to Hesiod, a Greek poet living at the same time as Homer, she "snorted raging fire, a beast great and terrible, and strong and swift-footed. Her heads were three: one was that of a glare-eyed lion, one of a goat, and the third of a snake, a powerful drakon..."[7]

Chimera proved a worthy opponent to many, finally being slain by Bellerophon, a mortal, who was a renowned hero and slayer of monsters, accompanied by Pegasus, the winged horse, a hybrid animal that Bellerophon had tamed. The term *chimerism* is used today in science and medicine to mean an entity containing two genetically distinct types of cells. A bone marrow transplant, for example, results in chimeric properties and can change the recipient's blood type.[8] Hybrids and chimeras are biologically different. A cell from a chimera contains the genetic material of either one parent species or the other. A mule is an example of a chimera, being the offspring of a horse and donkey.[9]

As cultures developed and formed new religions—Christianity in particular—they gave further proof to the importance that tissue replacement played in people's thinking. Jesus has been recorded by the Four Gospels as having performed over thirty-seven miracles, including replacing the severed ear of a high priest's slave, Malchus, which was sliced off by an over-protective Simon Peter. As disciples sought to spread Christianity throughout the world, many were slaughtered for their beliefs. These martyrs achieved sainthood because of their legendary powers to perform cures, induce healing or carry out tissue repair.

Two such saints were the Arabian twins Cosmas and Damian (ca. 270 CE), the patron saints of medicine. They practiced medicine in various parts of the Arab world and were highly respected and revered for their powers to cure maladies in both humans and animals. Known as "the silverless," they accepted no pay for their services. Both were brutally tortured for several years, then killed, for failing to denounce Christianity. Several reports of miraculous healings are attributed to them, the most significant being the story of the sacristan to whom they appeared in a vision while he slept alone in a church in Rome. Cosmas and Damian are reported to have removed his cancerous leg and replaced it with one from a Moor, representing the first real transplantation, since it grafted two different people's body parts. Dr. Jean-Paul Squifflet, in his publication *The History of Kidney Transplantation: Past, Present and Future*, writes that the twins' unprecedented influence spread beyond the Middle Ages, even into the modern era.[10]

Even as myths and legends abounded, real transplantation was being performed. Both Indian and Chinese civilizations had developed surgical techniques long before other cultures. Records exist of actual medical procedures around 1,000 BCE in India. In 800 BCE, in the Ganges region, an Indian surgeon named Sushruta or Susruta, known as the father of Indian surgery and often referred to as the father of plastic surgery, as well as creator of Ayurvedic medicine, used reconstructive surgical techniques to repair damaged tissue.[11] He wrote detailed instructions for transplanting a tissue flap from an area of a patient's body that was in close proximity to the one requiring the repairs. Today this is called an autograft.

Ayurvedic medicine refers to the use of holistic methods to prevent illness from developing and to promote the body's own capacity for maintenance and balance. It incorporates detoxification using herbal remedies, yoga, meditation and massage therapy.

Sushruta's treatise, entitled *Sushruta-samhita*, a medico-surgical compendium, was the main source of information about surgery in ancient India. It described various different methods of surgery such as cutting, opening, scratching, piercing, inserting and stitching. He was both a practitioner and teacher. Sushruta was most notable for rhinoplasty, the repair of the nose, but he also removed dead fetuses and removed bladder stones. Indian students practised suturing on fruit and leather. Students first used dummies to practise bandaging. They further extended and perfected their knowledge of anatomy by dissecting cadavers. With an increasing lean towards the creation of the caste system in India, surgical practices were soon regarded as performing manual labour and no longer considered appropriate to be carried out by professional classes. There was also a growing distaste for actually touching human flesh. This is pertinent to tissue transplantation, which soon lost its appeal. When Sushruta's practices were rediscovered in the 19th century, they were often performed by bricklayers and potters.

Sushruta primarily performed surgery on those whose disfigurement was caused by disease, violence or warfare from sword wounds. At the time, sword injuries were the most common cause of dismemberment and of disfigurement to soft tissues from head to feet and continued to be so until the introduction of modern firepower. Brutal leaders used the practice of cutting off noses both as a deterrent and as a form of punishment. Rhinoplasty was practiced not only in India, but also in ancient Africa, where records show that anaesthetic was used during the treatment of wounds, as well as during operations centuries before it was used in Europe.[12] In Egypt, ancillary to skin-grafting surgery, finely crafted, gold metallic noses were used to replace lost ones. Other parts of the face and body were similarly mutilated. Those afflicted would live the rest of their lives, not only as outcasts and treated as criminals, but also as disgraced individuals, who prevented from going to their deaths unsullied were therefore unlikely to be resurrected, according to traditional thought.

During the Italian Renaissance, a revival in interest in the classical scholars of Rome and Greece created awareness of ancient medical practice. Medical progress was on the map again. Three Sicilian surgeons, Gustavo Branca, his son Antonio Branca and Gaspare Tagliacozzi, are noteworthy. Gustavo Branca, a surgeon from Catania, initially performed nasal repair using what was known as the "Indian method," referring to the practices used by Sushruta. He removed a flap of skin from the cheek to restore a man's nose. The man had lost his orifice in a duel with his son. Antonio Branca, however, improved upon his father's method. Instead of taking a skin flap from a location near the nose, he used a flap of skin from the upper arm.[13] It caused scarring and required the patient to hold their arm behind their head for twenty days, something that must have been incredibly uncomfortable. Both father and son kept their methods secret.

The third surgeon, Gaspare Tagliacozzi, at the University of Bologna, one of the greatest medical centres of the 1500s, explored the Brancas' practices. He felt he could improve upon their surgical techniques and was certain he could do so, since he had had a university education. Tagliacozzi had gained prominence for his wound management. When he began nasal repair, he initially performed his surgeries at night because facial disfigurement was offensive to Renaissance people. A nose's shape, size and appearance were extremely important to a person, often a determining factor in how that person was judged and viewed. Also, it seems that women accused of adultery would be punished by having their noses clipped off and most likely sought repair in the seclusion of darkness.[14] Tagliacozzi not only performed surgical replacement therapy on those who had acquired injuries to noses, ears or lips, he also operated on those afflicted by syphilis, which had become increasingly common. Tagliacozzi would only operate on people with syphilis who had first tried cures with mercury. When this failed and the disease had progressed to its third stage, it eroded the inner nose. He described his surgical practices in a book entitled *De Curtorum Chirurgia* per Instionem (On the Surgery of Mutilation). His thinking was remarkably modern: "We restore, rebuild, and make whole those parts which nature hath given, but which fortune has understood away. Not so much more than that it might delight the eye, but that it might buoy up the spirit, and help the mind of the afflicted."[15] Tagliacozzi is considered to be the father of plastic surgery.

Tagliacozzi improved upon the Brancas' autografting methods by incorporating careful pre- and post-surgery management. Tagliacozzi's "Italian method" cut a flap of skin on the arm and with the flap still attached to the arm, sewed part of it to the face in preparation for creating a new nose. The patient sat upright, arm bandaged, until this new skin was successfully attached to the face, which usually took twenty days. Once the skin had been successfully grafted, the new nose skin was severed from the arm, and the newly attached skin was shaped so that it resembled a nose. Unlike other surgeons, Tagliacozzi also used specially designed shields to protect the nose.[16]

Tagliacozzi was one of the first to acknowledge that not all grafts could be successfully performed and that rejection could occur. He observed that taking tissue from one individual and replacing it in another may not work effectively.

Literature suggests that the many conflicts among countries, civil war in England and the switch to fire-powered weaponry led to fewer grafting procedures being carried out in the mid-1600s. There were fewer soft-tissue injuries as a result of the transition to guns and cannons, and fewer cases of syphilis being reported. Following Tagliacozzi's death, the Italian Method lost its appeal amidst debate concerning the efficacy of his grafting technique and discussions revolving around the suggestion he had used flesh for his repairs from live donors. The established practitioners were not always in favour of performing Tagliacozzi's methods. While legal mutilations still existed, surgeons preferred to use false prosthetics such as those employed by the Egyptians centuries earlier.[17] False noses were often made from gold or silver. Interestingly, the Italian method was used during the World War II to repair a wounded serviceman's damaged nose.

Some progress did continue in small areas. Additionally, there was a slow and moderate movement towards the study of experimental methods as opposed to relying on the surgeries recorded in ancient texts. Scientists were interested in collecting and studying data. They wanted to try more investigative types of medicine through research and practice. This research was based on direct and indirect observation of symptoms and surgical results that could be analyzed both quantitatively and qualitatively. It became known as the empirical "scientific method."

Other physicians and surgeons were developing medical procedures that would have considerable impact upon later surgeries and transplantations. In 1616 Dr. William Harvey (1578–1657), studied blood circulation in the body and published what was at that time a very controversial book *Exercitatio Anatomica de Motu Cordis et Sanguinis in Animalibus* (An Anatomical Study Concerning the Motion of the Heart and Blood in Animals). He described how the blood flowed from the heart and recirculated around the body.

A later experimenter, Richard Lower (1631–1691), performed a transfusion on dogs using sheep's blood. This was followed by the personal physician to King Louis XIV, Frenchman Jean-Baptiste Denis (1643–1704), who is credited with carrying out the first blood transfusion in a human in 1667. The transfusion was done on a fifteen-year-old boy who had bled so profusely that he required an infusion of blood. Interestingly enough, the blood used was that of a sheep. The boy survived. Unfortunately, a later attempt ended in the patient's demise. As a consequence, further transfusions were banned in France and later by Parliament in England.[18] It wasn't until 150 years later that transfusions were once more explored and used. In early kidney transplants, before EPO injections, transfusions were widely used to restore blood.

A century later, the Scottish physician and surgeon John Hunter (1728–1793) successfully transplanted the spur of a young chicken from its leg to its comb, and in so doing, he noticed that the spur on the comb grew more quickly and larger than the one left on the chicken's other leg. He conjectured this could be attributed to the fact that the comb was stronger than the hair on the leg, in spite of them being in relatively close proximity. He felt that the position of the comb favoured rapid growth since the veins of the spurs in the leg and head were the same and neither the leg nor its head had been affected. Hunter performed other experiments on chickens with some degree of success. He concluded that those that were unsuccessful were so because of the incompatibility between the two affected areas of the animal. He tried to graft a spur from a young cock onto the leg of a hen. He observed that, although it took root and the chicken grew to be a hen, the grafted spur grew slowly on the hen, while the spur that had been left on the other leg of the cock grew normally. He concluded that the cock's spur did not grow because the cock and hen were two distinct animals with two different types of tissues.[19] In stating this he had concurred with Tagliacozzi, who in the 16th century, had surmised different tissues would not necessarily match.

Hunter also practiced dentistry. He often extracted teeth from poor people and transplanted them into rich people's mouths. This practice—selling body parts for money—is entirely frowned upon today in western culture, but continues in some countries. Hunter's work is considered the vanguard of modern transplantation.[20]

To the route

Kidneys were the first organ to be transplanted. The reasons are threefold. First, the kidney consists of a relatively simple blood supply as opposed to other organs. Second, the ability to measure the flow of urine in the ureter from the grafted kidney means that successful outcomes can be monitored easily. Third, because the kidney is a paired organ, transplanting one kidney does not impair the ability of the remaining one.[21]

In our fast-paced, technologically driven world, where routine surgery is performed with minimal invasion, where more complex surgery is conducted with precise, high-tech tools, and where an iPhone application can test blood pressure, it is easy to forget just how cutting edge medical science was in the early 20th century. Landmark innovations that are today's commonplace practices were then considered revolutionary. What is even more remarkable, though, is that some of the original methods are still in use today. Advances in medicine, as in most scientific endeavours, occurred incrementally. What one physician or surgeon achieved led to improved methods by another, as is the case today.

The route to a successful transplant began in Austria in 1902—March 2nd to be precise. By the end of the 19th century, transplantation medicine had been an important topic at many medical conferences. There had been a number of attempts to transfer renal tissue to various locations on the body to alleviate kidney failure, but the whole organ had never been used. Who would be the first to unlock the key to the door, to the house, turn on the light and perform the first successful transplant?

Hungarian-born, Erich Ullmann (1861–1937), practising surgery in Vienna, was the first to perform a solid-organ transplant, as we now understand it. He first wanted to find out how much kidney tissue was needed to sustain the life of a dog. He was the first to use whole kidneys. He removed the whole kidneys from a goat and transplanted them into the groin of a dog. Ullmann, however, was concerned about the possibility of infection caused by the dog's constant licking and scratching of the organ's site. To obtain better protection for both his efforts and for the dog, he next transplanted a kidney under the skin of a dog's neck. He connected the kidney to the dog's carotid artery and jugular vein while suturing (sewing) the ureter to the skin.

A few days later, he reported his experiment and demonstrated how it worked, showing the dog to a group in the lecture hall of The Society of Physicians in Vienna. Those in attendance observed the urine dripping off the ureter. It can only be imagined what the impression of seeing this most novel experiment must have been on those present. The audience may well have sat either silently transfixed or else twitching in disbelief at the medical marvel taking place before their eyes. The surgery site healed well; however the dog did not. It died five days later.

Ullmann performed autotransplants (transplants of a body part from one place to another in the same individual) and homotransplants (transplants from one individual to another individual of the same species). Ullmann performed the first xenograft or heterograft, transplanting tissue from one species to another when he transplanted a pig's kidney into the left elbow of a woman who had experienced kidney failure, but reported, "I could not overcome the difficulties." The woman survived for five days.[22] Ullmann, through his experimental efforts with kidney transplantation, essentially placed a key in the door of the house. What would happen next to unlock it, and further extend experimental procedures, is intriguing.

Ullmann published descriptions of his work in a book, as well as in the weekly Austrian clinical journal *Wiener Klinische Wochenshrift*, the same journal in which Austrian-born American Karl Landsteiner (1868–1943) had published a report about the breakthrough discovery of blood group compatibility a few weeks earlier.[23] Landsteiner concluded that the success of blood transfusion from one individual to another depended upon the compatibility of the blood itself. As a result, he developed a system for categorizing blood into ABO (A, AB, O) types. This discovery would have considerable significance in later kidney transplantation. He received the Nobel Prize in 1930 for Physiology or Medicine. He also received the Lasker-DeBakey Clinical Medical Research Award in 1946.[24]

Coincidentally, a French physician Alexis Carrel (1873–1944), while unaware of Ullmann's work, in 1902 published an article in the *Lyon Médecine* entitled "The Operating Technique for Vascular Anastomosis and Organ Transplantation." He described a technique for the end-to-end connection or anastomosis of blood vessels. The article also contained his opinions regarding the importance of the future of transplantation. He wrote, "From a clinical standpoint, the transplantation of organs may become important ... and may open new fields in therapy and biology."[25]

Carrel had become interested in surgery of the blood vessels about 1894 following the death of the French president, Sadi Carnot, who had been assassinated. The assassin's bullet had severed a major artery. Wounds of this calibre could not be repaired. Carrel developed extraordinarily fine needles and devised a method of turning back the ends of cut vessels, similar to the way in which we turn back cuffs on sleeves, so that he could join the smooth lining of the vessels end-to-end without exposing the circulating blood to any other tissue. He coated his instruments, needles and thread with paraffin jelly to prevent blood clots from forming after he had sutured an artery or vein. He was rigorous in his attempts to avoid any bacterial infection, using only the most antiseptic techniques.[26]

After becoming disenchanted with the French establishment when he failed to secure a position at Lyons Hospital, Carrel immigrated first to Montreal, then to Chicago in 1904 where he worked in a variety of hospitals. He was primarily interested in researching the surgery of tissue and whole-organ transplantation. He worked in close association with the well-known physiologist Charles Guthrie (1880–1963), with whom he published thirty-three papers describing the basis of modern transplantation surgery: "The ability to sew blood vessels together, to reattach severed limbs, and to transplant organs (including kidneys and hearts) into dogs and cats."[27] In 1908, Carrel had devised methods for the transplantation of whole organs. Later, in 1910, he demonstrated that blood vessels could be kept for long periods in cold storage before they were used as transplants in surgery. This procedure greatly influenced the practice of further transplantation techniques, and he was awarded the Nobel Prize for Medicine or Physiology in 1912 based on his work on cellular structure.

What Carrel apparently failed to recognize was that transplanted organs would never be permanently accepted by the body, because the immune system could not support the existence of a foreign body. Neither he, nor anyone else, understood the existence of an immune system.

In 1935 Carrel formed a partnership with Charles Lindbergh, the noted transatlantic aviator. Lindbergh had approached Carrel to find a way of saving his sister-in-law who was dying from heart disease brought on by rheumatic fever. Carrel wanted to find a way of cultivating whole organs. Lindbergh devised a sterilizable glass pump to circulate culture fluid through an excised organ. Lindbergh was successful, enabling Carrel to keep organs such as the thyroid gland and kidney alive and, to a certain extent, functioning for days or weeks. This was a pioneering step in the development of apparatuses now used in surgeries of the heart and great vessels,[28] those large vessels that carry blood to and from the heart (the venae cavae, pulmonary artery, pulmonary veins, and aorta).

Carrel, in conjunction with Lindbergh, wrote *The Culture of Organs,* discussing the implications of their machine. Carrel not only received the Nobel Prize, but was also honoured by many countries such as France, Belgium and Sweden, receiving their most prestigious awards, as well as receiving tremendous recognition from other countries such as Serbia, Spain and Great Britain, as well as the Holy See.[29] He is best remembered for his suturing methods that, after having undergone some alterations in 1962, remain in use today.[30]

In 1905, around the same time as Ullmann was working on transplants, a French doctor living in Bordeaux, M. Princeteau, further explored the possibility of using animal tissue in humans. A sixteen-year-old with end-stage renal failure had been admitted hospital. Princeteau inserted slices of rabbits' kidneys into the teen's kidney. At first, according to his reports, "The immediate results were excellent. The volume of the urine increased; vomiting stopped... On the 16th day the child died of pulmonary congestion."[31] The key was yet to be turned to unlock the secret to successful kidney transplantation.

Another renowned French surgeon, Matthieu Jaboulay (1860–1913), head of the Lyon School of Medicine and one of Carrel's teachers, also worked on kidney transplantation. On January 24, 1906, he transplanted a pig's left kidney into the left elbow of a forty-eight-year-old woman with kidney failure. Unfortunately his patient died nine days later from early vascular thrombosis. Undaunted he next transplanted a goat's kidney into a fifty-year-old woman who died three days later. He documented his work, but Jaboulay, like Ullmann, may have felt the road to a successful transplant was too thorn-ridden. He turned his attention to innovative intestinal surgery. Some of the techniques he developed are in use today. He had also developed a reputation for delivering riveting lectures, attended by many doctors and students alike, on his experimental surgery. Jaboulay died rather tragically in a train accident in Melun, France, in 1913 without being able to turn the ever-elusive transplant key.[32,33]

In 1907 an American medical researcher, pathologist and first Director of the Rockefeller Institute, Simon Flexner (1863–1946), delivered a paper entitled "Tendencies in Pathology" at the University of Chicago. He declared, "that it would be possible in the 'coming future' for diseased human organs to be surgically substituted for healthy ones—these would include arteries, stomach, kidneys and heart."[34] The key that had been moved further into the transplant lock by Carrel was now turning even further in America.

Three years later, in Berlin, Ernst Unger (1875–1938), starting kidney transplantation in Germany, transplanted a complete pair of Macaque monkey[35] kidneys into the thigh of a girl dying of renal failure. The transplant did not produce any urine, so Unger concluded that the immunity defenses, or in medical terminology the biochemical barrier, were insoluble. What Unger did not realize was that the graft had been rejected by the patient's own immune system. In his first paper, published in 1909, he illustrated for the first time the methods used in his experimental kidney transplant surgery.[36,37]

In 1910, in his second paper, Unger further elaborated on his views regarding the biochemical barriers he had encountered. In this paper he was the first to illustrate a human kidney transplant. He must have become disheartened by his failure because he did not pursue further experimental procedures. He may, however, have been the first to place a long intravenous line, passing it from his own leg into his inferior vena cava—the vein that returns blood to the heart from the lower part of the body.[38]

The mystery remained unsolved. No further attempts were made between 1910 and 1922. Although the lock had been sprung, the door remained impenetrable. The reason for this is purely speculative, open to anyone's guess. It may have resulted from the barriers already encountered. They repeatedly seemed daunting and impossible to overcome. The medical community may have felt the task posed too great a challenge. Equally, growing world turbulence may have had a dampening effect on medical research, and the muddied, blood-drenched fields of Flanders could well have put a stop to any efforts, with the ensuing years required to recover from the catastrophes and wastelands caused during the war years. Physicians and surgeons like Carrel also may have been involved in treating war casualties. Indeed many promising medical practitioners may have been felled during the numerous battles, creating a vacuum of knowledge and expertise.

Whatever the reasons, efforts were renewed in 1923. A surgeon, Harold Neuhof (1875–1954) working at Mount Sinai Hospital, New York, attempted to perform a kidney transplant on a patient with kidney failure. The patient's condition had resulted from mercury poisoning, mercury being a pharmaceutical component at the time. Antibiotics had yet to be developed. Neuhof wanted to perform a heterotransplant, transplanting a human kidney. To his chagrin, he was unable to obtain a human kidney and instead chose a lamb's kidney to transplant into the patient. The patient lived for nine days. Neuhof was not totally discouraged by the transplant's failure. He wrote, "[This case] proves, however, that a heterografted kidney in a human being does not necessarily become gangrenous and the procedure is, therefore, not necessarily a dangerous one, as had been supposed. It also demonstrates that thrombosis or hemorrhage at the anastomosis (connection between blood vessels) is not inevitable. I believe that this case report should turn attention anew."[39] He appeared to be more optimistic about the future of transplantation than Unger.

Still in America, in 1926, Carl S. Williamson, working with the Division of Experimental Surgery and Pathology at the Mayo Foundation in New York, grafted two kidneys from two goats into two dogs. Both dogs died within minutes, but this surgery was the first to cause the medical community to begin to consider the rejection phenomenon and opened the door to using human grafts. Would the door now be opened soon?

In 1928, Serge Voronoff (1866–1951), a Russian surgeon at the Collège de France in Paris, already well known for his monkey-to-human testis transplantations, was ready to transplant a young girl who had renal tuberculosis. The organ donor was a murderer condemned to be beheaded. He was willing to offer his organs after his death. However, the surgery was not to be, because the Prosecutor of the Republic opposed it.[40] While Voronoff was ready, society was not. No further progress yet.

Who could have predicted that five years later, in 1933, another Russian surgeon, Yuri Yurijevich Voronoy (1895–1961), a relatively unknown doctor working in the Ukraine, would perform the first-ever renal homotransplant in a human? The patient, a twenty-six-year-old woman, had been admitted to hospital in a comatose state. She was diagnosed with severe end-stage renal failure and had apparently tried to commit suicide by swallowing mercury chloride. Voronoy used a kidney from a sixty-year-old man who had died six hours earlier from a fracture in the base of his skull. Using Landsteiner's method, Voronoy tested the blood compatibility and found the patient's blood type was O and the deceased man's was B. Voronoy placed the kidney into the woman's groin. He measured kidney function using a connection between the kidney and skin. Although the blood types were incompatible, urine output was good until the second day, when the woman died. An autopsy showed the graft blood vessels had not been impaired. Voronoy carried out a further six human homotransplants between 1933 and 1949 and reported that, "No significant long term renal function occurred in any of them."[41,42] While the door had been opened ajar, the room had yet to be penetrated. As a consequence, Voronoy's contribution was more than a mere footnote on the bottom of a page. He had become famous.

A further dimension was added to the transplantation story when, in 1943, a young Dutch physician, Willem Kolff (1911–2009), introduced an entirely new treatment for people suffering from kidney failure. He had invented the first modern drum dialyzer, essentially an artificial kidney. Its use remained the standard practice for the next decade. Its invention enabled people to survive without transplant intervention. This slowed transplantation experimentation for several years. Dr. Kolff's goal had been to help kidneys recover, and in so doing, he developed one of the most important life-saving devices in the history of medicine. He is considered the father of dialysis.[43]

Kolff first became inspired to create a machine that could do the work of the kidneys after he watched helplessly as a young man slowly died of renal failure on a small ward at the University of Groningen Hospital in the Netherlands. He was inspired to find a way of creating a machine that could do the work of the kidneys. Searching diligently through the hospital's library for information on removing toxins from the blood, he happened to come across an article about hemodialysis with animals published in 1913 by John Abel, a well-known pharmacologist at Johns Hopkins University. Kolff was now thoroughly committed to his cause and embarked on his mission.

The world does not always cooperate with scientific endeavours. World War II was on the brink of changing people's lives. The Netherlands were invaded, and Dr. Kolff found himself working in a remote Dutch hospital. Times were hard, but Kolff a true inventor, used sausage skins, orange juice cans, a washing machine and other common items to improvise a method for removing toxins from the blood. All the while he was doing this, the long vengeful eyes of the Nazis kept careful scrutiny of his work. He forged documents and enlisted the help of his wife and colleagues, who put their lives in jeopardy on his behalf so he could complete his task. They must have lived a life of cautious tiptoeing and secretive whisperings, in a stealth-like manner as they sought to achieve their desired results. By 1943, Kolff had completed his invention, crude though it was. From 1943 to 1945, he treated sixteen patients with end-stage renal failure, but with little success.

In 1945 Kolff had his first successful outcome: a sixty-seven-year-old woman in uremic coma regained consciousness after eleven hours of hemodialysis using Kolff's machine. Her first words on regaining consciousness were, "I'm going to divorce my husband!" She did and lived seven more years before dying of another ailment. That year, Kolff donated the five artificial kidneys he had made to hospitals around the world.[44] In the 1950s he was invited to visit America, where he worked with a Dr. Merrill, to redesign his dialysis machine. Dr. Kolff later acquired American citizenship.

Up to this time, conventional thought held that preventing rejection was a matter of surgical skill, not one of immunological incompatibility. Treatment methods developed during World War II, however, proved this incorrect. In Britain, the severity of burns received in bombing raids by both military personnel and civilians alike led to the establishment of a number of burn treatment centres throughout the country. Research produced remarkable treatment methods; it also led to an entirely new area of knowledge.

In 1943, a highly respected British doctor born in Brazil of Lebanese extraction, Peter Medawar (1915–1987), had been appointed by the War Wounds Committee of the British Medical Council to work with surgeon Thomas Gibson (1915–1993) at the Burn Unit of the Glasgow Infirmary. Together they produced a paper, "The Fate of Skin Homografts in Man," in which they described a series of skin grafts Gibson had performed on burn victims, and their subsequent discoveries.

Gibson had transplanted a set of autografts onto the back of a patient. The first set came from the patient's own skin and the second set from another burn victim. The grafts from the second victim are called homografts or, in the newer lexicon, allografts. At intervals, some of the small "pinch grafts" were removed and studied by Medawar, who observed that the autografts initially successfully bonded but the allografts did not. They failed after originally adhering. Importantly, he found the second set of allografts were rejected more rapidly than the first. To Gibson and Medawar, the rejection process appeared to have characteristics of an immunological response.

Following his work with Gibson, Medawar returned to his home base at Oxford and continued to study allograft rejection using rabbits for his tests. He produced a number of papers for the War Wounds Committee that confirmed the existence of the delay before rejection began, possibly explaining why some of the previous transplant recipients had survived the length of time they had before dying. Using different groups to further study graft survival times, he described what he thought was an invasion by lymphocytes, a sub-type of white blood cells and the main type of cell found in lymph, thus strengthening the case for rejection being due to an immune reaction.

To combat or slow rejection, Medawar first used steroids and then, together with several other doctors, began examining the effects of injecting cortisone under the skin on graft success. This treatment considerably lengthened the grafts' survival rate. This discovery provided the basis for subsequent successful attempts to enhance kidney graft survival using corticosteroids in later years. Medawar continued studying and redefining his knowledge and understanding of the theory of immunology through various research projects in both England and America.

In 1960 Medawar and Australian researcher Frank Macfarlane Burnet were awarded the Nobel Prize for Medicine or Physiology. Their introduction stated that "[I]mmunity is perhaps our most important defense against a hostile surrounding world. By penetrating analysis of existing data and brilliant deduction, and by painstaking experimental research you have unveiled a fundamental law governing the development and maintenance of this vital mechanism."[45]

A clue to the puzzle that had confounded medical experimenters and researchers for decades had been revealed, but it would be many years before this discovery would lead to the development of immunosuppressant medicine that would help resolve kidney transplant rejection. The door had been opened a little more.

It is difficult to say who performed the first successful human renal transplant. For their work in 1945 at the Peter Bent Brigham Hospital in Boston, the recognition could go to the following three pioneers: Charles Hufnagel (1916–1989), staff surgeon; Ernest Landsteiner (1917–2007), chief resident in urology; and David Hume (1917–1973), then-assistant surgical resident. Landsteiner was the son of Karl Landsteiner who had received the Nobel Prize for Medicine or Physiology in 1930 for developing the ABO blood classification scheme.[46]

Although Kolff had created a dialysis machine, none was available that could be used, so the doctors attempted to save the life of a twenty-nine-year-old woman suffering from end-stage renal failure with a kidney transplant. They obtained a kidney from an elderly patient who had just died during surgery. The doctors, using Voronoy's surgical techniques, attached the donor kidney to the recipient's elbow veins so that it rested outside the skin. They then covered the kidney with a plastic bag and watched as the patient's urine drained into a jar. This basic transplant lasted four days. The patient, however, recovered renal function and was discharged. This may have also been the first successful deceased cadaver donor transplant outside the abdomen.[47] A light switch had been found in the room, but it had not been turned on.

The next attempt was five years later on June 17, 1950, when Richard Lawler (1895–1982) performed a successful transplant on a forty-four-year-old woman named Ruth Tucker with polycystic kidney disease at a hospital in Illinois. The donated kidney came from a patient who had died of liver disease. The transplanted kidney was rejected ten months later, removed and found to be shrunken and discoloured. The woman who had also had one of her own kidneys removed during the surgery, however, lived for another five years because the intervention had enabled her own surviving kidney the time to recover its function. Dr. Lawler said of the donor, "Not the most ideal patient, but the best we could find," in an interview after the surgery.

Lawler never performed another transplant surgery although he had been asked to by numerous doctors wanting to learn from him, as well as patients seeking his assistance. Lawler never offered a reason as to why he chose not to. His explanation was, he said in 1979, "I just wanted to get it started."[48]

Then, in 1951, a breakthrough occurred in kidney transplant surgical technique. In Paris, the French School, also referred to as the French Transplantation Club, comprising Doctors Dubost, Œconomos, Servelle and Rougeulle, used kidneys procured from guillotined murderers. What differentiated The French School from others was that they had developed a method whereby the transplanted kidney was inserted into the right iliac fossa, the space in the pelvis or ilium and connected to the iliac vessels. This was a most innovative technique and is the method widely used today.[49] The French doctors performed a total of nine transplants. All nine patients rejected their grafts.

Other French doctors—Küss, Teinturier and Millez—performed transplants using kidneys from another patient. René Küss (1913–2006) published a now-famous article in 1951 in *Memoires, Academie de Chirurgie* in which he stated, "... in the present state of knowledge, the only rational basis for kidney replacement would be between monozygotic twins." The concept of immune-related rejection established by Medawar was widely embraced by this time and would later pave the way for a groundbreaking transplant in 1954 in America.[50] The light switch had been turned on.

The story shifts to Toronto, Canada, in 1951 when Gordon Murray (1894–1976) performed a series of four deceased donor kidney transplants in the pelvis area, but using a method he had discovered to be effective in dogs. He connected the ureter to the bladder so urine would flow internally rather than ectopically in the usual manner. Of the first three recipients, the longest survivor lived twelve days. On May 2, 1952, Murray's fourth patient was a twenty six-year-old woman who had been diagnosed with chronic nephritis eighteen months previously. She had hypertension and severe edema, carrying fifty pounds of excess fluid, along with various other symptoms. The young woman made a spectacular recovery, losing the swelling, and she showed signs of increased urine output. Her native kidneys were not functioning. She lived for a further twenty-one years, and the kidney was never removed. In his report Murray admitted that while, "this patient might have returned to this sort of good health independently," he remained convinced of the importance of the transplant in achieving that state. This may have been the first long-term success in renal transplantation.[51] The light was beginning to grow brighter in the room.

There are varying schools of opinion concerning Murray's work, but it is felt his place in history was overshadowed by the news of the successful kidney transplant between twins in Boston in 1954. To Murray's credit, he had, like Kolff, invented a hemodialysis machine that remains in use today.[52]

In France at the Necker Hospital, later in 1952, nephrologist Jean Hamburger (1909–1992) performed the first successful transplant between two unrelated people and in the following year performed the first transplant between two related people. Marius Renard, the recipient, a sixteen-year-old carpenter, had already had one kidney removed after having fallen off a ladder and now required a kidney following failure of his other kidney. A kidney from Marius Renard's mother was used following her death in a road accident.

The transplanted kidney performed well for the first three weeks until rejection occurred and Marius died. Rejection probably occurred due to the absence of immunosuppressant medication. At that time, the principal ingredients of organ transplantation: "Immunosuppression, tissue matching, organ procurement and preservation were still unknown or undeveloped, and would remain so for another decade," writes Dr. Squifflet.[53]

Hamburger, who founded French nephrology, has been recognized as possibly having coined the term "nephrology." He also established the International Society of Nephrology, which created an award in his name. (Interestingly, from a Canadian point of view, the president from 2015 to 2017, was Dr. Adeera Levin, head nephrologist practising at St. Paul's Hospital in Vancouver.) Dr. Hamburger identified a number of previously unrecognized syndromes and diseases, including water intoxication, hereditary renal disorders and illness involving the kidney's filtering system.[54,55] There were now several lights glimmering in the room.

Visitors flocked to France in the early 1950s to learn first-hand from this experience. Among them was John Merrill (1917–1984), who observed the French School surgical technique, and who, together with David Hume, is considered to be one of the pioneers in successful transplantation. In 1955 they wrote about the first clinical trials they had carried out at the Peter Bent Brigham Hospital, now the Brigham and Women's Hospital in Boston. Between 1951 and 1953, Merrill, together with his mentor George Thorn (1906–2004) and Hume, carried out a series of nine kidney transplants in patients with chronic renal failure.[56]

The first of these kidneys was transplanted internally in the recipient. The next eight renal allografts were placed in the patients' thighs. Urine drainage was through the skin. Hume's description of this experience is deemed to be one of the most outstanding accounts recorded in the 20th century. It provides a nearly complete clinical and pathological description of renal allograft rejection in an untreated human recipient. The only examples of probable allograft function, through 1954, were provided first by one of the non-immunosuppressed patients transplanted by Hume whose graft in the thigh location functioned for five months.

Although several of these grafted kidneys did function for several months, Hume and Merrill were forced to conclude that, "at the present state of our knowledge, renal homotransplants (known now as "allografts") do not appear to be justified in the treatment of human disease."[57] Clearly there were many conflicting views regarding the efficacy of kidney transplants. It would take yet another experiment for the views to coalesce. A temporary flicker in the room's lights occurred.

Interestingly, although Dr. Merrill's initial clinical interests were in cardiology, his special skills and attributes were recognized by his mentor, Dr. Thorn. Thorn asked Merrill to spearhead the efforts to develop the artificial kidney at the Brigham Hospital in Boston. Merrill began his studies with the artificial kidney dialysis machine, which, in collaboration with surgical colleagues, was modified from Kolff's original design. The artificial kidney developed by Merrill and his associates, now named the Brigham-Kolff dialyzer, was highly successful, especially in the treatment of acute renal failure and subsequently in the management of chronic renal failure. The first patient Merrill and Hume transplanted in 1951 had been undergoing short-term dialysis using the modified hemodialysis machine. Merrill was a prime mover in establishing the National Kidney Foundation in America and promoted the use of dialysis centers throughout the United States. He also persuaded the US Congress to provide funding for patients requiring long-term dialysis and kidney transplantation. This was a remarkable achievement.

Hume's career lasted well into the next era of transplantation. His untimely death occurred due to a private plane crash in May 1973 near Los Angeles. John Merrill drowned off the beach of a Caribbean island in 1984. It is believed that had Merrill survived he would have received a Nobel Prize for Medicine or Physiology.[58]

In 1954, Merrill led a multidisciplinary team that included J. Hartwell Harrison (1909–1984) and Joseph Murray (1919–2012) in a transformative kidney transplant operation. The procedure captured the attention of the local press and refocused the world's attention on the potential of kidney transplantation. It had been precipitated by a number of factors. First of all, Medawar's theory of immunology was fully supported by this time. Secondly, Dr. Küss's prophetic thoughts suggesting that the only successful transplant would be one performed between monozygotic twins was still in medical specialist's minds. And thirdly, the doctors at Brigham Hospital in Boston had been looking for twins with whom they might have greater success than they had previously had. As luck would have it, a set of twins had been found.

Richard Herrick, a twenty-three-year-old former coast guard, was suffering from an inflammation of the kidneys that was potentially fatal. He had been admitted to a hospital in Massachusetts. As Herrick lay dying, surrounded by his family, his doctor told them of the work by doctors at

Brigham Hospital to devise ways of transplanting healthy kidneys into those whose kidneys had failed and that they were looking for twins who could possibly help them with their research. The family immediately responded to this new piece of information. Richard's twin brother, Ronald, had two fully functioning, healthy kidneys. Could he help, and in turn, could the doctors help his family?

The doctors at Brigham thought they had everything to gain but not before they had thoroughly debated the pros and cons of transplanting one of Ronald's kidneys into his brother. Although it was widely known at the time that a healthy individual could live normally with a solitary kidney, the doctors knew the outcome of the contemplated operation was uncertain. They fully understood the implicit risk attached to any surgery. Aside from these medical challenges, it also raised significant ethical questions. It was the first time in America that a healthy person, while willingly consenting, would be participating in a surgical procedure entirely for the benefit of another. Would the doctors be actively harming or weakening one person in order to help another? Many discussions took place between the family and their doctors and most likely other doctors and the clergy, as well. In the end the doctors were satisfied the ethical questions had been satisfactorily resolved, and both recipient and donor had not only endorsed this experimental surgery but also desired it.

On Christmas Eve of 1954, the surgery was carried out. While Dr. Harrison removed Ronald's kidney in one OR, Richard was waiting, anaesthetized, close by in another. Having removed Ronald's kidney Harrison placed it in a cold storage case and ran quickly to Richard's OR where the two other doctors were waiting to transplant it. The surgery was a success. Both donor and recipient recovered well. Richard did not reject his brother's kidney and ended up marrying his nurse and fathering two children. He died eight years later from a recurrence of his chronic kidney disease. Ronald lived a full life, dying in 2010 at the age of seventy-nine.[59] Dr. Murray received the Nobel Prize for Physiology or Medicine in 1990. Not all in the medical community were completely supportive of the work Murray and his team had been doing. They were referred to "as a bunch of fools" for their efforts.[60] How wrong the medical community was in their description of this group. Not only had the lights been refurbished but also they were shining brightly, and would now never burn out!

The consequences of this successful transplant shortly led to similar work in other countries including Britain. The first kidney transplant in Britain took place in 1955 at St. Mary's Hospital, Hammersmith. It was performed by Charles Rob (1913–2001) and William James Dempster (1918–2008) using a deceased donor's kidney, but it was not successful. The second attempt, in 1959, performed by a urologist in Leeds, "Fred" Peter Raper, was successful. The doctors used an immunosuppressant called cyclophosphamide, possibly one of the first times such a medication had been used. The patient's transplanted kidney continued functioning well for eight months, until sadly the patient died from a viral infection totally unrelated to the kidney.

Five years later, in 1960, two doctors—Sir Michael Woodruff (1911–2001) and James A. Ross—carried out the first successful living kidney transplant on forty-nine-year-old identical twins at the Royal Infirmary of Edinburgh. Oscar, suffering from advanced chronic kidney disease, was operated on by Woodruff, while his brother, the donor, was operated on by Ross. The surgery was performed in October. All went well. The donor returned to work after three weeks and Oscar, fifteen weeks later. Oscar survived a further six years before dying from an unrelated disease.

Across the Atlantic, Gordon Murray performed the first successful non-twin sibling transplant in 1959 in Toronto. The first successful living transplant between non-twin siblings took place in France at the Koch Hospital in Suresnes in 1960. The surgery was performed by a team led by Dr. René Küss.[61]

Xenotransplantation—the transplantation of organ or tissue between members of two different species—had not been performed since the early part of the century, but was revived by Keith Reemtsma (1925–2000) at Tulane University in New Orleans under the direction of Thomas Starzl (1926–2017). Between 1963 and 1964, Dr. Reemtsma transplanted chimpanzee kidneys into five patients and a sixth into a twenty-three-year-old teacher. The first recipients died from infection between eight and sixty-three days later. The sixth recipient lived for nine months before succumbing to an overwhelming infection. Through his surgical attempts, Dr. Reemtsma was the first to show that non-human organs could be transplanted into humans and function for significant periods of time. He was, however, not only the first person to prove this could be achieved but also the last person in the

20th century to undertake this kind of transplantation.[62]

The 1960s saw a considerable expansion in kidney transplants; along with these came further challenges. There was a need to find a suitable way in which to preserve deceased organs for transplantation, to develop medication to prevent the transplanted kidney from being rejected and to find methods for matching tissue to the recipient's own tissue, ensuring the donor's organ transplant would bond easily. The 1960s also saw the first kidney–pancreas transplant in the United States, leading the way for further double transplants, which are now carried out more frequently.

Criteria regarding who were suitable candidates for kidney transplants was gradually introduced and is continually being revised as populations age and deceased organ donors become scarcer. The criteria for living donors were expanded from close relatives to friends and strangers. In 1984, the US Congress passed the National Organ Transplant Act to monitor ethical issues and address the country's organ shortage. A centralized registry for organ matching and placement was established. It outlawed sale of organs. Unfortunately, the sale of organs continues in many countries, leading to what is called "transplant tourism." In 2004, the World Health Organization passed a resolution asking its member states to take measures to protect the poorest and most vulnerable groups from the sale of tissues and organs to tourists.

As kidney transplants have become more commonplace, research has continued to be carried out in an effort to better protect transplanted kidneys, as well as the patients themselves. It is also being conducted in ways to prevent the need for kidney transplants. As well, new transplant procedures and experimental kidneys that may take the place of current human transplants are being developed. This experimental research includes the use of animals, thereby returning to xenotransplantation, mechanical kidneys and 3D printing to make kidney tissue function as real kidney tissue.

Much has happened since the early days, from the myths of the ancient world, to the beginning of tissue grafting in the medieval world, to the slow development of kidney transplantation at the start of the twentieth century, to modern kidney transplants. With the promise of future endeavours proving successful, current world shortages of donors may become a thing of the past. This bodes well for successive generations. Our children and those of tomorrow may have a brighter future than in the past. None of this would have been possible had it not been for the dogged determination of a few individuals in previous centuries who sought ways to help and treat ailing patients. To them, we owe today's successes and tomorrow's potential.

Appendix 2 | Some Milestones in Kidney Transplants: From Yesterday to Today to Tomorrow

The shell must break before the bird can fly.

—Alfred, Lord Tennyson, *The Ancient Sage*

The young woman caught my attention. She was slender and of moderate height, with a pleasant face and short, light brown hair. She seemed fairly healthy in comparison to many of the other patients attending the afternoon dialysis session. I was intrigued because it was uncommon for younger people to come during the daytime. If they did, it was either because they were new to dialysis or were transitioning to other facilities or sessions. Occasionally they might be having a top-up prior to a transplant. This young woman seemed to be a more regular attendee. I was curious to meet her. Luck was waiting in the wings. On my last afternoon before I switched to nocturnal dialysis, I noticed she was sitting in the waiting room, I presumed waiting to be picked up. I began to talk with her, and when I heard her story, my heart was moved.

Claire had already had a heart transplant, and now she had kidney failure. She spoke quietly and hesitatingly with a raspy, breathy voice, apologetically saying, "I am sorry, but I talk like this because my larynx has been damaged." I learned she had three young children. They were hardly school age and therefore required considerable nurturing. I asked her how she coped. Claire said it was hard but her family helped a bit, as did her husband. We patients are exhausted and worn out from our dialysis sessions and need considerable recovery time. Claire could have little of this, since as soon as she arrived home, she needed to tend to her children, and even with help, that can be difficult.

Mothers are expected to attend their children's activities and socialize with other parents. Claire could not easily do this. Remembering Roland, who was at the time considerably older than her children, and how my illness had affected him, I could only imagine how difficult it must have been for Claire. To have experienced two serious illnesses in her young life could only have been a great challenge for her and her family. None of this was evident during our conversation; she related her story calmly and objectively. My admiration for this stalwart young woman was incomparable. My hope for her is that she receives a kidney soon from a kind donor. This would improve her life enormously and give her the additional energy to care for her family as other mothers do.

Should she receive a kidney transplant, she would join the numbers who have had two transplants. Similarly, Rebecca has completed a consultation for a pancreas transplant. As with Claire, should this happen, she would become another person who has had two transplants.

Simultaneous transplants were performed in the 1960s. The first double kidney–pancreas transplant took place in the United States in 1966. Since then many simultaneous transplants have been performed. The following dates list some of the milestones in kidney transplants:

1950s, Paris: Possible first coining of the word "nephrology" and establishment of International Society of Nephrology. First successful transplant between two unrelated people.[1]

1952, Toronto: First long-term, successful kidney transplant in pelvis area. Twenty-six-year-old patient diagnosed with chronic nephritis received kidneys. Patient's native kidneys revived and patient lived for a further twenty-one years. Place in history overshadowed by following successful transplant in Boston.[2]

1954, Boston: Successful transplant between living twins paved the way for future transplants.

1958, Chicago: First baby born to kidney transplant recipient. Pregnancy at this time was considered a risk.

1962, Boston: First successful kidney transplant from a deceased donor.

1960, Pittsburgh: First kidney transplant since early part of 20th century using chimpanzee kidneys. Patient survived nine months. Surgery was carried out using chimpanzee kidneys due to shortage in human deceased donor kidneys. Surgeon performing operation completed further kidney transplants using animal parts several years later. In 1992 baboon kidneys were used and patient given an infusion of bone marrow. Patient died of an infection twenty-six days later. Surgeon performing operation was last one to use animal parts (xenotransplantation) in 20th century.[3]

1976, Belgium: An infusion of bone marrow into a patient following a kidney transplant.[4]

1989, Pittsburgh: First combination heart, liver and kidney transplant. A twenty-six-year-old was the recipient. She survived for four months.

1989, Belgium: First pediatric kidney transplant in Belgium.[5]

1989, Belgium: Arrival of third baby in the world to be born to a transplant recipient. The mother had received the world's 75th simultaneous pancreas–kidney transplant. In the same year, the first simultaneous liver and kidney transplant is performed, also in Belgium.

1989, Belgium: An infusion of bone marrow into a patient following a kidney transplant.[6]

1995, Miami: Doctors remove all abdominal organs from a patient with polyps in order to transplant a new kidney, pancreas, stomach, liver, large and small bowels and one iliac artery.

1999, Baltimore: Development of new procedures called High PRA Rescue (high panel reactive antibody rescue) to counteract the level of antibodies that lengthens waiting time for a kidney transplant.

2008, Ontario: Canadian Blood Services introduce Kidney Paired Donation and Living Paired Donor Exchange central registry.

2009, Minneapolis: Transplant recipient Chris Strouth receives kidney from donor who connected with him on Twitter. Believed to be first such transplant arranged entirely through social networking.

2014, Ontario: Canadian Blood Services introduce a national registry, High Sensitivity Program, for patients on the waiting list who have complications making it difficult for them to find matching kidneys.

2014, Vancouver: Aspect Biosystems starts using 3D bioprinting to develop human tissue. May eventually develop organs.[7] Other companies also working on 3D printing of organs.

2016, Leeds: Change in rules governing transplants creates the possibility of using kidney four-centimetres in size from a baby less than three months old who was deemed brain dead but with a beating heart. Kidney transplanted into forty-year-old woman. Kidney is capable of growing. Until 2015, when rules governing organs were changed, no organs could be retrieved from a baby younger than two months unless baby first certified brain dead as a result of heart having stopped.[8]

2017, San Francisco: Prellis begins working on 3D printing of organs. Company hopes to begin printing organs in next four to six years.[9]

Today, improved knowledge, advanced medical technique and newer immunosuppressant treatment, combined with follow-up care, have opened doors for kidney transplant recipients. Kidney transplants are considered the norm for people with kidney disease. An individual receiving a transplant has a better survival rate than an individual on dialysis. Figures suggest that even someone seventy-five years of age who receives a transplant will live four years longer than someone of the same age who does not.

Milestones will continue to be reached as laws change, scientific advancements occur and the general public's involvement increases. A promising but unknown tomorrow awaits patients affected by kidney failure. All changes and milestones can only create positive outcomes for every one of us.

Notes

Chapter 1

1. Definition provided by the Scleroderma Association of BC.

2. William Shakespeare (1564–1616): *Macbeth*, Act V, Scene 5, spoken by Macbeth after learning his wife has killed herself.

Chapter 2

1. John Constable (1776–1837), painter. The Hay Wain, painted in 1821, depicts an idyllic rural setting in Suffolk. It belongs to the Romantic School of painters and is currently exhibited in the National Gallery in London, England.

2. William Wordsworth (1770–1850), a Romantic poet. In 1799, he wrote, "Lines Written a Few Miles Above Tintern Abbey," an abbey that had been destroyed by Henry VIII following his break from the Catholic Church in Rome.

3. Scleroderma Association of BC (SABC): Courtesy of Bob Buzza and Joan Kelly, past president and vice-president, Scleroderma Association of BC.

Chapter 3

1. Hadfield, Christopher. *An Astronaut's Guide to Life on Earth*. Toronto: Random House Canada, 2013.

Chapter 4

1. *Spice It Up! Giving Zest To Your Renal Diet.* Recipe booklets for renal patients, published by Elke Henneberg, Ebmed Inc., Cowansville, Quebec. Retrieved from www.ebmed.ca. Last accessed November 12, 2015.

2. Ibid.

Chapter 5

1. New Kidney Research Focuses on Rare Disease – FSGS. Cision PR Newswire. Retrieved from www.prnewswire.com/news-releases/new-kidney-research-focuses-on-rare-disease-fsgs-300111634.html. Last accessed November 19, 2015.

2. National Kidney Foundation. Polycystic kidney disease (PKD). Retrieved from www.kidney.org.atoz/content/polycystic. Last accessed November 19, 2015.

3. National Kidney Foundation. Focal Segmental Glomerulosclerosis (FSGS). Retrieved from www.kidney.org/atoz/content/focal. Last accessed November 19, 2015.

4. *Spice It Up! Giving Zest To Your Renal Diet.* Recipe booklets for renal patients, published by Elke Henneberg, Ebmed Inc., Cowansville, Quebec. Retrieved from www.ebmed.ca. Last accessed November 12, 2015.

5. DaVita, Kidney Care. Kidney disease and dialysis information: Kidney-friendly recipes. Retrieved from www.davita.com. Last accessed November 12, 2015.

Chapter 6

1. BBC News. Firefighters have higher heart attack risk 'because of heat.' April 3, 2017. Aired December 5, 2012. Retrieved from www.bbc.com/news/health-39478080. Last accessed December 5, 2012.

2. National Institute of Diabetes and Digestive and Kidney Diseases. Mineral and Bone Disorder; What is mineral and bone disorder in chronic kidney disease? Retrieved from www.niddk.nih.gov/health-information/kidney diseases/chronic-kidney-diseases-ckd/mineral-bone-disorder. Last accessed December 5, 2012.

3. Kidney Foundation of Canada. 1 in 10 Canadians has kidney disease and millions more are at risk. Retrieved from www.kidney.ca/dcument.doc?id=242. Last accessed December 5, 2012.

4. Kidney Foundation of Canada. Retrieved from www.kidney.ca. Last accessed December 5, 2012; Head Clinical Nurse, St. Paul's Hospital, Vancouver, BC. Permission granted November 6, 2015.

5. Nichols, H. The top 10 leading causes of death in the United States.

Medical News Today, February 23, 2017. Retrieved from www.medicalnewstoday.com/articles/282929.php. Last accessed March 29, 2018.

6. American Kidney Fund. 2015 Kidney Disease Statistics. Retrieved from www.kidneyfund.org/assets/pdf/kidney-disease-statistics.pdf. Last accessed March 26, 2018.

7. St. Paul's Hospital nephrologists, Dr. Elizabeth Lee and Dr. Jane White. Personal Communication. July 15, 2016.

8. Williams, R. Canada still has a chance to reverse its diabetes epidemic. Huffpost, The Blog, November 24, 2016. Retrieved from www.huffingtonpost.ca/russell-williams/diabetes-in-canada_b_13201818.html. Last accessed March 26, 2018.

9. Wong, D. What you need to know about diabetes. *Vancouver Courier*, November 25, 2015. Retrieved from www.vancourier.com/living/health/health-what-you-need-to-know-about-diabetes-1.2119624. Last accessed November 25, 2015. Vuchnich, A. Canada's diabetes rate worse than US: report. Global News, November 4, 2015. Retrieved from globalnews.ca/news/2318187/canadas-diabetes-rate-worse-than-the-us-report. Last accessed November 4, 2015.

10. Oxford Advanced Learner's Dictionary. Diabetes blood sugar. Retrieved from www.oxfordlearnersdictionaries.com. Last accessed December 5, 2012.

11. Diabetes Canada. Kidney disease. Retrieved from www.diabetes.ca/diabetes-and-you/complications/kidney-disease. Last accessed November 19, 2015.

12. National Institute of Diabetes and Digestive and Kidney Diseases. Retrieved from www.niddk.nih.gov. Last accessed November 19, 2015.

13. Kidney Foundation of Canada. High Blood Pressure and Kidney Disease. Retrieved from www.kidney.ca. Last accessed November 19, 2015.

14. Canada Helps.org. Retrieved from www.canadahelps.org/en/charities. Last accessed November 19, 2015.

15. An extract from a patient's story. See page 145 in this book (*Warriors and Heroes of a Different Kind: Battling Kidney Failure*).

16. University of Michigan, Department of Internal Medicine, Division of Rheumatology, Scleroderma Program. Renal Involvement. Retrieved from

www.med.umich.edu/scleroderma/patients/renal.htm. Last accessed November 20, 2015.

17. Lupus Foundation of America. The history of lupus. Retrieved from www.lupus.org/answers/entry/what-is-the-history-of-Lupus. Last accessed November 20, 2015.

18. Lupus Foundation of America. What is lupus? Retrieved from resources.lupus.org/entry/what-is-lupus. Last accessed November 20, 2015.

19. Catherine Phung, personal communication in 2009 and information in C. Phung's personal Syndrome Assessment Manual, dated 2000. Permission granted to cite information.

20. Wegener's Disease. What's in a Name? Retrieved from www.wegeners-disease.co.uk/whats-in-a-name/. Last accessed November 19, 2015.

21. American College of Rheumatology. Granulomatosis with polyangiitis (Wegener's). Retrieved from www.rheumatology.org/I-Am-A/Patient-Caregiver/Diseases-Conditions/Granulomatosis-with-Polyangitis-Wegners. Last accessed November 19, 2015.

22. National Kidney Foundation. Focal segmental glomerulosclerosis (FSGS). Retrieved from www.kidney.org/atoz/content/focal. Last accessed November 19, 2015.

23. New Kidney Research Focuses on Rare Disease – FSGS. Cision PR Newswire. Retrieved from www.prnewswire.com/news-releases/new-kidney-research-focuses-on-rare-disease-fsgs-300111634.html. Last accessed November 19, 2015.

24. Brown, Melanie. Kidney Transplant and living kidney donation. Retrieved from www.bcrenalagency.ca/resource-gallery/Documents/Transplant%20and%20recipient%20eligibility.pdf. Last accessed March 26, 2018.

25. Kids Health. Infections: Recurrent urinary tract infections and related infections. Retrieved from kidshealth.org/en/parents/recurrent-uti-infections.html?ref=search&WT.ac=msh-p-dtop-en-search-clk. Last accessed November 19, 2015.

26. National Kidney Foundation. Urinary Tract Infections. Retrieved from www.kidney.org/sites/default/files/uti.pdf Last accessed November 19, 2015

27. The Kidney Foundation of Canada. Some facts about *E. coli* bacteria.

Retrieved from: www.kidney.ca/document.doc?id=3485. Last accessed November 19, 2015.

28. National Kidney Foundation. Urinary tract infections. Retrieved from www.kidney.ca/document.doc?id=316. Last accessed November 13, 2015.

29. Turnbull, B. What Spain can teach us about the gift of life. *Toronto Star*, Monday September 30, 2013. Retrieved from www.thestar.com/life/health_wellness/2013/09/30/what_spain_can_teach_us_about_the_gift_of_life.html. Last accessed June 15, 2016.

30. Squifflet, J.-P. *The History of Kidney Transplantation: Past, Present and Future (with Special References to the Belgian History), Understanding the Complexities of Kidney Transplantation*. Jorge Ortiz (Ed.), InTech, 2011. Retrieved from www.intechopen.com/books/understanding-the-complexities-of-kidney-transplantation/the-history-of-kidney-transplantation-past-present-and-future-with-special-references-to-the-belgian. Last accessed May 5, 2015.

31. National Heart, Lung and Blood Institute. Atrial Fibrillation – What is. Retrieved from www.nhlbi.nih.gov/health-topics/atrial-fibrillation. Last accessed November 13, 2015.

32. CBC News. Child obesity at highest level in Canada and U.S. August 2015. Retrieved from www.cbc.ca/news/health/child-obesity-at-highest-level-in-canada-and-u-s-1.3203561. Last accessed November 13, 2015.

33. Keck School of Medicine, University of Southern California. Vascular Access. Retrieved from www.surgery.usc.edu/vascular/vascularaccess.html. Last accessed November 16, 2015.

34. US Postal Service. Postal Service Mission and "Motto." Retrieved from about.usps.com/who-we-are/postal-history/mission-motto.pdf. Last accessed November 16, 2015.

35. Kidney Research UK. Statement on dialysis vs transplantation as the form of renal replacement therapy. Retrieved from www.kidneyresearchuk.org/about-us/position-statement-dialysis-vs-transplantation. Last accessed November 16, 2015.

36. Chai, C. Kidney transplants could save health-care system millions: Report. Postmedia News, January 21, 2011. Retrieved from www.canada.com/health/Kidney+transplants+could+save+health+care+system+millions

+Report/4144445/story.html Last accessed March 2016.

37. BC Transplant spokesperson. Transplant longevity. Personal communication, February 20, 2016. Permission granted.

38. BBC News. Woman with 100-year-old kidney from mum 'still going strong.' August 10, 2016. Retrieved from www.bbc.com/news/uk-england-tyne-37025389. Last accessed August 10, 2016.

Chapter 7

1. Agar, J. Nocturnal Home Haemodialysis. Barwon Health, 2012. Retrieved from www.nocturnaldialysis.org. Last accessed December 1, 2016.

2. Ibid.

3. Malmgren, J.K. The Night Shift. Promise, Fall/Winter 2011. Retrieved from www.helpstpauls.com/app/uploads/2012/08/The-Night-Shift.pdf. Last accessed December 1, 2016.

Chapter 8

1. The National Kidney Foundation. Blood Tests for Transplants. Retrieved from www.kidney.org/atoz/content/BloodTests-for-Transplant. Last accessed December 5, 2016.

2. Tuller, D. Advances Expand Kidney Transplants. *The New York Times*, April 27, 2009. Retrieved from www.nytimes.com/2009/04/28/health/28kidn.html. Last accessed June 7, 2016.

3. Cedars-Sinai. Highly Sensitized Transplants. Retrieved from www.cedars-sinai.edu/Patients/Programs-and-Services/Comprehensive-Transplant-Center/Kidney-and-Pancreas/Conditions-and-Treatments/Highly-Sensitized-Transplants.aspx. Last accessed December 5, 2016.

4. Canadian Institute for Health Information (CIHI). Deceased Organ Donor Potential in Canada. December 2014. Retrieved from www.cihi.ca/web/resource/en/organdonorpotential_2014_en.pdf. Last accessed March 2016.

5. Ibid.

6. Eurotransplant: Cooperating Saves Lives. Various articles accessed: About Eurotransplant–Eurotransplant Aims; Projects and Themes–Participation

EU projects, Projects and Themes–ESP Program. Retrieved from www.eu-rotransplant.org/cms/. Last accessed June 15, 2016.

7. Bill C-223: Private member's bill: Canadian Organ Donor Registry Act. Retrieved from openparliament.ca/bills/42-1/C-223/. Last accessed June 15, 2016.

8. Canadian Institute for Health Information (CIHI). Treatment of End-Stage Organ Failure in Canada, Canadian Organ Replacement Register, 2005 to 2014. Retrieved from secure.cihi.ca/free_products/2016_CORR_Snapshot_EN(web).pdf. Last accessed March 17, 2016.

9. Ibid.

10. Canadian Transplant Society. Home page. Retrieved from www.can-transplant.ca/home/. Last accessed December 5, 2016.

11. AVRA Medical Robotics Inc. All about robotic surgery. Retrieved from allaboutroboticsurgery.com/roboticsurgeryhistory.html. Last accessed December 5, 2016.

12. BC Transplant. Spokesperson, personal communication, November 2015. Permission to cite granted. St. Paul's Hospital, Vancouver, BC. Transplant Department social worker, personal communication, November 9, 2014. Permission to cite granted.

13. BBC News. 83-year-old man becomes UK's oldest living donor. May 17, 2012. Retrieved from www.bbc.com/news/av/uk-18100028/83-year-old-becomes-uk-s-oldest-living-kidney-donor. Last accessed December 14, 2014.

14. Canadian Institute for Health Information. Canadian Organ Replacement Register, Annual Statistics 2016. Retrieved from www.cihi.ca/en/canadian-organ-replacement-register-2016. Last accessed June 7, 2016.

15. Rivero, E. Two altruistic donors launch rare kidney chains at UCLA. UCLA Newsroom, June 15, 2009. Retrieved from newsroom.ucla.edu/releases/two-altruistic-donors-launch-rare-94189. Last accessed September 11, 2017. This article refers to the first chain created in Toledo by Dr. Michael Rees in 2009.

16. Butt, F.K., H.A. Gritsch, P. Schulam, GM Danovitch, A. Wilkinson, et al. Asynchronous, out-of-sequence, transcontinental chain kidney transplantation: a novel concept. *American Journal of Transplantation* 9 (August 2009):

2180–2185. doi: 10.1111/j.1600-6143.2009.02730.x. Last accessed June 7, 2016.

17. Kidney Foundation of Canada. Facing the Facts 2016 (fact sheet). Retrieved from www.kidney.ca/our-publications. Last accessed June 7, 2016.

18. National Kidney Foundation. Focal Segmental Glomerulosclerosis (FSGS). Retrieved from www.kidney.org/atoz/content/focal. Last accessed November 19, 2015.

19. Quote taken from Hoffer, E. *The Passionate State of Mind: And Other Aphorisms*. Titusville: Hopewell Publications, 2006. Eric Hoffer (1898–1983) was an American moral and social philosopher. He was the author of ten books and was awarded the Presidential Medal of Freedom in February 1983.

20. Kidney Foundation of Canada. Facing the Facts.

21. Ibid.

Chapter 9

1. University of Michigan Transplant Center. FAQ, 23. How are donated organs preserved and transported? TransWeb.org: A resource on transplantation and donation. Retrieved from www.transweb.org/faq/923.shtml. Last accessed May 5, 2015.

2. Guibert, E., A.Y. Alexander, C.L. Balaban, A.Y. Somov, J.V. Rodriguez, and B.J. Fuller. Organ preservation: Current concepts and new strategies for the next decade. Transfusion Medicine and Hemotherapy 38 (March 2011): 125–142. doi: 10.1159/000327033 Last accessed May 5, 2015.

3. Starzl, T.E. Transplantation immunology: Tissue matching. University of Pittsburgh. Retrieved from www.starzl.pitt.edu/transplantation/immunology/tissue_matching.html. Last accessed May 5, 2015.

4. Squifflet, J.-P. *The History of Kidney Transplantation: Past, Present and Future (with Special References to the Belgian History), Understanding the Complexities of Kidney Transplantation*. Jorge Ortiz (Ed.), InTech, 2011. Retrieved from www.intechopen.com/books/understanding-the-complexities-of-kidney-transplantation/the-history-of-kidney-transplantation-past-present-and-future-with-special-references-to-the-belgian. Last accessed May 5, 2015.

Chapter 10

1. Research study: Effect of immunosuppressive medication use on patient outcomes following kidney transplant failure. March 2, 2011, to May 24, 2018. Principal investigators: John Gill and O. Johnston. Co-investigators: Jagbir Gill, D. Landsberg, and G. Nussbaumer. Funded by the Canadian Institutes of Health Research (CIHR). Retrieved from renal.providencehealthcare.org/research/studies. Last accessed March 7, 2018.

2. Research study: Dialysis patients interested in research to reduce cardiovascular morbidity and mortality registry. Principal investigator: A. Levin. Co-investigators: J. Jastrzebski, J. Antonsen, and D. Shwartz. Funded by the Canadian Institutes of Health Research (CIHR). Sponsored by the Population Health Research Institute, Hamilton, Ontario. Interested patients interested sign a consent form, and information is transferred to a database held by Population Health Research Institute in Hamilton, Ontario. Information is maintained in the database for at least 10 years.

3. Research study: Inter-rater reliability of exit site monitoring tool for hemodialysis catheters. Principal investigator: W. Lau. Co-investigators: M. Kiaii, S. Marchuk, R. Luscombe, and R. Shaw. In-house study.

4. Research study: A qualitative study of patient/family experience of health care quality improvement and safety initiatives from an ethical lens. Principal investigator: P. Rodney. Co-Investigator: B. Sawatzky-Girling. The study is part of a doctoral thesis by B. Sawatzky-Girling in the School of Population and Public Health, University of British Columbia.

5. Participant in postal survey conducted by BC Provincial Renal Agency, Vancouver, BC. May 2016. Purpose to evaluate patient care services.

6. Kidney Research UK. PIVITOL Trial. Retrieved from www.kidneyresearchuk.org/research/case-study-pivotal? Last accessed June 18, 2017.

7. Kidney Research UK. Searching for a way to save patients' kidneys from polycystic kidney disease (PKD). Retrieved from www.kidneyresearchuk.org/research/case-study-jill-norman? Last accessed June 18, 2017.

8. McGreevey, S. Researchers find drug that could halt kidney failure. *The Harvard Gazette*, November 15, 2013. Retrieved from news.harvard.edu/gazette/story/2013/11/researchers-find-drug-that-could-halt-kidney-failure/. Last accessed June 19, 2017.

9. Shcherbina, Y. A whole new way to treat diabetes? Canadian Stem Cell Foundation blog, April 24, 2015. Retrieved from stem-cellfoundation.ca/en/2015/04/24/a-whole-new-way-to treat-diabetes.

Last accessed June 19, 2017. Permission to use information granted.

10. Roberts, M. Lab-grown kidneys a step closer. BBC News Online, September 22, 2015. Retrieved from www.bbc.com/news/health-34312125. Last accessed September 22, 2015.

11. Gallagher, J. Human-pig 'chimera embryos' detailed. BBC News Online, January 26, 2017. www.bbc.com/news/health-38717930. Last accessed June 21, 2017.

12. Martin, A. Ray Owen and the history of naturally acquired chimerism. Chimerism. 6 (April 2016): 2–7. doi: 10.1080/19381956.2016.1168561. Last accessed June 21, 2017.

13. Wingfield-Hayes, R. Quest to grow human organs inside pigs in Japan. Retrieved from www.bbc.com/news/world-asia-25550419. Last accessed June 21, 2017.

14. Roberts, M. Lab-grown kidneys.

15. Reetsma, K. Xenotransplantation: a historical perspective. *ILAR Journal* 37 (January 1995): 9–12. doi.org/10.1093/ilar.37.1.9. Last accessed June 6, 2016.

16. Canadian National Transplant Research Program (CNTRP). Transforming transplant research in Canada. Retrieved from htps://www.cntrp.ca/about. Last accessed June 22, 2017.

17. Investigators show that age and sex of both the donor and the recipient may affect kidney graft outcomes. Media publication adapted from McGill University Health Centre, June 21, 2017. Retrieved from www.cntrp.ca/single-post/2017/06/21/CNTRP-Investigators-show-that-age-and-sex-of-both-the-donor-and-the-recipient-may-affect-kidney-graft-outcomes. Last accessed June 22, 2017.

18. Canadian National Transplant Research Program (CNTRP). Organ donation after medical assistance in dying – Understanding the challenges, issues and facts. Retrieved from www.cntrp.ca/single-post/2017/03/31/Organ-donation-after-medical-aid-in-dying---Understanding-the-challenges-issues-and-facts. Last accessed June 22, 2017.

19. University of Alberta. A breath of relief. Retrieved from www.ualberta.ca/giving/giving-news/2017/january/a-breath-of-relief. Last accessed March 7, 2018.

20. National Institute of Biomedical Imaging and Bioengineering. Tissue engineering and regenerative medicine. Retrieved from www.nibib.nih.gov/science-education/science-topics/tissue-engineering-and-regenerative-medicine. Last accessed June 23, 2017.

21. Van den Broek, A. Top surgeon tells us about the future of transplant medicine. *Vital Bonds, The Nature of Things*, CBC television documentary, September 16, 2017. Retrieved from www.cbc.ca/natureofthings/features/top-surgeon-talks-about-the-future-of-transplant-medicine. Last accessed November 23, 2017.

22. Canadian National Transplant Research Program (CNTRP). First successful human kidney transplant using the new Toronto ex vivo kidney device. February 6, 2018. Retrieved from www.cntrp.ca/single-post/2018/02/06/First-successful-human-kidney-transplant-using-the-new-Toronto-ex-vivo-kidney-device. Last accessed March 7, 2018.

23. Wolf, A. Dr. William Fissell's artificial kidney. VU Inside, Vanderbilt University. Retrieved from news.vanderbilt.edu/2016/02/12/vu-inside-dr-william-fissells-artificial-kidney/. Last accessed June 24, 2017.

24. Canadian National Transplant Research Program (CNTRP). New guidelines on the public solicitation of anonymous organ donors: A position paper by the Canadian Society of Transplantation. Retrieved from www.cntrp.ca/single-post/2016/10/20/New-guidelines-on-the-public-solicitation-of-anonymous-organ-donors. Last accessed June 24, 2017.

25. Rodgers L. Caring for kidneys. *Promise: Voice of St. Paul's Foundation.* Fall/Winter 2016. Retrieved from helpstpauls.com/app/uploads/2016/11/STP_Fall-2016_LR.pdf. Permission to reproduce article given by BC Renal Agency, Providence Health Authority, Dr. A. Levin, and Kidney Foundation of Canada, June 12, 2017.

Epilogue

1. Chao, L. and H.D. McCarthy. 2015. Is there an association between dietary protein intake, Nordic walking exercise, and sarcopenia risk factors?

British Journal of Sports Medicine 49:A3. Retrieved from bjsm.bmj.com/content/49/Suppl_2/A3.2. Permission to cite granted January 2016.

Appendix 1

1. The King James Bible. Genesis 5.21–27.

2. Hamilton, D. *A History of Organ Transplantation: Ancient Legends to Modern Practice.* University of Pittsburgh Press, 2012, pp. 1–30.

3. Johnson, M. Preserving the body Christian: the motif of "recapitation" in Ireland's medieval hagiography. The Heroic Age. Issue 10, 2007. Retrieved from www.heroicage.org/issues/10/johnson.html. Last accessed January 16, 2016.

4. Squire, C. *Celtic Myth and Legend.* Chapter VII, The Rise of the Son-God. Gresham, 1905. Retrieved from www.sacred-texts.com/neu/celt/cml/cml11.htm. Last accessed January 15, 2016.

Nuada was the supreme god of the Tuatha De Danem. He is also called "Nuada Airgetlam" because it is said he lost a hand in battle that was replaced with a silver one by the Dian Cecht, the father of Miach. It had become festered and painful and led to Miach replacing it with his original one. He later resumed his role as king after having battled with another warrior, Bres.

5. Doyle, A.M., R.I. Lechler, and L.A. Turka. 2004. Organ transplantation: Halfway through the first century. *Journal of the American Society of Nephrology.* 15(12): 2965–2971. doi:10.1097/01.ASN.0000145434.00279.DD. Last accessed January 15, 2016.

6. Kashgar. The Hindu God Ganesh. Retrieved from www.kashgar.com/au/articles/ganesh. Last accessed January 15, 2016.

7. Theoi Project. Khimaira. Retrieved from www.theoi.com/Ther/Khimaira.html. Last accessed January 15, 2016.

8. MedicineNet.com. Medical definition of c12himerism. Retrieved from www.medicinenet.com/script/main/art.asp?articlekey=8905. Last accessed May 5, 2016.

9. University of Minnesota, Center for Bioethics. Chimeras. Retrieved from www.ahc.umn.edu/img/assets/25857/chimeras.pdf. Last accessed May 5, 2016

10. Squifflet, J.-P. *The History of Kidney Transplantation: Past, Present and*

Future (with Special References to the Belgian History), Understanding the Complexities of Kidney Transplantation. Jorge Ortiz (Ed.), InTech, 2011. Retrieved from www.intechopen.com/books/understanding-the-complexities-of-kidney-transplantation/the-history-of-kidney-transplantation-past-present-and-future-with-special-references-to-the-belgian. Last accessed May 5, 2015.

11. Hindu Online. Sushruta Samhita. Retrieved from hinduonline.co/Scriptures/Samhita/SushrutaSamhita.html. Last accessed May 20, 2016.

12. Blatch, S. Great achievements in science and technology in ancient Africa. *ASBMB Today,* February 2013. www.asbmb.org/asbmbtoday/asbmbtoday_article.aspx?id=32437. Last accessed May 20, 2016.

13. Hamilton, D. *A History of Organ Transplantation: Ancient Legends to Modern Practice.* University of Pittsburgh Press, 2012, pp. 1–30.

14. Anderson, K. Gasparo Tagliacozzi. October 2013. Retrieved from prezi.com/lpbjmaggwahk/gasparo-tagliacozzi/. Last accessed January 17, 2016.

15. Santoni-Rugiu, P. and P.J. Sykes. *A History of Plastic Surgery.* Springer, 2007, p. 320; Hamilton, D. *A History of Organ Transplantation: Ancient Legends to Modern Practice.* University of Pittsburgh Press, 2012, p. 18.

16. Hamilton, D. *A History of Organ Transplantation*, p.18.

17. Ibid.

18. Mandal, A. History of blood transfusion. Retrieved from www.news-medical.net/health/History-of-Blood-Transfusion.aspx. Last accessed January 21, 2016.

19. Palmer, J.F. (editor). The Works of John Hunter, F.R.S. with Notes. Vol. III. London: Longman, Rees, Orme, Browne, Green, and Longman, 1835. Original from the Bavarian State Library; digitalized November 30, 2008. Retrieved from books.google.ca. Last accessed January 21, 2016.

20. Hunter, J. The natural history of human teeth. UT Health, San Antonio. Retrieved from library.uthscsa.edu/2015/03/the-natural-history-of-human-teeth-john-hunter/. Last accessed January 21, 2016.

21. Smith, S.L. 2002. Historical perspective of transplantation. Medscape Retrieved from www.medscape.com/viewarticle/436532_4. Last accessed April 26, 2016.

22. Druml, W and C. Druml. 2004. Emerich Ullmann (1861-1937): not only a pioneer of kidney transplantation. J. Nephrology 17(3):461–6. Retrieved from www.ncbi.nlm.nih.gov/pubmed/15365973. Last accessed April 17, 2016.

According to the authors, Ullmann, not only an extremely innovative surgeon, was also a broadly educated man and an international art expert and collector. His scientific work was that of an amateur. He neither created a "school" nor had students who could follow in continuing developing his methods. When he died his work was lost and further destroyed when the Nazis assumed power, shutting down the "Jews and Liberastic" Society of Physicians in Vienna.

23. Nobelprize.org. Karl Landsteiner – Biographical. Retrieved from www.nobelprize.org/nobel_prizes/medicine/laureates/1930/landsteiner-bio.html. Last accessed April 17, 2016.

24. Margreiter, R. (reviewer). History of renal transplant. RenalMed. Retrieved from www.renalmed.co.uk/history-of/renal-transplant. Last accessed May 1, 2016.

25. Encyclopedia.com. Carrel, Alexis. Retrieved from www.encyclopedia.com/people/medicine/medicine-biographies/alexis-carrel. Last accessed May 1, 2016.

26. Margreiter, R. History of renal transplant.

27. Squifflet, J.-P. The History of Kidney Transplantation.

28. Redman, E. To save his dying sister-in-law, Charles Lindbergh invented a medical device. Smithsonian. Retrieved from www.smithsonianmag.com/smithsonian-institution/save-his-dying-sister-law-charles-lindbergh-Invented-medical-device-180956526/. Last accessed May 1, 2016. Lindbergh's perfusion pump on display at the Smithsonian was also a popular exhibit at the World's Fair in New York in 1939.

29. Encyclopedia.com. Alexis Carrel.

30. Squifflet, J.-P. The History of Kidney Transplantation.

31. Margreiter, R. History of renal transplant.

32. Ibid.

33. Khan, F., S. Madaan, S. Sriprasad, and I. Dickenson. 2013. A tribute to the life and accomplishments of Mathieu Jaboulay. The Journal of Urology

189(4) Supplement: e455–e456. Retrieved from www.jurology.com/article/
S0022-5347(13)00981-6/fulltext. Last accessed May 2, 2016.

34. Revolvy. Simon Flexner. Retrieved from www.revolvy.com/main/index.php?s=Simon%20Flexner. Last accessed March 12, 2018.

35. Understanding Animal Research. Macaques in medical research. Retrieved from www.understandinganimalresearch.org.uk/resources/video-library/macaques-in-medical-research/. Last accessed March 18, 2018. Macaque monkeys are frequently used in research. They have been used in kidney transplantation since the 1950's. Macaque monkeys are often referred to as Old World monkeys having originated in Asia.

36. Margreiter, R. History of renal transplant.

37. Eigler, F.W. The history of kidney transplantation in Germany. *Zentralblatt fur Chirurgie*. 127 (November 2002): 1001–8. Retrieved from www.ncbi.nlm.nih.gov/pubmed/12476377. Last accessed May 3, 2015.

38. Margreiter, R. History of renal transplant.

39. Ibid.

40. Squifflet, J.-P. *The History of Kidney Transplantation*.

41. Margreiter, R. History of renal transplant.

42. Squifflet, J.-P. *The History of Kidney Transplantation*.

43. Davita.com. The history of dialysis: life, death and a "washing machine." Retrieved from www.davita.com/kidney-disease/dialysis/motivational/the-history-of-dialysis/e/197. Last accessed May 6, 2016.

44. Ibid.

45. Encylopedia.com. Medawar, Peter Brian. Retrieved from www.encyclopedia.com/people/medicine/medicine-biographies/peter-brian-medawar. Last accessed May 12, 2016.

46. Margreiter, R. History of renal transplant.

47. Ibid.

48. Ibid.

49. Squifflet, J.-P. *The History of Kidney Transplantation*.

50. Margreiter, R. History of renal transplant.

51. Ibid.

52. Ibid.

53. Squifflet, J.-P. *The History of Kidney Transplantation.*

54. McAlister, V.C. Clinical kidney transplantation: a 50th anniversary review of the first reported series. *American Journal of Surgery* 190 (September 2005): 485–8: Retrieved from www.ncbi.nlm.nih.gov/pubmed/16105541. Last accessed May 6, 2016.

55. Saxon, W. Dr. Jean Hamburger, 82, pioneer in kidney medicine and a writer. *The New York Times*, February 6, 1992. Retrieved from www.nytimes.com/1992/02/06/world/dr-jean-hamburger-82-pioneer-in-kidney-medicine-and-a-writer.html. Last accessed May 4, 2016.

56. Margreiter, R. History of renal transplant.

57. Ramsay, M. Advances in transplantation 1940–2014. *Anesthesiology Clinics* 31 (December 2013): 645–658. doi.org/10.1016/j.anclin.2013.08.001. Last accessed September 17, 2017.

58. Epstein, M. John P. Merrill: The father of nephrology as a specialty. *Clinical Journal of the American Society of Nephrology* 4 (January 2009): 2–8. Retrieved from cjasn.asnjournals.org/content/4/1/2.full. Last accessed May 1, 2016.

59. Powell, A. A transplant makes history: Joseph Murray's 1954 kidney operation ushered in a new medical era. *The Harvard Gazette*, September 22, 2011. Retrieved from news.harvard.edu/gazette/story/2011/09/a-transplant-makes-history/. Last accessed May 3, 2016.

60. Margreiter, R. History of renal transplant.

61. Ibid.

62. Reemtsma, K. Xenotransplantation: a historical perspective. *ILAR Journal* 37 (January 1995): 9–12. doi.org/10.1093/ilar.37.1.9. Last accessed May 4, 2016.

Appendix 2

1. Margreiter, R. (reviewer). History of renal transplant. RenalMed. Retrieved from www.renalmed.co.uk/history-of/renal-transplant. Last accessed May 1, 2016.

2. Squifflet, J.-P. *The History of Kidney Transplantation: Past, Present and*

Future (with Special References to the Belgian History), Understanding the Complexities of Kidney Transplantation. Jorge Ortiz (Ed.), InTech, 2011. Retrieved from www.intechopen.com/books/understanding-the-complexities-of-kidney-transplantation/the-history-of-kidney-transplantation-past-present-and-future-with-special-references-to-the-belgian. Last accessed May 5, 2015.

3. Reemtsma, K. Xenotransplantation: a historical perspective. *ILAR Journal* 37 (January 1995): 9–12. doi.org/10.1093/ilar.37.1.9. Last accessed May 4, 2016.

4. Squifflet, J.-P. *The History of Kidney Transplantation.*

5. Ibid.

6. Ibid.

7. Ibid.

8. Shaw, G. Vancouver company develops 3-D printing of human tissue. *Vancouver Sun,* Staff blog, October 16, 2014. Retrieved from vancouversun.com/news/staff-blogs/vancouver-company-develops-3-d-printing-of-human-tissue. Last accessed December, 2017.

9. Adams, S. and B. Marsh. Brain dead baby is kept on a ventilator so the child's kidneys can save an adult. Daily Mail, March 13, 2016. Retrieved from www.dailymail.co.uk/health/article-3489699/Brain-dead-baby-kept-alive-ventilator-child-s-kidneys-save-woman-40s.html. Last accessed December 21, 2016.

10. Business Wire. Human tissue engineering startup Prellis Biologics receives funding to create human organs with 3D printing. Retrieved from www.businesswire.com/news/home/20170913005487/en/Human-Tissue-Engineering-Startup-Prellis-Biologics-Receives. Last accessed September 13, 2017.

Glossary

Albumin: A protein made by the liver, making up about 60 percent of the total protein in the blood. Albumin is found in meat, milk products and eggs, as well as in beans, nuts and seeds. Its purpose is to keep fluid from leaking out of blood vessels, nourishing tissues and carrying hormones, vitamins, medications and matter such as calcium throughout the body. In kidney failure, albumin is lost through dialysis and requires monitoring.

Antibody: A protein produced by the body in response to the presence of an antigen. Various tests determine the type and number of antibodies in a person's blood.

Antigen: A substance that stimulates an immune response in the body. The immune system perceives an antigen as being foreign and produces an antibody against it.

Blood type: The classification system based on hereditary characteristics of the blood. There are four main blood types: A, B, AB and O.

Creatinine: A chemical waste in the blood; a natural by-product of normal muscle function that passes through the kidneys to be filtered and eliminated in the urine. It is measured to determine the effectiveness of kidney function. When damage to a kidney occurs or in kidney failure, the kidneys are no longer able to filter waste efficiently, causing the levels of creatinine to rise in the blood. In women the normal range is 60 to 110 micromoles per litre (μmol/L). In men the normal range is 70 to 120 μmol/L. Women frequently have lower creatinine than men because they have less muscle mass than men.

Dialysate solution: Chemical solution used during dialysis to cleanse the blood.

Dialysis: The artificial process in which waste products are removed from the blood when the kidneys no longer have the ability to perform this function effectively.

Dialyzer: The filtering unit on a hemodialysis machine. The dialyzer removes waste products and excess water from the blood.

Dwell time: The length of time solution is left in the body during peritoneal dialysis.

Fistula: An artificially created access point, usually in the wrist or arm, that directly connects an artery to a vein so blood can be cleansed and returned during hemodialysis.

Glomerular Filtration Rate (GFR): An estimate of the amount of blood passing through the glomeruli each minute. GFR is calculated from blood creatinine results, age, body size, weight, height and gender. In a healthy kidney, the rate is usually over 60 millilitres/minute per 1.73 m^2 (ml/min/1.73 m^2). Low GFR means less waste is filtered and often means medication effects such as antibiotics remain in the system longer. A measurement of 15 ml/min/1.73 m^2 denotes kidney failure.

Goal weight: An end-of-dialysis-session target weight.

Hemodiafiltration (HDF): A specially designed, faster-paced dialysis machine with the purpose of removing not only small molecules but also medium to large toxin molecules. It is used with patients who have experienced greater pain, stiffness, fluid in the joints, restless legs and possibly carpal tunnel syndrome (found in 50 percent of hemodialysis patients) due to an increase in toxin levels. A more porous artificial kidney is used to filter the blood. A higher volume of water is used. The machine's faster speed contributes to more toxin molecules being removed from the blood and the faster water flow draws more of the water from the blood, likewise removing more toxins. Because of the complexity of the process in removing more water than is required to reach the goal weight, the machine calculates and adds the amount of fluid required in the line returning blood to the body.

Hemodialysis machine: A form of dialysis that uses pressure to filter water from blood through a membrane called the "artificial kidney" found on the front side of the dialysis machine. Once through the artificial kidney, the water mixes with dialysate fluid supplied through tubes that is in turn discarded through waste drains. In the dialysis process, toxins no longer excreted through damaged kidneys are diffused through the artificial kidney and discarded along with the dialysate solution. There are two types of toxins consisting of large and small molecules. Hemodialysis removes small toxins. During a dialysis session, blood is removed through the venous tube for cleansing and returned to the body through the arterial tube.

Hemoglobin: A protein of red blood cells that contains iron and carries oxygen from the lungs to the tissues and carbon dioxide from the tissues to the lungs. Normal hemoglobin levels in women ranges from 120 to 160 grams per litre (g/L), and in men, from 140 to 180 g/L.

Neck catheter: An artificially created access point, usually in the lower neck area, that connects an insert tube to a heart artery to remove dirty fluid and return cleansed blood during hemodialysis.

Peritoneal dialysis: A form of dialysis in which the blood is cleansed inside the body through the peritoneum, a thin membrane that surrounds the outside of the organs in the abdomen. The peritoneum is very rich in small blood vessels. Waste products can pass through the peritoneum via a flexible tube called a Tenckhoff catheter that has been surgically sewn into the peritoneal membrane. Part of this tube remains outside the body so that waste fluid can be drained out. Dialysate solutions are used to cleanse the blood. Peritoneal dialysis fluid is a glucose solution containing other salts. There are two types of peritoneal dialysis:

1) Continuous Ambulatory Peritoneal Dialysis (CAPD) is completed throughout a day. Between 1.5 and 3 litres of dialysate solution is run into the body four times a day, once the cleansed waste solution has been drained out. CAPD provides an individual with more freedom to work, travel and consume a range of fluids, since waste is being continually removed.

2) Automated Peritoneal Dialysis (APD) is completed during sleep. A cycler machine is programmed to automatically run in dialysate and drain out waste solution. The machine can exchange 8 to 12 litres over eight to ten hours and leave 1 to 2 litres to dwell during the day. A dialysis patient requires training to use the machine effectively. It works in exactly the same way as CAPD does.

Phosphorus: An essential mineral necessary in aiding growth and re-pair of body cells and tissues. All body cells contain phosphorus, 85 percent of which is found in bones and teeth. Reduced production of calcium can contribute to phosphorus being stripped from bones and contribute to a condition called osteodystrophy. Surplus phosphorus, no longer filtered out through urination, can cause skin to be itchy. In kidney failure, foods containing high amounts of phosphorus are restricted. Most foods contain components of phosphorus. Protein foods containing high levels of phosphorus and calcium include dairy products, nuts, seeds, fish, meat, legumes, cereals and grains. Carbonated drinks also contain high levels of phosphorus. Phosphorus binders, usually taken with meals, are used to absorb the extra phosphorus.

Potassium: An essential mineral for maintaining good cardiovascular health, blood pressure and bone and muscle strength. One function of potassium is to soak up excess amounts of sodium, keeping blood pressure low. A deficiency can lead to fatigue, weakness and constipation. In its extreme, low potassium can escalate to paralysis, respiratory failure and painful gut obstruction. An excess can lead to high blood pressure and cardiovascular and musculature problems. Foods high in potassium include bananas, potatoes, beans, leafy greens and tomatoes. Healthy individuals usually require 4.7 grams a day to maintain good levels. Potassium solutions are used during hemodialysis to augment loss of potassium through dialysis and diet.

Tissue type: A set of inherited characteristics on the surface of tissue cells.

Toxins: Waste products that accumulate in the blood when not filtered out by the kidneys. A by-product of kidney failure.

Urea: A waste product that accumulates in the blood. The level of urea indicates how well or poorly the kidneys are working.

Sample of Emergency Diet Meal Plan

Reproduced with kind permission from BC Renal Agency.

Breakfast	• 1cup cold cereal (puffed wheat, puffed rice or 2 shredded wheat biscuits) • 1/2 cup (125ml) Rice Dream or ½ cup milk prepared from dry milk powder or ¼ cup evaporated milk mixed with ¼ cup purified or distilled water. • 5 low salt crackers + 2 Tbsp. jelly, jam or honey • 1/2 cup canned fruit * (packed in juice), drink the juice and count it as part of your daily fluid intake
Snack	• Hard candy
Lunch	• 15 low salt crackers & 6 Tbsp jelly, jam or honey • 1/2 cup canned fruit * (packed in juice), drink the juice and count it as part of your daily fluid intake • Hard candy
Snack	• 4 cookies • 1/2 cup canned fruit * (packed in juice), drink the juice and count it as part of your daily fluid intake
Dinner	• 1 can (85-170 grams) drained tuna or salmon (preferably no salt added or low salt), **or** 1 can (156 grams) "33% Less Salt" Flaked Chicken or Turkey • 15 low salt crackers & 4 tbsp. jelly, jam or honey • 1/2 cup canned fruit * (packed in juice), drink the juice and count it as part of your daily fluid intake

- If you are hungry, you can have another 10 low salt crackers and 6 cookies each day.
- You could also have 2 tbsp. peanut butter.
- Repeat this meal plan until dialysis in available.

* For example: Applesauce, pears, peaches, pineapple

Resources

Provincial Organ and Tissue Donation Organizations:

Alberta
Alberta Organ and Tissue Donation Registry
myhealth.alberta.ca/pages/otdrhome.aspx
Edmonton: 866.407.1970
Calgary: 403.944.8700

British Columbia
BC Transplant
www.transplant.bc.ca/health-info/organ-donation/living-donation
604.877.2240
800.663.6189

Manitoba
Transplant Manitoba
www.transplantmanitoba.ca/decide/how-do-i-become-an-organ-donor-in-manitoba
204.787.7001

New Brunswick
New Brunswick Organ and Tissue Donation Program
www2.gnb.ca/content/gnb/en/departments/health/Hospital-Services/content/organ_donation.html
506.643.6848

Newfoundland and Labrador

Eastern Health

www.easternhealth.ca/Give.aspx?d=1&id=323&p=53

709.777.6600

877.640.1110

Nova Scotia

Legacy of Life, Nova Scotia Organ and Tissue Donation Program

www.legacyoflife.ns.ca

902.473.5049

Northwest Territories

Northern Alberta and the Territories Branch

www.kidney.ca/page.aspx?pid=496

780.451.6900

800.461.9063

Nunavut

For information and telephone numbers, refer to myhealth.alberta.ca

Ontario

Trillium Gift of Life Network

www.giftoflife.on.ca/en/

416-363-4001

800-263-2833

Prince Edward Island

Health PEI

www.princeedwardisland.ca/en/service/register-organ-andor-tissue-donor

902.368.5920

Quebec

Transplant Québec

www.transplantquebec.ca/en/organ-donation

855.373.1414

Saskatchewan

Organ and Tissue Transplants and Donations

www.saskatchewan.ca/residents/health/accessing-health-care-services/organ-and-tissue-transplants-and-donations

Saskatoon: 306.655.5054

Regina: 306.766.6477

Yukon

Organ Donation Program, Yukon Health and Social Services

www.hss.gov.yk.ca/organdonation.php

867.667.5209

800.661.0408

Other Organizations with Kidney Information:

The Kidney Foundation of Canada

www.kidney.ca

www.kidney.ca/resources

Kidney Connect Canada

Connect with Kidney Patients Online

kidney.ning.com

Ontario Renal Network

www.renalnetwork.on.ca

Canadian Society of Nephrology

www.csnscn.ca

www.csnscn.ca/education/educational-resources

Canadian Transplant Association

www.canadiantransplant.com

Canadian Blood Services

blood.ca/en

organtissuedonation.ca/en

888.236.6283

BC Provincial Organizations:

BCGuidelines.ca (Clinical practice guidelines and protocols)

Chronic Kidney Disease – Identification, Evaluation and Management of Adult Patients

www2.gov.bc.ca/gov/content/health/practitioner-professional-resources/bc-guidelines/chronic-kidney-disease

BC Renal Agency

www.bcrenalagency.ca

National Organizations and Societies for Chronic Illnesses:

Diabetes Canada

www.diabetes.ca

Heart and Stroke Foundation of Canada

www.heartandstroke.com

Lupus Canada

www.lupuscanada.org

Polycystic Kidney Disease, The Kidney Foundation of Canada

www.kidney.ca/polycystic-kidney-disease

Scleroderma Canada

www.scleroderma.ca

Vasculitis Foundation Canada (Formerly Wegener's Granulomatosis Support Group of Canada)

www.vasculitis.ca

Acknowledgements

A book of this nature is never the work of a single person. Just as it takes a village to raise a child, so it took a host of individuals to create my completed manuscript. I am deeply indebted to the following individuals, organizations and agencies for their contributions, assistance and expertise in helping me craft this work.

First of all, I am extremely grateful to the patients who contributed their stories and trusted me to record them accurately, albeit with alterations to their names and sometimes gender. To you, I owe a considerable amount. Without your input, my book would have been a shadow lurking in the background. I am also incredibly impressed by your spirit, determination and courage to live full lives despite challenging circumstances. You, my fellow patients, are an inspiration and deserve many accolades. Your optimism and resolve have kept me moving forward. Thank you for sharing your tales with me and providing me with valuable insight.

Second, I would like to raise my cap to the multitude of nurses who have cared for me during my hospital sessions. You are dedicated to your work, approaching it with humour, warmth, kindness and grace. Never have I witnessed an unpleasant, uncaring nurse. You serve us well, fulfilling many requests for more blankets, water to drink, ubiquitous bed pans should the need arise and pain killers to ease our comfort, irrespective of how busy you are. A request is rarely denied and often fulfilled with, "It's a pleasure to do so." I am also appreciative of the interest in the progress of my book shown to me during conversations. Thank you for your care and concern and for being there for us.

Third, I am indebted to those who assisted me in gathering medical and technical details. Thanks go to Dr. Jagbir Gill who provided me with necessary information about kidney disease when I began writing this book. Thank you also to the various other nephrologists who likewise supplied me with background details. Special thanks to Drs. Elizabeth Lee and Jane White who spent hours reviewing a chapter and correcting my mistakes where I was amiss—quite a few, as it transpired. Hopefully, my knowledge has improved as I continued researching medical facts, terminology and statistics. I wish to thank Stan Marchuk, the unit's nurse practitioner, whom I frequently referred to as "my loyal reader" for being willing to review and critique a majority of my manuscript. In so doing, he forewarned me, "I will not hesitate to tell you if you are incorrect." Yes, I soon learned where I had erred. Your input was gratefully received.

Nationally, I am extremely appreciative of the assistance and support I received from sources such as the Canadian National Transplant Research Program (CNTRP), Canadian Blood Services (CBS), Canadian Institute for Health Information (CIHI) and Canadian Stem Cell Foundation. Thank you for providing me with invaluable information.

Internationally, I am extremely appreciative of being able to include material provided by Renal Med and Eurotransplant. Thank you to Dr. David Hamilton for critiquing a chapter. It was kind of you.

I am also indebted to Dr. Jean-Paul Squifflet who not only assisted me with medical information regarding kidney disease but also reviewed some of my written material, despite having a full schedule of commitments. Thank you indeed.

I am thankful, too, for the input provided to me by BC Transplant, as well as to Providence Health, BC Renal Agency and Dr. Adeera Levin for permitting me to cite their current renal project. Thank you to BC Renal Agency for granting me permission to include a copy of the emergency diet. Additional thanks go to Pain BC for their assistance.

I extend further thanks to Shohreh Vaezi for both her interest in and enthusiasm for assisting me with my manuscript, as well as introducing me to patients whose stories she felt would be of particular interest to me. As a result I made more connections with fellow dialysis patients and in so doing acquired further friends. Similarly, I would like to thank Catherine Phung, too, for giving me access to her training manual as a way of contributing to my background information. Thank you to Leonora Chao for information supplied and for supporting my venture. I have learned a great deal from your contributions.

Fourth, I am more than appreciative of those who read and reviewed my manuscript and provided me with feedback. Thanks go to my dear friends Natalie Loubiere and Sarah Brydon who followed me along every step of my journey. Your input was invaluable and your feedback most useful. Thank you also to the following, who likewise took time to read various chapters: my cousin Mary Nicolls, friends Rosemary Mansell, Rolf Lippelt, Debby Vollbrecht and Anne-Marie Klasson who told me, "keep it real"—hopefully I have—and long-time friend, Elizabeth Abbott, a published author, with whom I discussed the craft of writing and creating a book. Your wisdom was really helpful.

Thank you to SABC for all the support and interest taken in my book's progress; in particular to Joan Kelly and Rosanne Queen for permitting me to share your story, as well as Bob Buzza and Robyn Buzza Fox who likewise waded through various chapters. Robyn continued to provide me with feedback until she was diagnosed with leukemia that has thankfully been successfully treated. Thanks to my many friends who often inquired as to how my writing was progressing and to those like Casey Dorin and Cal Finley whose advice I sought regarding aspects of my content.

Fifth, closer to the home front, I wish to give heartfelt thanks to my pain specialist, Dr. Roger Shick, who continues to support me through my trials and who from the outset believed I possessed the ability to write and encouraged me to do so. I am tremendously appreciative of his time invested in reading my entire manuscript and for advice I received. An avid reader himself, he would read through sections of books he thought particularly well written in order to stimulate my creative juices. He soon became my "Literary Advisor" as well as my mentor, healer and supporter during manifold occasions of doubt. Without your assistance and support, my manuscript may have long been abandoned.

Without a designer, proofreader and editor even the best-written piece of work loses something. Thank you to those whom I refer to as "my production team." To Lucilla Girotto, designer, for your expertise in designing the book's interior, and to Jazmin Welch for designing the outstanding cover. To Rowena Rae, my heartfelt thanks for proofreading the finished copy prior to it being published. Your input was invaluable. My book has been vastly improved with the help, advice and hours of support provided by my editor, Trevor McMonagle. How I must have frustrated you with my slow delivery, procrastination, stubbornness and need for reassurance. Thank you for your much-required assistance and literary talents. My book has been all the better for it. Last, but in no way least, I thank Megan Williams for helping me bring together the final threads and get the book uploaded to distribution and printing channels.

Few books are written without the support of family and close kin. Mine is no different. To my brother, Robert, who, often having dropped by for a visit, would find himself having to proofread my latest draft, thank you for graciously accepting this task. I owe considerable amounts of gratitude to my former husband and friend, Christopher, who was one of my most ardent supporters. He spent many hours critiquing my writing and printing out copies for me to read until cancer stole his mind and body. His last few words to me were, "I would like to see your book in every library before I die." A desire not achieved. RIP, Christopher, and so many thanks to you in memoriam. To my son, Roland, who told me, "Mum, you can do this," hundreds, no, probably thousands, of times when I felt my ability lacking. My dearest love and heartfelt thanks for being there.

About the Author

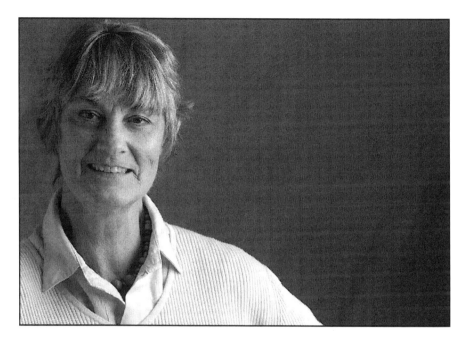

Priscilla Stanbury taught in the post-secondary education sector in London, England, and Vancouver, British Columbia. She was diagnosed with an autoimmune disease, scleroderma, in 1990. Her kidneys failed a year later. Following nine months of dialysis, she received a kidney transplant that functioned well for over twenty-two years. She is currently a hemodialysis out-patient in Vancouver.

Made in the USA
San Bernardino, CA
17 May 2018